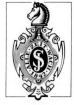

R. Texhammar   C. Colton

AO/ASIF Instruments and Implants

A Technical Manual

Contributors   F. Baumgart J. Buchanan J. A. Disegi
R. Hertel A. Murphy S. M. Perren

Foreword   M. E. Müller

Completely Revised and Enlarged
Second Edition
With Approx. 3000 Figures

Springer-Verlag   Berlin Heidelberg New York
London Paris Tokyo
Hong Kong Barcelona
Budapest

Rigmor Texhammar, RN
Former Director of Nurse Education
AO International
Fatbursgatan 18 A
11828 Stockholm, Sweden

Christopher Colton
M. B., B. S., L. R. C. P., F. R. C. S., F. R. C. S. Ed.
Professor in Orthopaedics and Accident Surgery
at Nottingham University
Senior Orthopaedic Trauma Surgeon and
Consultant Paediatric Orthopaedic Surgeon
at Nottingham University Hospital
Nottingham NG7 2UH, Great Britain

The first edition appeared under the title:
F. Séquin/R. Texhammar, AO/ASIF Instrumentation
© Springer-Verlag Berlin Heidelberg 1981

ISBN 3-540-56895-6 2nd Edition Springer-Verlag
                    Berlin Heidelberg New York
ISBN 0-387-56895-6 2nd Edition Springer-Verlag
                    New York Heidelberg Berlin

ISBN 3-540-10337-6 1st Edition Springer-Verlag
                    Berlin Heidelberg New York
ISBN 0-387-10337-6 1st Edition Springer-Verlag
                    New York Heidelberg Berlin

Library of Congress Cataloging-in-Publication Data
Texhammar, R. (Rigmor): AO/ASIF instruments and implants : a technical manual / R. Texhammar , C. Colton ; with contributions by F. Baumgart . . . [et al.]. ; with a
foreword by M. E. Müller. – Completely rev. and enlarged 2nd ed. p. cm. Rev. ed.
of: AO/ASIF instrumentation / F. Séquin, R. Texhammar. 1981. Includes bibliograph-
ical references and index. ISBN 3-540-56895-6 (alk. paper). – ISBN 0-387-56895-6
(alk. paper). 1. Internal fixation in fractures. 2. Surgical instruments and apparatus.
I. Colton, Christopher L. II. Séquin, F. (Fridolin) AO/ASIF instrumentation. III.
Title. IV. Title: AO/ASIF instruments and implants. [DNLM: 1. Fracture Fixation,
Internal – instrumentation. WE 185 T 355 a 1994] RD 103. I5S47 1994 617.1'5 –
dc 20 DNLM/DLC for Library of Congress 93-21299 CIP

© Springer-Verlag Berlin Heidelberg 1981, 1994
Printed in Germany

Typesetting: Data conversion by Aprinta, Wemding

Printing and binding: Appl, Wemding

24/3130 – 5 4 3 2 1 0 – Printed on acid-free paper

Foreword

The original *AO/ASIF Instrumentation* manual presented a concise and complete description of the AO instruments. Thoughtfully developed by Fridolin Séquin and Rigmor Texhammar, the manual discussed in a clear fashion the purpose and care of the various AO instruments that are handled by the operating room staff. One important feature of the first edition was a detailed checklist of the instruments required for the more common operative procedures for treating fractures. Fridolin Séquin was well-suited to author the first edition: his 15 years of experience as a technical engineer for the AO gave him in-depth knowledge of AO instruments, and he drew on the clinical knowledge of Rigmor Texhammar, a consultant and director of the AO courses for nurses. Its original feature of combining a column of text with a column of illustrations meant the manual quickly became accepted as a standard. By 1981, translations could be found in English, French, Spanish, and Italian. Not surprisingly, the manual was very popular.

The success of the first edition and the development of new AO/ASIF techniques led to plans for a second edition. Unfortunately, Fridolin Sequin's passing meant the original team could not carry on with the project, but Chris Colton of Nottingham, England, stepped in where Fridolin Séquin left off. As director of one of the strongest orthopaedic trauma units in Great Britain, he was well-suited to take on this difficult task. The combined forces of Chris Colton and Rigmor Texhammar led to a new focus of emphasis for the second edition, which evolved around providing a reference not only for the operating room staff, but also for the increasing numbers of young surgeons who, it was noticed, used the first edition to aid their understanding of the operative care of fractures.

Operative fracture care is not only a worthwhile and rewarding experience for new surgeons, but also a difficult and demanding task. For this reason, a readily available text outlining both AO instruments and techniques was needed. The aims of this manual, however, are broader than merely providing a description of AO instruments and techniques. In chapters written in collaboration with S.M. Perren and other clinicians and researchers with comprehensive knowledge in the field, the principles and the history of the AO are updated. A further chapter, by J. Disegi and F. Baumgart, describes the materials used for AO/ASIF

The nature of the fracture pattern depends on the type of force which led to the fracture: if torque is applied (e. g. skiing), the fracture shows a spiral pattern. If, however, a bending force is applied (e. g. when the bumper of a car hits the leg of a pedestrian), then a transverse fracture is produced. Similarly, too large a tensile force may disrupt the patella or the olecranon or avulse a malleolar fragment. When a person lands hard, for example, after jumping from a balcony, the bone is compressed and the fractured limb will probably be shortened.

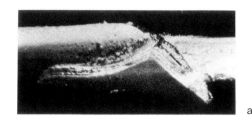

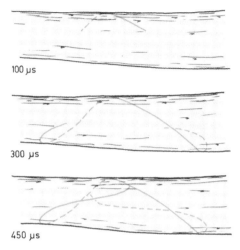

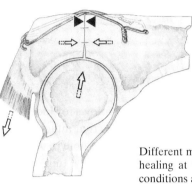

Different mechanical conditions and types of healing at the same fracture site. Different conditions at a fracture site at different times of observation (tension band wiring of the olecranon). The preload exerted by the wire is shown by *black triangles* (static compression); the changing load due to function, i.e. pull of the triceps muscle and related articular compression producing additional compression of the fracture surface, is shown by *open arrows*.

The bone fracture. The sequence of events resulting in a spiral fracture with additional (butterfly) fragment analysed using high-speed cinematography. A human cadaver tibia was fractured using axial torque. The process, which resulted in a butterfly fracture, was recorded at 10 000 frames per second (Moor et al. 1989). **a** Tissue trauma. When the applied torque reaches the limit of the strength of the bone, the bone fractures and a gap opens up abruptly. A temporary vacuum is created. This is succeeded by implosion, the effect of which can be compared to that of cavitation in high-velocity gunshot wounds. Marked tissue trauma in the areas of cavitation results. **b** Sequence of events and timing. The schematic diagram shows the sequence of events in the process of fracturing. Within 400 s the fracture is fully developed. The sequence leading to the dissolution of the butterfly fragment is also shown.

4.1.1 Reduction

The first specific action in the treatment of a fracture consists of reducing the fragments to reinstate the shape of the bone before it fractured. This process is called "reduction". Reduction basically reverses the forces that led to the displacement: if the fracture was produced by an external rotation of the foot, then reduction will involve applying a moment to produce internal rotation. This neutralises the displacement brought about by the external rotation. The reduction may be achieved using one of the following procedures.

4.1.1.1 External Reduction

A fracture dislocation may be reduced by applying a force "by hand". The problem with this procedure is that it is difficult to achieve optimal reduction. Very often massive manipulation results in considerable trauma of the soft tissues. Furthermore, if soft tissues such as tendons are caught within the fracture, reduction may be impossible.

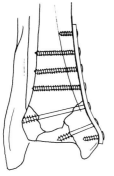

Precise anatomical reduction is required. Fractures which compromise articulating surfaces of joints result in post-traumatic arthrosis due to overload following the loss of even stress distribution.

4.1.1.2 Direct Surgical Reduction

When external reduction is impossible or insufficient, then the reduction may take place by surgical fixation after exposure of the fracture fragments. These fragments are manipulated using special forceps and the fragments are reduced. Such reduction normally results in perfect restoration of the original shape. Perfect restoration may be required when treating articular fractures, although it is not mandatory for optimal function in the case of shaft fractures.

4.1.1.3 Indirect Surgical Reduction

Indirect reduction is a process of reduction whereby the fracture fragments are not directly manipulated by the hands of the surgeon or with forceps. A classic example of indirect reduction is the insertion of pins, such as those used for external fixation, into the bone. The free end of these pins is then guided by a special device called a distractor or by an implant such as a plate. The mere application of distraction, i.e. pull along the axis of the bone, results in an astonishingly good reduction of a multifragmentary fracture. Mast and coworkers (1989) have provided the first systematic description of "indirect reduction". Since the fracture displacement usually results from the compressive forces arising from the pull of the muscles, the application of distraction is frequently appropriate. Very often the fragments of a comminuted fracture are still connected to the soft tissues. Under these conditions, the application of traction by indirect means, for example, by the distractor, plates or nails, reduces the fracture sufficiently to ensure good function later on. Considerable traction can be applied with the distractor without causing the kind of soft tissue damage which results from the application of external force by hand.

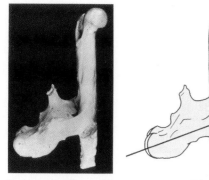

Fracture healing without treatment. The fractured femur of a dog united solidly without treatment; however, marked malalignment resulted. The fracture was not reduced or splinted. (Courtesy of G. Sumner-Smith).

4.1.1.4 Surgical Reduction and Bone Healing

A fracture in a wild animal may heal solidly even if it remains untreated. It can be assumed, however, that an untreated fracture will unite with more difficulty under conditions of malalignment because the displacing forces to be overcome by the healing process are greater if the bone is bent than if it were straight. The speed and quality of bone healing is influenced by the damage due to manipulation in external reduction and/or by the exposure necessary in internal reduction. For example, callus formation in open reduction and i.m. nailing is least at the surface where surgical intervention damaged the periosteum. Indirect reduction as proposed by Mast and coworkers represents a major breakthrough in the improvement of fracture treatment.

4.1.2 Fixation

The fracture displaces the bone fragments and the surgeon reduces the fragments, but once the fragments are in place again, they must be maintained in this position. This can be achieved by external splinting, traction or internal fixation.

4.1.2.1 Stability and Lack of Tissue Irritation

The movement of fracture fragments in relation to each other is painful. The stability resulting from fixation suppresses the motion of these fragments and thus alleviates pain. The stability of fixation is therefore an important element in preventing irritation and dystrophy (i.e. swelling, pain and reduced articular mobility).

4.1.2.2 Stability and Direct Tissue Differentiation

The stability of fracture fixation determines the amount of callus that is formed. An unstable fracture site will soon be surrounded, bridged and stabilised by a cuff of bone called callus (scar). In general, one can state that the more movement there is, the more callus is produced. The appearance of callus indicates a reaction which helps the fracture to unite. Therefore, although the surgeon in general likes to see callus, in some cases of internal fixation the appearance of callus is a sign of unwanted instability. This explains the paradox that the surgeon may not like to see callus, but the callus will help heal the fracture.

4.1.2.3 Stability and Painless Function

Once a certain degree of stability of fixation has been attained the injured limb can be moved without pain. Immobilisation of the joints of a limb results in stiffness of those joints, and this may bother the patient more than the fracture itself. Early function prevents joints from becoming stiff. Since stable internal fixation allows for early movement of the joints, the major advantage of internal fixation is early and complete recovery of limb function.

4.1.2.4 Stability of Fixation and Bone Healing

Stability of fixation is synonymous with prevention of movement at the fracture site. Movement of the fracture fragments induces callus formation and, as we will see later, induces bone surface resorption of the fracture fragments and enhances indirect bone formation. Thus, stability of fixation has a very important influence on the healing pattern of bone. In the rare case of absolutely stable fixation without any motion at the fracture site, the fracture may unite without callus formation. This type of healing was preferred for several decades. Today we know that this type of healing is of little importance as long as the fracture unites early and without complication.

4.1.3 Immediate Function

It has been mentioned above that the primary goal of fracture treatment is to achieve early and completely undisturbed limb function.

4.1.3.1 Avoidance of Dystrophy

Dystrophy, which consists in swelling, pain and stiffness of the joints, must be avoided whenever possible. It was shown by a study of the Swiss National Insurance company that the greatest loss of work capacity following bone fracture is not due to retardation of healing but to dystrophy.

4.1.3.2 Maintenance of Articular Mobility

The best means of avoiding dystrophy is full movement of the articulations as soon as possible after fracture. Today fracture treatment also deals with the soft tissues as part of the early restoration of limb function.

4.1.3.3 Psychological Health

Early restoration of limb function plays an important role in the psychological health of the patient. The injured patient who can function normally soon after the injury and care for himself and his daily needs, such as taking a shower, will overcome the mental injury of being temporarily handicapped sooner.

4.1.3.4 Immediate Function and Bone Healing

Blood circulation is at the basis of bone healing, which means that anything which improves or maintains blood circulation to the bone is a top priority.

4.1.3.4.1 Bone Structure

As we will see later the uninterrupted blood supply to the bone is important for preventing bone porosis, i.e. a loss of bone with the appearance of small pores within the bone.

4.1.3.4.2 Induction of Bone Formation

In the long term, bone reacts to unloading with loss of structure. In this respect bone can be understood as a structural material which reinforces itself under increased load and loses structure under conditions of lack of mechanical stimulation.

4.1.3.4.3 Bone Healing Pattern

Immediate function is more important for maintaining the integrity of the locomotor system than for the pattern of bone healing. Indirectly, the bone healing process is enhanced by a perfectly functioning blood supply resulting from optimal recovery of limb function soon after the fracture and its treatment.

4.1.4 The Principle of Soft Tissue Care

In the early days of internal fixation, the surgeon approached the bone without paying much attention to the soft tissues. It was assumed that the periosteum had little to do with fracture healing. In contrast to this outdated attitude, we now know that every detail is important, the incision, the approach to the bone, avoidance of stripping the periosteum, the fixation of the implant and its contact to bone. These are all factors which contribute to the recovery of function and to undisturbed bone healing. Any tissue from which the blood supply is cut off, be it soft tissue or bone, will be liable to infection.

4.1.5 The Principle of Biological Fixation

Clinical results of a procedure called biological internal fixation have recently proved very successful. Biological internal fixation is a term which points to the fact that this procedure tries to preserve the biological reactivity of tissue as much as possible. The less the blood supply to the bone fragments is disturbed, the better the formation of callus and the better the resistance to infection.

The term "biological internal fixation" does not mean that now for the first time fracture healing is biological. However, it does indicate that for the first time special care is given to both the soft tissues and the bone. Characteristic of biological internal fixation is that it does not view technical fixation as more important than the biological milieu of the healing fracture.

Biological internal fixation means very careful dissection, indirect reduction and a minimum of fixation. For example, special care is taken not to devascularise the bone fragments far from the plate. One would expect the lack of "medial support" to result in implant failure due to fatigue. This danger is offset by the fact that a bone bridge is formed early on and supports the "medial" cortex, thus unloading the implant.

Bone healing after "biological" internal fixation is seen to follow the well known course of indirect bone healing. With flexible fixation, one would expect the deformation of the soft tissues to impede fracture healing, but the fact that the fracture is not simple but multifragmentary and that exact adjustment is not imperative reduces critical tissue deformation. This all helps to explain why fracture treatment using biological internal fixation seems to be exceedingly successful.

4.2 Aims of the AO Technique: Stability and Biology

By R. Hertel

The aim of fracture treatment is to restore full function and integrity. The best possible long term function of the injured tissues including their cosmetic appearance should be obtained. Treatment methods are customised to the given injury. Possible pitfalls, time off work and global costs have to be considered.

The basic problem which led to the development of skeletal fixation systems has remained unchanged: dissatisfaction with the functional outcome of some conventionally treated fractures. Increasing experience has helped us recognise the importance of soft tissue trauma. Indeed, a given radiologic fracture pattern may be treated by different fixation methods, depending upon the nature of the soft tissue injury. It is essential to focus attention on the global musculo-skeletal injury pattern, which definitively determines the practical approach to any given fracture.

The challenge is to reach the overall aim of restoring full function and integrity, carefully avoiding any potential serious complications. Since the inception of AO teaching, atraumatic, or better oligotraumatic, tissue handling has been given high priority. Poor planning and rough surgery may lead to additional devascularisation. The resulting necrosis is prone to infection. Necrosis and/or infection may lead to nonunion and to skeletal and soft tissue defects which are difficult and time consuming to remedy. Avoiding ischaemia and necrosis should therefore be our principal short term objective.

There are circumstances where iatrogenic damage is inflicted by a lack of treatment. The missed compartment syndrome is one example. Ischaemia due to high intracompartmental pressure (swelling of the contused muscle) may lead to total muscle necrosis. Inadequate initial debridement, in combination with additional devascularisation by poor fixation technique, may lead to irreparable damage. As a general rule, only living tissue, including bone, has the capacity to heal. We will refer to this as the biological potential of the tissue. Alongside this, there is the undoubted need for some degree of stability for a fracture to heal. How much stability is needed does, curiously enough, not depend as much on the type of fracture itself as on the type of fixation. A theoretical explanation can be sought in Perren's cell strain theory. The essential message is that the smaller the fracture gap, the higher the strain on the interposed cells. Thus, plate osteosynthesis which leaves very small fracture gaps is vulnerable in this regard. In fractures with minimal additional soft tissue trauma and no major endosteal or periosteal devascularisation, a simple cast (provided that alignment and length are correct) leads to reliable and rapid bone union, leaving no permanent functional impairment. In the presence of a poor biological potential, the fixation needs to be more long standing, although additional devascularisation must be minimised.

The practical aims of internal fixation have been gradually revised in the light of experience and adapted to different fracture situations. For intra-articular fractures anatomical reduction is mandatory, but reduction and internal fixation must preserve their vascularity. For meta- and diaphyseal fractures, although correct length and spatial alignment are necessary, anatomical reduction of all fragments is not considered mandatory. Reduction and internal fixation must preserve the healing potential, which is easily destroyed by too aggressive surgical exposure of the fracture. The degree of stability needed is adapted to the fracture pattern. Optimal, not maximal, stability is required. The biological status of the injury site must never be compromised to achieve a mechanical goal.

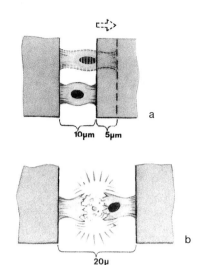

Large strain in small gaps. The elongation of cells or tissue is critical. Above the critical value a disturbed function or even rupture will occur. **a** A small displacement in the gap is tolerated by the cell. **b** A slightly larger displacement results in rupture of the cell.

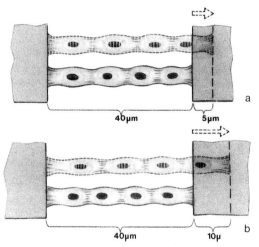

Small strain in large gaps. The strain on the individual cell can be reduced by widening the fracture gap. The global displacement is shared by multiple tissue elements (e. g. cells). **a** A small displacement in the gap is tolerated by the cell. **b** A larger displacement is still tolerated.

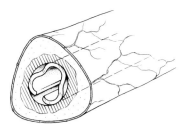

Reamed intramedullary nailing. Reaming destroys the endosteal vascularity by direct stripping of the vessels, by microembolisation and by heat. This results in ischaemia of the central part of the cortex (*slotted area*).

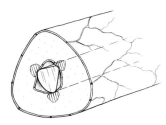

Unreamed intramedullary nailing. The introduction of a nail without reaming leads to minimal circulatory disturbance of the cortex.

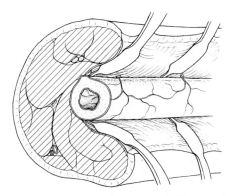

Nonevascularising surgical approach. The bone is exposed trough generous skin incisions, but the periosteal circulation is respected. Epiperiosteal exposure leaves a thin layer of tissue over the exposed part of the bone, thus preserving most of its circulation. At least half of the bone circumference is left untouched. It is important to be extremely careful with Hohmann retractors to avoid involuntary soft tissue stripping.

4.2.1 Technique

Medullary nailing fulfils many of the criteria for biologically successful osteosynthesis. When performed as a "closed" procedure, it is minimally invasive and yields sufficient stability. Unfortunately, reaming of the medullary cavity greatly impairs bone circulation. In a sense there is an antagonism between biology and mechanics. Recently a new generation of unreamed nails has become available, which leave the cortical circulation relatively undisturbed. Improved design will hopefully yield optimal stability, whilst preserving a maximum of biological potential.

In plate osteosynthesis, mainly indicated for epi-, metaphyseal or multilevel fractures, two main considerations remain the key for biological osteosynthesis: the surgical approach and the technique of reduction. The surgical approach must be chosen according to the soft tissue condition. As a general rule, it is wise to include any traumatic laceration in the surgical approach; this allows debridement of contused tissue and preserves the integrity of the remaining tissues. The bone should be minimally exposed. Subperiosteal exposure of bone must be abandoned for epiperiosteal dissection. Not more than half of the bone circumference should be epiperiosteally exposed. Generous lengths of incisions will help to avoid inadvertent stripping during manipulation.

The technique of reduction is of paramount importance since periosteal stripping is frequently due to repeated unsuccessful reduction manoeuvres. The surgeon's frustration leads to a more aggressive handling with forceful reduction, followed by an even stronger devascularisation of the bone. Conventional manual reduction is often cumbersome and time consuming. The worst aspect is the repeated application of bone clamps for unsuccessful reduction manoeuvres, which may lead to massive, circumferential stripping of the periosteum and devitalisation of the fragments. Indirect reduction techniques will help to avoid these errors and are always applicable.

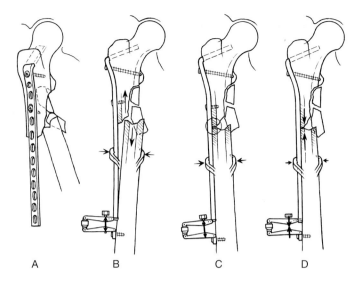

A   B   C   D

Indirect reduction technique.
A A long condylar plate is fixed to the proximal main fragment, regardless of the position of the distal fragments. **B** Indirect reduction of the main fracture plane, utilising the plate to distract and reduce the fracture, is prepared. The articulated tension device is mounted in the distraction mode and a critically positioned Verbrügge clamp is applied. **C** Simultaneous distraction and tightening of the clamp leads to approximative reduction in slight overdistraction. Length, axis and rotation are controlled. **D** Compression of the main fracture plane with the articulated tension device leads to high primary stability. Finally, the critical screws are introduced (two on each main fragment). Reduction and stabilisation of the medial fragments is not attempted to avoid additional vascular damage.

The first step after epiperiosteal exposure is to identify the key fracture plane. Next, preliminary plate fixation to a major proximal or distal fragment in the expected axial alignment is performed. Approximate reduction and placement of a reduction clamp to hold the plate is followed by distraction either with the articulated tension device or a conventional distractor.

The second step of reduction, carefully controlling the major fracture plane for rotational and axial alignment, is carried out using a pointed bone clamp applied carefully to strategic points. Finally, compression is applied with the articulating tension device to at least 1500 N (green ring) and the crucial screws inserted. The exact site of compression is relatively unimportant. It is certainly not necessary to fill all the screw holes. Judicious use of screws helps avoid unnecessary additional necrosis, known to occur after drilling and insertion of screws (cylindrical sequestrum due to heat and crush). The minimum number of screws is at least two on each side of the main fracture. For better leverage rather longer plates are advocated.

In some instances, a combination of external and internal fixation is preferable. This is especially true for comminuted epimetaphyseal fractures of the proximal tibia since the use of bilateral plates can seriously jeopardise bone and skin circulation. The combination of a unilateral plate and an external fixator (buttress), which temporarily replaces the contralateral cortex, is one possible way to satisfy both biology and mechanics.

In extensive, combined trauma it is occasionally preferable to opt for a staged procedure. In the acute phase, debridement is followed by external fixation to avoid additional trauma associated with the application of an internal stabilising device. After soft tissue recovery, generally a few weeks, definitive internal fixation can be safely performed.

Another aspect of "biological osteosynthesis" is the refinement in implant design and material. Plates, for instance, have

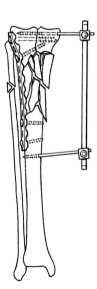

Combination of plate and external fixator. The use of an external fixator, as a substitute for an additional plate, has proven very effective in diminishing surgical trauma.

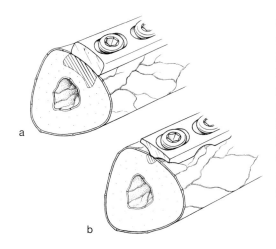

DCP (dynamic compression plate) and LC-DCP (limited contact dynamic compression plate). **a** The conventional plate has a wide contact area with the bone. In the underlying cortex a zone of ischaemia is created. **b** The LC DCP minimises the contact area and thus the zone of cortical ischaemia. Note the position of the plate over the periosteum.

evolved from a broad contact area with the bone to a limited contact design. Limited contact plates produce less circulatory disturbance of the underlying bone than full contact plates. Nails have evolved to the unreamed design since reaming was recognised as potentially harmful due to the destruction of the medullary vascular network, in addition to causing microembolisms and direct thermal lesions. External fixation is being improved. A "radial preload" Schanz screw promises reduction of pin track problems. A newly designed "pinless" fixator is clamped on the bone surface, thus avoiding the perforation needed for the insertion of standard Schanz screws.

4.3 Biomechanical Aspects of the AO/ASIF Technique

By S. M. Perren and J. Buchanan

It is obvious that the process of bone fracture changes the bone's mechanical conditions. It is suddenly no longer intact but broken up into two or more pieces, it is no longer capable of carrying load, its fragments are unstable and produce pain. As we pointed out in Sect. 4.1, there is a close relationship between the degree of mobility (instability) of the fracture and the amount of callus produced. The mechanical conditions obviously control the biological reaction: In the context of our work "biomechanical" refers to the biological reaction to mechanical input.

The mechanical input may be motion or force. The weight of a person loads the bone and thus produces internal stresses. If excessive load is applied to the bone, the bone breaks. If, on the other hand, a bone is unloaded, it loses its structure and becomes porotic, i.e. small holes appear within the unloaded bone.

As we will see later, the reaction of bone to loading is less important than the reaction of bone to instability. The surface of bone does not tolerate motion well. Instability (motion at the fracture site) induces resorption and shortening of the fracture fragment. This is a process which under normal conditions enables bone to heal in spite of instability. Since the resorption increases the width of the fracture gap, the repair tissues in the fracture gap are less deformed and it is less likely that they will be disrupted. In internal fixation, motion between bone fragments and between an implant and bone induces surface resorption, which results in loosening of the fracture fixation and may therefore result in initial microinstability turning into gross instability, which might impede fracture healing. These are examples of the relation between mechanical input and the biological reaction of bone. This relation determines to a great extent the type of fracture healing resulting from the different mechanical conditions that may prevail when a variety of internal fixation techniques are used. We will now discuss these techniques with special reference to the reaction they induce in fractured and intact bone.

When a surgeon reconstructs a patient's broken leg, he puts the fractured pieces back into place, holds them together with forceps and inserts a screw that catches in only one fragment of the fracture while the other fragment is held by the head of the screw resting against the surface of the bone. This technique is called the lag screw technique. The important feature of this technique is that of the two fracture fragments only one is in contact with the thread of the screw. The other fragment, namely, the one near the head of the screw, can glide along the screw. This can be achieved either by using a shaft screw or more commonly by drilling the hole in the bone the same size as the outer diameter of the screw thread (gliding hole). One single excessive load applied to the lag screw pulls the screw out of its tight connection to the bone and the screw "strips". One overload will permanently negate the function of the screw. This means that the lag screw technique is not forgiving.

In the conventional AO/ASIF technique, plating was used exclusively to bridge a fracture which had been fixed using a lag screw. The plate acts like a splint in the same way as an external splint (plaster cast). The rigid device applied to the bone takes a major part of the load off the fracture, thus protecting the lag screw fixation from overload. The term "neutralisation plate" or better "protection plate" indicates that the plate should prevent overloading of the lag screw and thus stripping.

A plate used without a lag screw acts, when bent, as an elastic but rigid spring. Any load applied to the plate will always deform the plate somewhat, which in turn causes the fracture to undergo some movement. This then induces callus and resorption at the fracture site.

Some improvement in the stability achieved using plates may be attained by applying the plates under tension, which compresses and stabilises the fractured bone. When the AO/ASIF technique was first started, the plates were tensioned using the removable compressor. The so-called dynamic compression plate (DCP) permits application of compression by taking advantage of a specially designed screw hole. This hole has an inclined surface, which means that the plate compresses the fracture when the screws are inserted in a somewhat eccentric position. Furthermore, the spherical geometry of the DCP permits insertion of the plate screws at an angle in order to avoid fracture lines and improve their function as lag screws.

Thus, while in the conventional AO/ASIF technique plates were not used without lag screws, in the newer techniques of internal fixation (biological internal fixation) plates are often used without lag screws; in these cases, callus formation is not an unwanted side effect but the goal of the treatment. The conventional plates are made of a rectangular piece of metal with screw holes and a rounded undersurface. The disadvantage of the close contact between the plate undersurface and the bone surface was damage to the blood supply to bone. Efforts to overcome this disadvantage led to the development of the so-called limited contact DC plate (LC-DCP) (Perren et al. 1991). The LC-DCP permits continued blood supply to the bone and is much easier to contour than its older counterpart, the DCP.

A nail may also function as a splint, in the same way as a plate. While the plate is applied to the external surface of the bone, the nail is inserted inside the bone marrow cavity – a so-called intramedullary nail (i.m. nail). This is an elastic but rigid body which maintains the shape of the bone to allow the fracture to heal in a well reduced position. Similar to a splinting plaster cast or a splinting plate, the splinting i.m. nail does not completely prevent movement at the fracture site. It resists bending load well, but is relatively inefficient in resisting torque. This means that the fragments can rotate about the long axis of the bone, i.e. a nail does not protect against inward or outward rotation of the foot. Furthermore, a conventional i.m. nail will not efficiently resist forces, such as compression, which tend to shorten the bone. Consequently, only those bone fractures can be well treated using the i.m. nail which are more or less transverse or short oblique. To prevent rotation and shortening of multifragmentary fractures, so-called locking bolts are inserted above and below the fracture (Küntscher, Klemm and Schellmann, Grosse and Kempf). These locking bolts provide a close connection between the bone fragments and the nail, thus allowing the i.m. nail to be used for the treatment of comminuted (multifragmentary) fractures. This technique, called interlocked nailing, has extended the indications for the i.m. nail.

A new development in i.m. nailing is the "unreamed nail", i.e. a small solid nail is inserted without first reaming the medullary cavity. The AO/ASIF unreamed nail is based on experimental findings in animal research by Klein and has been developed by Frigg at the AO/ASIF development institute (Klein et al. 1990). The nail is relatively small and does not by itself provide good fixation. Therefore, it can only be used as an interlocked nail and only under conditions of limited loading. Due to its interesting biological characteristics, the unreamed nail is especially well suited for the initial treatment of open fractures.

Another technique to provide splinting of a fracture is the one using an "external fixator". Here, as with the interlocking nail, a splint is fixed to the bone using bolts. The splint of the external fixator is the connecting tube, the bolts are the Steinmann pins or the Schanz screws. The external fixator provides semi rigid flexible fixation and is preferentially used in open fractures where the surgeon does not wish to use massive implants for reasons of maintaining good resistance to infection. The disadvantage of the external fixator is its pins, which connect the medullary cavity with the splint outside the body. Since this connection to the outside may precipitate an infection of the medullary cavity, the latest development replaces the transosseous pin with a forceps-type clamp,, which greatly minimises the amount of damage to the bone (see the reports on the pinless external fixator by Swiontkowski, 1992, and Frigg, 1992).

Long spiral fractures were previously treated using "cerclage wire", i.e. a wire that was put around the bone and tensioned by applying a so-called quirl. Cerclage wires are well suited for holding fragments with longitudinal fracture lines together during surgical intervention. They do not provide long-term stability and only little strength. Therefore, cerclage wires can very rarely be used alone. The combination of cerclage wire and plaster cast has not offered enough advantages and has therefore disappeared. Today cerclage is no longer used for permanent fixation.

Fractures of small bones or of metaphyseal bones are often temporarily fixed using Kirschner wires (K wires) or small pins with or without threaded pins. Today such pins are mainly used for temporary fixation preceding stable internal fixation using plates, for example, for metaphyseal fractures.

The following list provides an overview of the different techniques in relation to the amount of stability achieved.

1. *Absolutely Stable Fixation.* Absolute stability of fixation, i.e. no movement of the fracture under dynamic functional loading, is uniquely achieved by the use of compression applied between the fracture fragments (interfragmentary compression). The lag screw is a classical example of an implant providing absolute stability. It produces around 3000 N within the fracture plane, a force which holds the fragments together to resist traction as a result of bending and shear produced by twisting of the bone. The first principle is called stabilisation by preload; the second, stabilisation by friction. The plate produces less compression (about 600 N) and the compression produced acts asymmetrically, i.e. it compresses the fracture on the side near the plate, but tends to open the fracture at the cortex far from the plate. The nail (AO/ASIF universal nail and unreamed nail) may cause compression, but it will only last if locking bolts are placed within cortical bone. The external fixator allows compression of the fracture, but its eccentric placement is the cause of a very asymmetric compression, which is not usually very effective. The cerclage wire may produce compression when it is tightened, but once the quirl is released and bent to avoid protrusion the wire completely loses pre-tension. K wires and pins do not produce compression but splint the fragments so that the functional compression may act upon the fracture surfaces without displacement.

2. *Rigid But Not Absolutely Stable Fixation.* Such fixation depends on the use of rigid splints such as large diameter medullary nails. Functional loading of the fracture splinted with a rigid splint will produce very little displacement and in most cases the nail is able to carry body weight.

3. *Flexible Fixation.* Flexible splint fixation as provided by a small medullary nail (such as the unreamed nail) maintains the position of the fracture while allowing intermittent flexion or twist. Such fixation and fixation using plates with extensive undercuts to reduce the contact area at the bone–plate interface are at the basis of biological fixation.

4.4 Glossary

By S. M. Perren and J. Buchanan

Absolute Stability: The compressed surfaces of the fracture do not displace under applied functional load. The definition of absolute stability applies only to a given time and place of observation. While under certain conditions some areas of a fracture do not displace in relation to each other, other areas of the fracture may do so simultaneously and vice versa. Practically the only method to achieve absolute stability is to apply interfragmental compression. Compression stabilises by preloading and by producing friction (Perren 1972).

Biological Internal Fixation: Also known as biological plate fixation and biological fixation (Mast et al. 1989): In internal fixation there is a delicate balance between the degree of stabilisation and that of surgical trauma. The benefits of each must be taken into account. Biological fixation favours the preservation of the blood supply and thus optimises the healing potential of bone and soft tissues. It provides sufficient stability for multifragmentary fractures to heal in correct alignment. To protect the implants from overload, it relies on early biological reaction (callus formation).

If simple fractures are plated, stable fixation to prevent induction of bone surface resorption is required. In single fractures with closely adapted fracture surfaces, minimal motion generates high strain, which in turn induces bone surface resorption in contact areas. When locking or nongliding splints are used for fracture fixation, reliable results are produced by stability which prevents loosening. Surgical exposure required for stabilisation of a simple fracture is limited and therefore less detrimental to the blood supply and healing of the fracture.

Multifragmentary fractures and complex fractures are less demanding in respect to stability. Here, instability produces small amounts of strain due to (a) larger fracture gaps and (b) distribution of strain over several, serially located fracture gaps. The operative procedures required for stable fixation of multifragmentary fractures are extensive and cause considerable subsequent disturbances to blood supply. Consequently, when plating a single fracture stability is the prime goal, while in multifragmentary fractures biology takes precedence.

Blood Supply to Cortical Bone (or restoration thereof): Cortical bone which has been completely deprived of its blood supply for an extended period of time becomes necrotic. It may be revascularised by the regrowth of blood vessels without a marked widening of the Haversian canals (Pfister et al. 1979) or it may be revascularised by newly formed Haversian canals. The restoration of previous Haversian canals is a process with a marked lag period and is relatively slow (0.1 mm/day, Schenk

1987). Bone may be revascularised by resorption and replacement with newly formed, vascular bone (creeping substitution).

Buttress: If trauma results in impaction of a bone (e.g. at the distal metaphysis of the tibia), a defect remains after fracture reduction. An implant (plate, external fixator or interlocking nail) then temporarily carries functional load while it maintains the shape of the bone.

Callus: A reparative tissue made of connective, cartilaginous or bony tissue (or any combination thereof). Callus formation may be induced by any irritation due to chemicals (Küntscher 1970), infection and/or instability (Hutzschenreuter et al. 1969) and other factors. In internal fixation the appearance of callus is therefore a little appreciated sign of an unwanted condition. Callus is, however, always welcome as a repair tissue.

Cancellous Bone: While the shaft of the long bones consists of cortical, i.e. dense bone, the proximal and distal ends (metaphysis and epiphysis) consist mainly of a less dense, trabecular bone, cancellous bone. Cancellous bone has per volume a much larger surface area and is, therefore, more readily receptive to blood supply as well as to osteoclasts for resorption.

Complete Articular Fracture: The articular surface is completely dissociated from the diaphysis

Complex Fracture: Fracture in which after reduction there is no contact between the main fragments.

Compression: The act of pressing together. It results in deformation (shortening as of a spring) and in an improvement or creation of stability. Compression is used, first, to provide stability of fixation where motion induced resorption must be prevented and, second, to protect the implants and to improve the efficiency of the implants by unloading them. Unloading is achieved through restoration of the load-bearing capacity of the bone. Any fixation taking advantage of the load bearing capacity of fragments of a fractured bone can withstand appreciable amounts of load without mechanical failure or temporary micromotion within the fracture. This is the main reason for using careful reduction and application of compression. Compression furthermore helps to restore dynamic loading of the bone fragments, a process for which stable contact of the fracture fragments is a prerequisite.

If the implant (screw, plate) bridging the fracture is applied under tension, the fracture focus undergoes an equal amount of compression The compression is used to help stabilise the fracture. We have not observed any "magic biological effect" of compression.

Compression Plate: When a plate is applied to produce compression, i.e. when the plate is tensioned, it is called a compression plate. The tension in the plate is produced by the application of one plate end to the bone and by the use of a removable compressor or by eccentric placement of the screws within so-called compression holes in the DCP or LC-DCP, for example. The fracture line in between will then be compressed (interfragmental compression). The compression produced by the compression plate acts outside the fracture, and is therefore asymmetric and produces high local stress in the cortex immediately below the plate. The amount of compression produced by the plate is about 60 kp.

Compression Screw: This term does not describe a special implant but rather the special use or application of an implant. When a screw is applied to produce compression, i.e. when the screw is tensioned, it is called a compression screw. The tension in the screw is produced by the combined effect of a screw with a threaded pilot hole and a smooth gliding hole. When such a screw is tightened, the thread presses the bone fragment against the head of the screw, compressing the fracture line (interfragmental compression). The compression produced by the screw acts from within the fracture surface and is therefore most efficient. The amount of compression produced by a 4.5 mm cortex screw is around 250–300 kp.

Contact Healing: Healing which occurs between two fragment ends of a fractured bone at circumscribed places which are maintained in motionless contact. The fracture is then repaired by direct internal remodelling.

Contact healing may also be observed where the gap is only a few micrometers wide.

Cortical Bone, Cortex: The dense bone within the diaphysis (middle part) of long bones is called cortical bone; the dense shell of the cancellous bone is called cortex. The two terms are often used synonymously.

Debricolage: A French term to signify the process of mechanical failure of an internal fixation prior to the onset of solid bone bridging.

Diaphysis: The cylindrical part between the ends of a long bone is called the diaphysis.

Direct Healing: A type of fracture healing observed in stable internal fixation. It is characterised by (a) the absence of callus formation specific to the fracture site, (b) absence of bone surface resorption at the fracture site and (c) direct bone formation, i. e. without intermediary repair tissue. Direct fracture healing was formerly called "primary" healing in some countries. Today we avoid the term primary in order not to grade the quality of fracture healing. Two types of direct healing are distinguished: contact healing (see above) and gap healing (see below).

Dynamisation: The mechanical load can be increased at a certain stage to enhance bone formation or to promote "maturisation" of the bone. Examples are the removal of some screws in plate fixation or the opening of some clamps in fixation using an external fixator. Early dynamisation, i. e. dynamisation before solid bridging of the bone, results in stimulated callus formation. The value of late dynamisation is less obvious.

Epiphysis: The ends of a long bone are called epiphyses. The epiphysis carries the articular component of a long bone.

Extra-Articular Fractures: The fracture does not involve the articular surface, but may be intracapsular.

Far (Trans-) Cortex: The cortex away from the plate is called the far cortex. It may also be called the trans-cortex. The consequence of a defect within the far cortex is much more important than that of a defect in the near cortex. The difference is due to the larger lever arm of the far cortex.

Flexible Fixation: Generally, internal fixation according to AO/ASIF methods means stable fixation possibly using close adaptation and compression. Recently, a less stable fixation (flexible fixation using splinting plates, nails or fixators) has been observed to yield very good results under conditions in which the fragments are well vascularised. Given best preservation of the viability of the fragments, flexible fixation induces abundant callus formation. It must be pointed out that the combination of instability and necrosis may be deleterious.

Fracture: A sudden rupture of a structure which starts whenever the internal stress produced by load exceeds the limits of strength. Depending on the type of load – compressive, flexural, torsional, shear and any combination thereof – a typical fracture pattern can be observed (impaction, transverse fracture, spiral fracture, avulsion, etc.). The complexity of the fracture depends mainly upon the amount of energy stored prior to fracture.

Fracture Disease: A condition characterised by pain, swelling and other signs of dystrophy such as patchy bone loss and stiffness of joints (Lucas-Championniere 1907). Fracture disease (synonym, Sudeck's atrophy) can best be avoided by stable fixation to reduce irritation, by early active movement and, whenever possible, by immediate or at least partial weight bearing on the injured limb (Allgöwer 1978)

Gap Healing: The healing process taking place between two fragment ends kept in stable relative positions with a small gap between the fragment ends. Gap healing progresses in two phases: (a) the filling of the gap with lamellar bone of different orientation than the bone of the fragments, and (b) the subsequent remodelling of the newly filled bone from within the gap into the fragments (plugging) or crossing from one fragment through the newly filled bone into the other fragment (remodelling)

Gliding Hole: When a fully threaded screw is used as a lag screw, the cortex under the screwhead should not engage. This can be accomplished by overdrilling the near cortex screw hole to at least the size of the outer diameter of the screw thread.

Gliding Splint: A splint (e.g. conventional nail) which allows for axial shortening. Such a splint offers the possibility of coaptation under conditions of fragment end shortening due to bone surface resorption.

Goal of Fracture Treatment: According to M. E. Mueller et al. (1963): "To restore optimal function of the limb in respect to mobility and load bearing capacity." The goal is furthermore to avoid early disturbances such as Sudeck's atrophy ("fracture disease") and late sequelae such as post-traumatic arthrosis.

Haversian System: The cortical bone is composed of a system of small channels (osteons) about 1/10 of a millimetre in diameter. These channels contain the blood vessels and are remodelled after a disturbance of the blood supply to bone.

Healing: Restoration of the original integrity. Theoretically the healing process after a bone fracture would last many years, even after internal fracture remodelling has subsided. For practical purposes, healing is considered completed when the bone has regained its normal stiffness and strength.

Impacted Fracture: A fracture in which the cortex or articular surface is driven into the cancellous bone.

Indirect Healing: Bone healing as observed in nontreated or unstably treated fractures. Callus formation is predominant, the fracture fragment ends are resorbed and bone formation results from a process of transformation of fibrous and/or cartilaginous tissue into bone.

Interfragmental Compression (Effect of): Static compression applied to a fracture area stabilises the fragments and thus reduces irritation. Bone surface resorption is then absent. No proof has been found that compression per se has an effect upon internal remodelling of the cortical bone (Matter et al. 1974).

Interlocking Nail: A nail provides some degree of stability mainly by its (flexural) stiffness. Since a conventional nail allows the fragments to slide along the nail, the fracture must therefore provide a solid support against shortening. For the treatment of complex fractures, the nail can be interlocked to prevent shortening and rotation.

Lag Screw: The lag screw produces interfragmental compression by compressing the bone under the screw head against the fragment in which the screw threads are anchored. Interfragmental compression can be reduced by wedging the screw threads against the walls of the gliding hole. Anchorage in the near fragment can be avoided by the use of a shaft screw. This method is required to maintain efficient compression when the lag screw is applied through the plate in an inclined position.

Locking Splint: An implant (e. g. plate) acting as a splint, which when somewhat loosened by interface resorption, does not allow coaptation. Therefore when using a locking splint for fixation of a simple and adapted fracture, interfragmental displacement should be avoided to prevent bone surface resorption with subsequent biological loosening of the fixation. Such loosening without possible coaptation may result in a mechanically induced nonunion. This is a problem after plating, whereas after locked nailing the mere removal of the locking pins allows for maintenance of the splinting while gliding along the long axis of the nail is permitted.

Metaphysis: The segment of a long bone located between the end part (epiphysis) and the shaft (diaphysis). It consists mostly of cancellous bone.

Multifragmentary Fracture: A term reserved usually for extra-articular and articular fractures which have one or more completely dissociated intermediate fragments.

Near (Cis-) Cortex: Within the plated segment of bone the screws cross two cortices, the one near the plate is called the near cortex. For this cortex, the term "cis-cortex" is used as well. In respect to bending, the near cortex contributes little to stability of fixation. When, for example, in a wave plate application, the distance between the plate and the near cortex is increased, the bone and the repair tissues gain better leverage.

Neutralisation: An implant (plate, external fixators or nail) which acts based upon its stiffness is said to neutralise the effect of the functional load. The implant carries a major part of the functional load and thus protects, for example, a screw fixation. It does not actually neutralise but does minimise the effect of the forces (see protection).

Osteoblast/Osteoclast: Cells that form or destroy bone. The osteoblasts line a bone surface where bone apposition occurs. The osteoclasts rest in the Howship lacunae (a small well within the bone surface). They are typically found at the tip of the remodelling osteons (see above).

Overbending (of plate): See Prebending.

Partial Articular Fracture: The fracture involves only part of the joint while the remainder remains attached to the diaphysis.

Pilot Hole: If a fully threaded screw is to function as a lag screw, the screw is anchored in the fragment near the tip of the screw within a threaded hole. This is called the pilot hole. Within the fragment near the head of the screw, the thread of the screw should not anchor but glide (gliding hole). A pilot hole is prepared when inserting a Schanz screw or Steinmann pin.

Pin Loosening: The pins of external fixator frames serve to stabilise the fragments of a fracture. The stability provided depends, amongst other things, on the contact between pin and bone. If bone surface resorption at the pin–bone interface occurs, stability is reduced. Pin loosening is less important in respect to loss of stability but is important in respect to its deleterious effect on pin track infection.

Prebending of Plate: Exactly contoured plates produce asymmetric compression, i.e. the near cortex is more compressed than the far cortex. The latter may not be compressed at all. In respect to stabilisation against torque and bending, the compression of the far cortex is more important than that of the near cortex. To provide compression of the far cortex the plate is applied after exact contouring but with an additional bend of the plate segment bridging the fracture. The bend is such that the mid-section of the plate is elevated from the bone surface prior to fixation to the bone. Prebending is an important tool in increasing stability in small and/or porotic bones.

Precise Reduction: The exact adaptation of fracture fragments (hairline adjustment). It should result in complete restoration of anatomy and optimal late function. It should be noted that overall stability does not depend on precise reduction, but precise reduction more reliably results in stability and increased strength of fixation.

Preload: The application of interfragmental compression keeps the fragments together until a tensile force exceeding the compression (preload) is applied.

Protection: While the term neutralisation has often be used in plate and screw fixation, the term protection should replace it. In reality nothing is neutralised (which would mean that a force, for example, is counteracted in its effect by an equal but opposite force). In plate fixation, the plate reduces the load placed upon the screw fixation. It therefore protects the screw fixation from overload.

Pure Depression: An articular fracture in which there is a pure depression of the articular surface without a split.

Pure Split: An articular fracture in which there is an articular split without any additional cartilaginous lesion.

Radial Preload: To prevent pin loosening (see above), the contact zone between the implant and bone can be preloaded, i.e. a static compressive force is applied. Hitherto, preloading was achieved by applying a permanent bending moment to the pins. Today it is radial preload, i.e. a tight fit produced by insertion of a pin slightly larger than the drill hole. The effect of radial preload is to minimise pin loosening and to seal the pin track such that a possible infection from outside cannot reach the medullary cavity. The amount of misfit between the hole diameter and the pin diameter should not exceed 0.05–0.1 mm. Such a difference can only reliably be established using self-cutting tips.

Refracture: A fracture occurring after the bone has solidly bridged, at a load level otherwise tolerated by normal bone. The resulting fracture line may coincide with the original fracture line or it may be located remote from the original fracture but within the area of bone undergoing changes due to fracture and treatment.

Glossary

Relative Stability: An internal fixation construct that allows small amounts of motion in proportion to the load applied. This is the case with a fixation which depends only on the stiffness of the implant (such as a nail bridging a fracture without exerting compression). It will always show deformation or displacement which is inversely proportional to the stiffness of the implant. Such motion is always present but harmless in nail fixation. According to the philosophy of the AO/ASIF group, plate fixation is more reliable if motion is prevented. (Callus as a sign of unwanted instability is then absent.)

Remodelling (of bone): The process of transformation of external bone shape (external remodelling) or of internal bone structure (internal remodelling, or remodelling of the Haversian system).

Resorption (of bone): The process of bone removal includes the dissolution of mineral and matrix and their uptake into the cell (phagocytosis).

Rigid Fixation: A fixation of a fracture which permits only little deformation under load.

Rigid Implants: In general, implants are considered to be rigid when they are made of metal. The implant geometry is more important than the stiffness of the material. Most implants made of metal are much more flexible than the corresponding bone.

Rigidity: This term is often used synonymously to stiffness. According to Timoshenko (1941), it should be used when related to shear (e. g. at the interface of plate and bone).

Simple Fracture (or single fracture): A disruption of bone (diaphyseal, extra articular, articular) with two main fragments.

Splinting: The action of reducing the mobility of a fracture based upon a stiff body being coupled to the bone fragments. The splint may be external (plaster, external fixators) or internal (internal fixation plate, i.m. nail).

Split Depression: A combination of split and depression.

Spontaneous Healing: The healing pattern of a fracture without treatment. Most often, solid healing is observed but frequently malalignment results.

Stable Fixation: A fixation which keeps the fragments of a fracture in motionless adaptation at least for joint movement. While a mobile fracture produces pain with any attempts to move the limb, stable fixation allows early painless mobilisation. Thus stable fixation minimises irritation, which may eventually lead to fracture disease.

Stability of Fixation: This is characterised by the lack of motion at the fracture site (i. e. little or no displacement between the fragments of the fracture), while in technical terms stability characterises the tendency to revert to a condition of low energy.

Stiffness: The resistance of a structure to deformation. The higher the stiffness of an implant, the smaller the deformation of the implant, the smaller the displacement of the fracture fragments, and the greater the strain reduction in the repair tissue. Reduced but not abolished strain promotes healing.

Stiffness and Geometrical Properties: The thickness affects the deformability by its third power. Changes in geometry are therefore much more critical than changes in material properties. This fact is often overlooked by non-engineers. Thus, the goal of flexible fixation can be achieved better by a small change in dimensions than by using a "less rigid" material.

Stiffness and Material Properties: The stiffness of a structure depends on its Young's modulus of elasticity. An increasing Young's modulus affects the deformation of the material by its first power.

Strain: Relative deformation of repair tissue. Not the motion at the fracture site but the resulting relative deformation, called strain, is the important characteristic. As strain is a relative unit (displacement of the fragments divided by the width of the fracture gap), very high levels of strain may be present within small fracture gaps under conditions where the amount of displacement may not even be visible. Under these conditions invisible displacement producing strain must be taken into consideration.

Strain Induction: Tissue deformation – amongst other things – may result in induction of callus. This is an example of a mechanically induced biological reaction. For reactions triggered by strain, such as callus formation and bone surface resorption, a lower limit of strain, the minimum strain is to be considered.

Strain Tolerance: Determines the tolerance of the repair tissues to mechanical conditions. No tissue can be formed under conditions of strain which exceed elongation and cause rupture of the tissue. Above the critical level, the strain on the recently formed tissues will destroy them once formed or even prevent their formation.

Strength: The ability to withstand load without structural failure. The strength of a material can be reported as ultimate tensile strength, as bending strength or as torsional strength. The local criterion for failure of a bone or implant is expressed in units of force per unit area, i.e. *stress*, or as (equivalent) deformation per unit length, strain or elongation at rupture.

Stress Protection: This term, initially used to describe bone reaction to reduced functional load (Allgöwer et al. 1969) is used today mainly to express the negative aspects of stress relief of bone. The basic assumption is that bone deprived of necessary functional stimulation by changing mechanical load becomes less dense or strong (Wolff's law, Wolff 1893, 1986). Stress protection is often used synonymously with stress shielding, i.e. in a purely mechanical sense. It is often used to characterise bone loss, implying a negative reaction to stress shielding. In respect to internal fixation of cortical bone, stress protection seems to play a fairly unimportant role compared to vascular considerations.

The early bone loss which was hitherto attributed to stress protection can be explained by a temporary lack of blood supply. The necrotic area is then remodelled by osteons which originate from the area with good blood supply. Remodelling goes along with temporary osteoporosis.

Measurements of late bone loss under clinical conditions of internal fixation in the human using quantitative computed tomography show very little bone loss at the time of implant removal (Cordey et al. 1985).

In summary, bone may react to unloading but this plays a minor role in internal fixation of cortical bone fractures.

Stress Shielding: If internal fixation relies upon screws and plates, as maintained by the AO/ASIF group, the stability of fixation is achieved by interfragmental compression exerted mainly by the lag screws. Such stabilisation using lag screws is very stable but only provides safety under functional load in some special situations (long spiral fractures, metaphyseal fractures, etc.). A plate providing protection (or neutralisation) is therefore often added. The function of such a plate is to reduce the amount of peak load applied to the screw fixation. Protection is provided based upon the stiffness of the plate. The plate shields the fractured and temporarily fixed bone.

Tension Band: An implant (wire or plate) functioning according to the tension band principle. The bone carries tensile force when it undergoes flexural load and the implant is attached to the convex surface; the bone, and especially the cortex far from the plate, is then dynamically compressed. The plate is able to resist very large amounts of tensile force, so that the bone in turn can best resist compressive load.

Vascularity: A tissue is vascularised if it contains blood vessels connected to the main circulatory system. Blood vessels may be shut off temporarily from the circulatory system. We consider a tissue to be nonvascular if either there are no vessels, as in cartilage, or the vessels present are not functioning, for example obliterated by thrombosis.

Wedge Fracture: Fracture with a third fragment in which there is some direct contact between the main fragments after reduction.

4.5 Principles of Bone Grafting

By C. Colton

In 1668, Job van Meekeren, a Dutch surgeon, filled a cranial defect in a soldier with a portion of a dog's skull. The patient was promptly excommunicated and later asked for the bone to be removed. This was not possible as it is said that it had by then incorporated.

This would have to be regarded as unusual, as normally only the patient's own bone – an autograft – will incorporate and not suffer rejection. Bone from another subject of the same species – an allograft – contains elements which may stimulate an immune response by the recipient (host) but certain methods of processing the graft can destroy them and allow an allograft to be accepted, still retaining some power to stimulate new bone formation. Such a process is freezing at very low temperatures, this being the basis of most bone banks. MacEwen of Liverpool, England, was probably the first to use a human bone allograft, in 1880, to replace the humeral shaft of a young boy, destroyed by infection.

The function of a bone graft is either to stimulate healing of an ununited fracture or to fill a bony defect left by trauma, infection or congenital deficit. The graft acts by providing a "scaffolding" for the new bone (osteoconduction) and also by stimulating osteogenesis, or new bone formation (osteoinduction). Bone containing haemopoietic marrow cells is the best osteoinductive tissue; cortical bone is much less effective. Small fragments of graft are better than solid blocks, because the graft dies soon after transplantation, but is then revascularised, replaced and incorporated by the ingrowth of blood vessels from the graft surface (creeping substitution). The greater the surface for any given volume, the more rapid the incorporation and healing will be. It is for these reasons that small chips of the patient's own cancellous, marrow-containing bone make the best bone graft material. The commonest sites for harvesting such bone are the greater trochanter of the femur and the iliac crests. See also Sect. 6.18

Specialised bone grafts consisting of blocks of bone together with a vascular pedicle are occasionally transplanted using microvascular anastomotic techniques. These vascularised grafts are less successful than was originally hoped, and their use is declining.

4.5.1 Immunology of Bone Grafting

Any foreign biological material introduced, or finding its way, into the body may contain chemical components specific to itself which the host recognises as foreign and potentially noxious (antigens). This may cause the host to produce antibodies which neutralise or destroy the antigens – the immune response.

An antigen–antibody interaction may simply cause an inflammatory state with the local release of histamine, e. g. an allergic skin reaction to contact with a plant or inflammation of the upper respiratory mucous membranes in allergic reactions to pollen (hay fever). The release of histamine may be greater and have systemic effects, e. g. anaphylactic shock. Alternatively, as in tissue grafting, the action of antibodies in attacking the material that released the antigen may result in a slower process of destruction of the graft tissue – a slower immunological rejection.

The individual's own grafted tissue (autograft) will not, of course, be seen by the body as a foreign invader and will not excite such an immune response. On the other hand, an allograft will be detected by the host's immune system as an invader, by virtue of the antigenic components of the graft tissue, and is likely to result in rejection unless the tissue types of the host and donor are identical or very similar. There are methods, such as freeze drying, which destroy the antigenic material in allograft tissue and thereby render it more acceptable to the host's immune system. The deep freezing of bone allografts is the basis on which bone banks operate.

Nowadays, a greater danger than potential rejection of the allograft is the possibility that the human donor may have acquired the human immunodeficiency virus (HIV) or some other virus, such as a hepatitis virus, which the graft then transmits to the host. When bone is donated to a bank, the donor is usually screened for HIV and hepatitis virus at the time of donation and 3–4 months later, before the bone graft can be used. The second test is, of course, not possible in the case of cadaveric material. Screening protocols vary from centre to centre, and some countries are stricter than others in the range of tests undertaken on donors and donated tissue.

4.5.2 Bone Banking

Bank bone is foreign material and may be rejected; this also reduces its osteogenic potential. It may also be contaminated with pyogenic organisms. The risks are of rejection and/or infection. Bank bone is only used as a last resort, when a graft is needed in quantities greater than the patient can provide, either because vast amounts of graft are required as in filling large defects or extensive spinal fusions, or because the patient's donor sites are exhausted due to previous failed bone graft surgery. Bank bone is rarely used in acute fracture surgery.

4.5.3 Glossary

Allograft: Graft of tissue from another individual of the same species.

Antibody: A substance produced by the host in response to the detection of an antigen. The antibody is "designed" to attack and destroy the antigen.

Antigen: Component of transplanted tissue which causes the host to mount an attack on the graft by producing antibodies which destroy the antigen and in so doing may result in failure of the graft to incorporate.

Autograft: Graft of tissue from the same individual. Same as homograft.

Creeping Substitution: The process of incorporation of a bone graft by vascular ingrowth from the host bed, removal of the dead graft bone by osteoclasis and its replacement with living bone by a process of osteoblastic activity.

Heterograft: Graft of tissue from another individual of the same species.

Homograft: Graft of tissue from the same individual. Same as autograft.

Xenograft: Graft of tissue from an individual of a different species.

4.6 References

Aebi M, Regazzoni P (eds) Bone transplantation. Springer, Berlin Heidelberg New York

Allgöwer M (1978) Cinderella of surgery – fractures? Surg Clin North Am 58: 1071–1093

Allgöwer M, Ehrsam R, Ganz R, Matter P, Perren SM (1969) Clinical experience with a new compression plate "DCP". Acta Orthop Scand [Suppl] 125: 45–63

Cordey J, Schwyzer HK, Brun S, Matter P (1985) Bone loss following plate fixation of fractures? Helv Chir Acta 52: 181–184

Frigg R (1992) The development of the pinless external fixator: from the idea to the implant. Injury 23 [Suppl 3] : 3–8

Hutzschenreuter P, Perren SM, Steinemann S, Geret B, Klebl M (1969) Some effects of rigidity of internal fixation on the healing pattern of osteotomies. Injury 1: 77–81

Klein MPM, Rahn BA, Frigg R, Kessler S, Perren SM (1990) Reaming versus non-reaming in medullary nailing: interference with cortical circulation of the canine tibua. arch Orthop trauma Surg 109/6 : 314–316

Küntscher G (1970) Das Kallus-Problem. Enke, Stuttgart

Lucas-Championnière J (1907) Les dangers de l'immogilisation des membres – fagilité des os– altération de la nutrition du membre – conclusions pratiques. Rev Méd Chir Pratique 78: 81–87

Mast J, Jakob R, Ganz R (1989) Planning and reduction techniques in fracture surgery. Springer, Berlin Heidelberg New York

Matter P, Brennwald J, Perren SM (1974) Biologische Reaktion des Knochens auf Osteosyntheseplatten. Helv Chir Acta [Suppl] 12 : 1

Moor R, Tepic S, Perren SM (1989) Hochgeschwindigkeits-Film-Analyse des Knochenbruchs. Z Unfallchir 82: 128–132

Müller ME, Allgöwer M, Willenegger H (1963) Technik der operativen Frakturenbehandlung. Springer, Berlin Heidelberg New York

Perren SM, Klaue K, Frigg R, Predieri M, Tepic S (1991) The concept of biolgical plating: the limited contact dynamic compression plate, LC-DCP. Orthop Trauma

Schenk R (1987) Cytodynamics and histodynamics of primary bone repair. In Lane JM (ed) Fracture healing. Churchill Livingstone, New York

Swiontkowski M (1992) Pinless fixation – Part I: introduction. Injury 23 [Suppl 3] : 1–2

Timoshenko S (1941) Strength of materials. Van Nostrand, Princeton

Wolff J (1986 [1893]) The law of bone remodeling. Springer, Berlin Heidelberg New York

5 Clinical and Special Assessment

By C. Colton

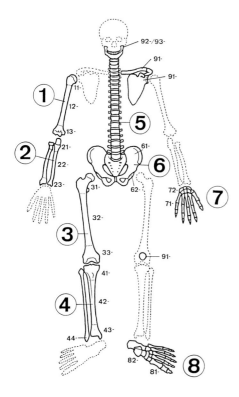

5.1 Classification of Fractures

The need to classify fractures is an expression of the requirement to categorise all the myriad different patterns of failure of all the bones of the body. Surgeons must somehow speak a common tongue when they communicate facts about individual fractures or groups of fractures, either as part of the sharing of clinical information or for research purposes. Especially for the latter, the computer has become such a basic information processing tool that the "surgical language" must be recognisable by these devices.

This necessity led to the evolution of the AO classification of fractures, the brain child of Prof. M. E. Müller. Basically each long bone group, as well as the spine and the pelvis, is allocated a number as follows):

– Humerus	1		– Spine	5
– Radius/ulna	2		– Pelvis	5
– Femur	3		– Hand	7
– Tibia/fibula	4		– Foot	8

For the long bones, each is divided into three zones:
1. Proximal metaphyseal/epiphyseal
2. Shaft
3. Distal metaphyseal/epiphyseal

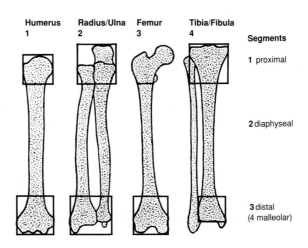

Thus a shaft fracture of the femur would fall into group 32 (3 for femur and 2 for shaft), and by the same token a fracture of the distal radius at the wrist would be a 23.

An exception is made for the ankle joint mortise with its malleoli, because of the special nature of this joint. For it there is a fourth zone, so that malleolar fracture complexes of the ankle are group 44 (4 for tibia/fibula and 4 for the malleolar zone).

For each zone of each bone the fractures are divided into three groups – A, B and C, A being the less severe and less difficult to manage and C being the more serious injuries. It is therefore logical that a complex intra-articular fracture of the distal humerus with many joint fragments will be a 13-C injury).

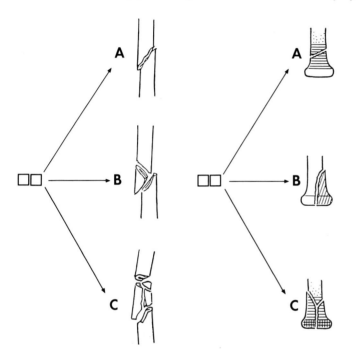

Furthermore, within each A, B or C group there are three additional subgroups, 1, 2 and 3. The severe elbow fracture of the type just mentioned would be a 13-C3).

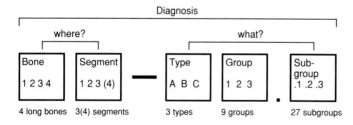

There are even further subdivisions for even more precise coding of fracture types, such as 13-C3.3, a horrendous, multifragmentary joint fracture of the elbow.

The spinal classification has not yet been fully decided on, but there is near agreement on the pelvic and acetabular classifications.

Clinical and Special Assessment

5.2 General Assessment in Fracture Care

5.2.1 Clinical Diagnosis of Fractures

The clinical features of a fracture are:
- History of trauma
- Pain
- Swelling
- Deformity
- Loss of function
- Tenderness
- Abnormal movement
- Crepius

Not all these features will be present in every case. Clinical suspicion of a fracture will be confirmed by the appropriate radiographs. Specialised imaging techniques may be needed to define precisely the anatomical nature of the injury, knowledge of which is necessary in order to develop a logical treatment plan.

5.2.2 Assessment of Soft Tissues

The degree of force required to break a bone (the energy transfer) very often also results in damage to the adjacent soft tissues, including the skin and fat (integuments), the muscles and tendons, the major blood vessels and the nerves. The damage may be such that the fracture site communicates with the exterior – an open fracture. Such fractures were previously called compound fractures, the closed fractures without breach of the integuments being called simple fractures. No fracture should ever be regarded as "simple", and furthermore this outdated terminology fails to emphasise the importance of the distinction being drawn, namely that some fractures are "open" to the risk of infection.

Assessment of the associated soft tissue damage is an integral and necessary part of the evaluation of any injury.

5.2.2.1 Classification of Soft Tissue Injury

Gustillo and Anderson (1976) graded the wounding of the soft tissues into:

Grade 1 Small exit wound <1 cm in length and clean
Grade 2 Significantly larger wound of the integument without extensive damage to the underlying muscles, flaps or avulsions
Grade 3 Open segmental fractures, fractures with major soft tissue damage or traumatic amputation

It soon became evident that the definition of grade 3 was too wide, and Gustillo et al. (1984) subdivided grade 3 into groups A, B and C, 3C denoting major vascular damage requiring arterial and venous repair.

As the techniques for limb preservation have developed and we have progressed from almost universal amputation for any significant open fracture at the turn of this century, to the complex reconstructive potential of modern surgery, it has become necessary to categorise soft tissue injuries even more precisely. The aim of this is to assist in predicting the survivability of a limb.

5.2.2.2 Salvage Versus Amputation

The Mangled Extremity Severity Score (M. E. S. S.) of the Tampa and Seattle trauma groups defines a point scoring system for injured limbs in such a manner that a score of up to 6 usually means that attempts at limb salvage are likely to be rewarding, whereas scores of 7 or more usually indicate the need for amputation.

In some ways this scoring system is also not ideal and tends to concentrate on open injuries. It does not correctly indicate the severity of a number of injuries in which, even though the integument is intact and therefore there is technically not an open fracture, there is massive crushing of the interior of the limb; in these cases the severity is masked by the intact skin. Tscherne, of Hanover, emphasised this important consideration and, building upon his work, the AO coding of soft tissue injury was devised.

In this AO system the letter C is used if the injury is closed and O if it is open. A score of 1–5 (1 indicates normal, except tiny wounds of minimally open fractures; 2–4 denote increasing severity and 5 refers to something special) is then allocated to each of the following:

– Integument: IC (closed) or IO (open)
– Muscle/tendon: MT
– Nerve/vessel: NV

A moderately severe open injury with extensive muscle damage but no neurovascular injury would be coded IO2-MT4-NV1. Associated with a multifragmentary midshaft fracture of the femur, this would then be coded 32-C2.1-IO2-MT4-NV1. This may appear cumbersome but to a computer it is instantly recognisable. All such precisely defined injuries can be analysed as a group, for example to study the results of different forms of management (including amputation rates). Furthermore, it is international – a sort of musculo-skeletal Esperanto! This is how accurate knowledge is gathered and grows. For more information, see Müller et al. (1991).

5.2.3 General Medical Overview of Patient

Although most patients with fractures, whether single or multiple, are young and fit, a significant number may have a pre-existing pathology, either a medical illness, congenital problems (such as congenital heart disease) or even the aftereffects of previous trauma. It is of vital importance that the patient's status be viewed as a whole. It is all too easy to become narrowly focused upon a dramatic injury and to neglect to appraise the overall status. A careful medical history must be obtained from the patient, relatives or friends, or from available medical records. There may be factors, such as those mentioned above, that will affect resuscitation, anaesthesia, the choice of treatment method and the postoperative medical and nursing care.

5.2.4 Priorities in Polytrauma

Polytrauma, or multiple injury, is a major challenge to the physiology of even the young and healthy. Polytrauma is usually defined on the Injury Severity Score (ISS) scale as more than 16[1]. There is frequently a threat to life, either immediate or potential. Multiple fractures, especially of the femur, pelvis and spine, have a profound effect and often lead to life-threatening complications. In the phase immediately after injury, fractures, particularly open ones, cause major blood loss (a closed femoral fracture can easily result in 1–1.5 litres of blood being hidden in a swollen thigh, and a closed pelvic fracture can result in massive occult haemorrhage of many litres) Sadly, many a patient has bled to death because the hypovolaemia from a pelvic disruption has been grossly underestimated. The stabilisation of fractures, even by simple splinting in an emergency, is part of the resuscitation. Sir Robert Jones, the father of British orthopaedics, noted that the introduction of battle-front splinting of femoral gun shot wounds (using the Thomas's splint) in 1916 during the First World War reduced mortality from this injury from nearly 80% to 15%!

Obviously, also in the immediate postinjury phase, the skilled management of hypoxia from chest injury is a matter of extreme urgency, as is the diagnosis and treatment of head injury.

Over the last three decades, it has come to be appreciated that death in the first few days after injury from adult respiratory dis-

---

[1] The Injury Severity Score scale is a point scoring system which allocates a score of 0–5 to each of seven body zones or systems, then takes the three highest scores – the worst injured zones – and adds their squares. The maximum score would of course be $5^2+5^2+5^2 = 75$, which would be fatal. The ISS reflects the extent of the anatomical injury and is widely used to predict outcome and to audit trauma care.

tress syndrome (ARDS) and a little later from multiple system organ failure can very dramatically be reduced by surgical stabilisation of all major fractures in the first 24 h after injury. Indeed, fracture fixation, internal or external, is regarded as a continuation of the primary resuscitative measures, and the seriously injured patient should proceed directly from the emergency room to the operating suite for immediate total surgical care, all surgical procedures – thoracic, neurosurgical, abdominal and musculo-skeletal – being undertaken at a single sitting. With a skilled anaesthetist using good ventilatory control and modern techniques of monitoring blood gases and intracranial pressure, the patient is safer under surgery than anywhere else in the hospital.

5.3 Imaging Techniques

5.3.1 Radiography

As indicated above, after the initial clinical suspicion of a fracture, radiographs confirm (or refute) the diagnosis. Films must be of good diagnostic quality, taken in at least two planes perpendicular to each other (usually antero-posterior and lateral projections) and the full length of each bone imaged. If a joint is involved, views centred on the articulation are mandatory. It is negligent to make management decisions about an intra-articular fracture on the basis of a full length film of a bone with the joint at the very edge of the image – as is so often done! In certain situations, e. g. at the tibial plateaux and the pelvis, oblique views can help.

Special radiographic projections are helpful in many sites – e. g. axillary views of the shoulder and acromio-clavicular joints, the Judet–Letournel iliac and obturator views of the acetabulum and inlet/outlet films of the pelvic ring. Other techniques of enhancing plain radiographs include load-bearing views, such as the gripping views of the scaphoid and weight carrying views to elucidate acromio-clavicular joint instability. Stress views for ligamentous discontinuity are also used at the ankle and sometimes the knee.

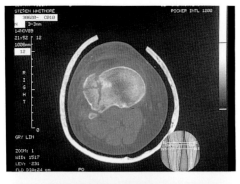

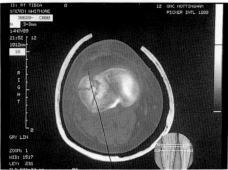

5.3.2 Tomography

Tomography is a radiographic technique which by "trickery" produces an image of a slice of tissue. The film and the X-ray source are both moving as the film is shot. The complex trajectory of each is such that only a thin slice of the body is in focus, the rest being blurred by the movement. By adjusting the positions of the film and the source, a series of slices at different depths through the part being examined can be produced. Their interpretation, however, requires considerable experience; yet tomography can be a great adjunct to standard radiographs in difficult fractures, for example anterior-posterior (A-P) and lateral tomography of the tibial plateaux is most valuable.

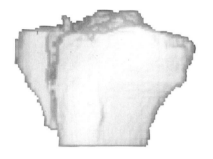

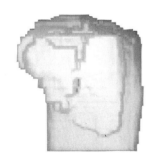

5.3.3 CT Imaging

This is a complex technique in which an X-ray beam is shot through the body repeatedly in a transverse direction but aimed at a different angle each exposure, rather like a sword being stabbed through from many points around the body, but always passing through its centre. This produces multiple sets of information about the various structures in the path of the beam for each "stab". These data are then processed by a computer to construct an image which looks like the cut end of the body after it has been chopped in half transversely.By further complex processing of the data of many slices, three-dimensional images can be reconstructed , which give invaluable information, for example in complicated pelvic and acetabular fractures.

5.3.4 Magnetic Resonance Imaging

When living tissue is subjected to an intense magnetic field, the tissue emits faint radio waves (magnetic resonance). The characteristics of these radio emissions vary according to the chemical composition of the tissue. By passing the patient in graduated steps through a circular magnetic coil and monitoring the radio emissions, it is possible to build images of the tissues. These are very different from radiographic images, and the detection equipment can be tuned in to the radio waves in different ways so as to select which tissue is being imaged. Magnetic resonance imaging (MRI) is very useful for imaging tissues which do not show on standard X-rays, such as cartilage, menisci, intervertebral discs, and soft tissue tumours. It can even indicate the vascularity of tissues. Very fine resolution images of selected areas can be produced by using surface magnetic coils.

The materials of which AO implants are made, namely 316L stainless steel and unalloyed titanium, are essentially nonmagnetic, even after cold working (bending and contouring), and therefore will not cause heat effects or become magnetically deformed by MRI. They will, however, produce artefacts on the images, although titanium is less problematic in this respect. There are methods of modifying the imaging technique to reduce this "star burst" effect.

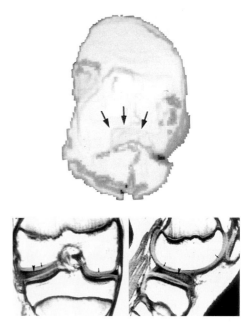

MRI lateral discoid meniscus of the right knee in a 14-year old boy. On sagittal and coronal T1 slices the extent is well visible: increased signal intensity (arrowhead) compared with the normal medial meniscus (small white arrow). The hyaline normal cartilage (small black arrow) has a normal signal intensity.

5.3.5 Arthrography

By injecting a radio-opaque dye into a joint cavity and taking standard X-rays, negative images of the relationships of cartilaginous and other intra-articular structures can be made. Such imaging of cruciate ligament damage is an aid in planning reconstructive surgery. To a certain extent, arthroscopy and high resolution MRI have superseded arthrography. It is extremely valuable in the diagnosis of elbow injuries in children and in the investigation of congenital displacement of the hip. Arthrography of the injured adult ankle sometimes aids in the diagnosis of lateral ligament ruptures.

5.3.6 Ultrasound

Ultrasound (extremely high frequency sound, inaudible to the human ear) bounces off tissues to a varying degree, according to the density of the tissue. This can be used as a safe noninvasive investigation of soft tissue abnormalities. It is a highly sophisticated form of the echo-sounding used by ships to scan for underwater objects, either the floor of the ocean or submarines.

Medical ultrasonography, in skilled hands, is useful for detecting effusions of the hip joint and deep haematomas, and of course, its use in foetal scanning is widely known. Its application in trauma is currently limited.

5.4 Treatment Options Closed Fractures

5.4.1 Conservative Treatment

Many single, closed and uncomplicated fractures can be treated by some form of external splintage. The commonest is of course the plaster of Paris cast – so called as a major source of the gypsum used for plaster was the Mount of Martyrs (or Montmartre) in Paris. Plaster has been used for centuries in architecture and art: the technique of fresco painting (see Michaelangelo's ceiling in the Sistine chapel in Rome) consists of plastering the surface then painting on the damp plaster so that the colour seeps into the material and retains its brightness for hundreds of years. It was not until Mathysen, a Dutch military surgeon, described the plaster bandage in 1854 that modern casting techniques started to develop. Recently, resin-based casting materials have partly replaced plaster of Paris, although nothing beats it for the ability to mould the setting cast to reduce a fresh fracture.

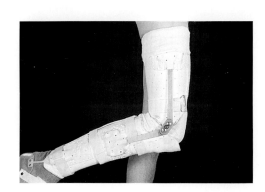

The concept of functional bracing was reintroduced in the 1970s by workers such as Mooney and Sarmiento, although the concept was first described by Gooch in 1776! Basically after a week or so of traditional casting, which always immobilises the joint above and the joint below a fracture, an articulated brace, made either of standard casting material or of heat-mouldable (thermoplastic) sheet plastic, is constructed with joint hinges to permit joint motion whilst still maintaining control of fracture position. This has proven to be of particular value in tibial and lower femoral fractures. It is also of use in the early mobilisation after internal fixation of certain joint fractures, especially tibial plateau injuries.

Another form of noninvasive fracture treatment is traction. This has been traditionally used for femoral fractures, with or without additional splintage such as Thomas' splint. It is also sometimes used to gain temporary control of an unstable fracture whilst swelling and soft tissue problems prevent surgery, although external fixation is usually preferred nowadays in this situation. Traction has to be continued for several months before femoral fracture union is secured, although attempts to reduce this period by functional bracing have met with some success when surgery has been inappropriate for various reasons.

Traction for femoral fractures in the polytrauma patient has been shown to be associated with a high incidence of potentially life-threatening complications.

The disadvantages of external casting, and to a certain extent traction, are that the adjacent joints get stiff, the muscles waste and the unloaded bones lose mineral and become osteopoenic. In addition, changes may take place in the vascular and lymphatic capillary systems leading to prolonged oedema.

Conservative fracture care is sometimes regarded as being a simpler alternative to surgical management. To obtain good functional results from closed fracture treatment requires great skill and experience, with a constant review of progress and adjustment of the splintage; it is not a question of less skill being required, it is just that the repertoire of necessary skills is different from that required for good surgical care.

5.4.2 Surgical Treatment

The surgical treatment of a fracture may be by internal fixation, directly bridging the skeletal elements with an implant of one type or another, or by external fixation, in which the skeletal elements are attached to implants, usually away from the fracture site itself, and external "scaffolding" is used to bridge the space between these implants (pins or screws projecting out of the integument).

The disadvantages of surgical fixation are:
1. The potential for the introduction of infection
2. The requirement for specialised surgical skills
3. Instrumentation and the increased need for inpatient facilities

The positive advantages of modern surgical fracture treatment are that union occurs without deformity in the majority of cases and that the limb function can be regained more rapidly and, indeed, more predictably. The disasters of osteosynthesis usually result from surgical enthusiasm and bravado, untempered by basic education and experience. Education in fracture surgery is of paramount importance in reducing such disasters to a minimum. Surgical treatment of a fracture should be chosen only when certain criteria are fulfilled:

1. The predicted outcome will be better than the closed option.
2. The fracture is amenable to stable fixation.
3. The fixation will permit early functional aftercare.
4. The patient is fit for surgery.
5. The appropriate surgical skills and experience are available.
6. The appropriate surgical facilities are available.
7. The full range of instrumentation to cope with any eventuality is available.
8. The necessary aftercare can be delivered.

Any compromise of one or more of these criteria can lead to a less than optimal result. The greatest disaster is to expose the patient to the disadvantages of surgery and then fail to reap the benefits of osteosynthesis – the worst of both worlds.

Tile (personal communication) refers to "the personality of the fracture problem" which must be assessed before fracture surgery is undertaken. He means the totality of:

– The nature of the fracture
– The nature of the soft tissues
– The nature of the patient
– The nature of the hospital
– The nature of the surgeon!

There are many different techniques of internal fixation and external fixation of fractures, the principles of which have been considered in Sect. 4.3 and which will be discussed in detail, as they are applied to individual fractures, in Chap. 7.

5.5 Treatment Open Fractures

The assessment of the soft tissue injury associated with open fractures is discussed above.

5.5.1 Soft Tissue Surgery

The surgical management of any open fracture is an emergency. It is generally agreed that the fracture site must be regarded as being infected (rather than just contaminated) 6 hours after the injury and that primary surgery must be undertaken before that deadline.

The open wound must be extended so that the whole injury zone can be visualised (Dessault described this in the nineteenth century as "débridement", meaning unbridling) and all devitalised and heavily contaminated tissue removed. Even bony fragments with no soft tissue attachment must be sacrificed in an open fracture. The injury zone, after débridement and surgical excision, should then be copiously washed with large volumes of fluid, usually Hartmann's or Ringer lactate solution (not normal saline, which is cytotoxic on prolonged contact with tissue); pulsed jet lavage is probably even better if available. Rojczyk (1981) showed that swabs taken from the open wounds of 199 consecutive open fractures were sterile in only 49 cases on arrival at hospital, but 129 were sterile after surgical wound excision and 168 yielded no growth when taken just prior to the conclusion of primary surgery. This demonstrates very clearly the efficacy of good surgery in reducing the bacterial population of the fracture site.

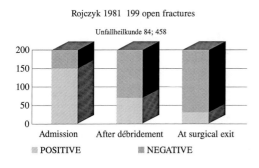

Rojczyk 1981 199 open fractures

Unfallheilkunde 84; 458

43 ∎

Lacerated major nerves may be considered for direct repair after skeletal stabilisation, but if in doubt they should be tagged with a coloured suture material for subsequent reconstruction or grafting.

Major vessel anastomosis or grafting must be undertaken after skeletal stabilisation, if necessary to restore viability of the limb. Although the extensions of the surgical wound débridement may be closed, the original open wound should never be sutured primarily, as this greatly increases the chances of infection.

In general, definitive soft tissue cover, either by delayed primary closure, split skin graft, local soft tissue flap (muscular or fascio-cutaneous) or free tissue transfer by microvascular techniques, should be achieved by 7 days from injury. This is of course greatly aided by stabilisation of the skeleton.

5.5.2 Skeletal Stabilisation

Stabilisation of the fractures greatly aids soft tissue healing in open injuries. External cast immobilisation is inadequate because fracture movement still occurs and risks continuously disturbing the delicate healing tissues. Furthermore, access to the wounding, even through windows in casts, is grossly inadequate. It is also difficult to monitor for muscle compartment syndromes with the limb encased.

Most open fractures in the hands of modern fracture surgeons will be stabilised surgically. Perhaps the commonest method is the use of external fixation. This, as it were, puts the fracture "on the back burner" whilst attention is rightly devoted to the care of the soft tissue injury. The aim is to achieve stable soft tissue cover by 7–10 days from the injury. The external fixator may later be changed to another method of skeletal care if mechanical and/or biological considerations so dictate.

The configuration of the external fixator assembly will be chosen according to the needs of the fracture complex but also with a view to permitting appropriate access to the wounds for whatever soft tissue reconstruction is foreseen as possibly becoming necessary. The planning of the external fixation with these factors in mind on day 1 is the mark of a good fracture surgeon.

Plating of open fractures is usually safe in skilled hands, provided the surgical wound care has been impeccable. It is desirable that the placement of the implants be planned so that they may be covered at the time of surgical exit. Although other methods, such as external fixation or intramedullary nailing, are superseding plating for the tibia and the femur, plating still has a place in the humerus and the forearm and for combined diaphyseal/articular injuries in upper and lower limbs.

Intramedullary nailing of open fractures, once condemned, is achieving a certain currency. Although there still remain concerns over the effect of medullary reaming upon the endosteal blood supply, especially when the periosteal vascularity is compromised by the wounding, there are emerging reports of satisfactory results for reamed nailing of open tibial and femoral fractures (even Gustillo grade 3 fractures) in very skilled hands. The advent of unreamed locked nailing, with the theoretical preservation of the medullary vascularity, has broadened the appeal of nailing for open fractures.

The "second look" procedure in the first 48 hours after open fracture treatment is mandatory to check the efficacy of the surgical wound excision, and in extensive wounding, especially crushing injuries, serial wound excision often proves to be necessary.

5.5.3 General Measures

The general physiological support of the patient is of vital importance and the avoidance of complications in these very serious injuries is assisted by maintaining the comfort and nutritional status of the injured person. Where an open fracture is part of a polytrauma complex, then full intensive care, with prophylactic intermittent positive pressure ventilation, nasoduodenal feeding and intravenous antibiotic prophylaxis, is required.

The whole question of prophylactic measures against thromboembolic complications remains unresolved at the present time. Certainly it is contraindicated in the early stages after multiple injury, especially with pelvic and spinal fractures, and where suspected visceral haemorrhage is being treated nonoperatively.

Broad spectrum, systemic antibiotic prophylaxis is used for most open fractures, but must *not* be regarded as a substitute for the most immaculate surgical wound excision and aftercare. It is totally erroneous to believe that a short course of antibiotics can compensate for fundamental surgical inadequacies.

5.6 Compartment Syndromes

The swelling of muscles after injury, especially crushing injury, or haemorrhage into a closed osseofascial muscular compartment will rapidly raise the intracompartmental pressure to critical levels. If that pressure exceeds the capillary critical closing pressure, then muscle ischaemia supervenes. Muscle at body temperature necroses after 2 hours or more of ischaemia, and failure to recognise and relieve a compartment syndrome can result in death of muscle with the consequence of, at least, se-

vere paralysis of the affected group leading to ischaemic contracture, and even worse, the dead muscle may become infected and anaerobic organisms can produce life-threatening toxins.
The diagnosis of muscle compartment syndrome is suspected in any injured patient where the level of pain is more than expected, with tenderness and induration of the muscle compartment, loss of active function of the muscle group and pain on passively moving the distal parts in such a way as to stretch the affected muscle group. If compartment pressure measuring equipment is available, emergency monitoring is performed, and if the pressure is suspiciously high, then fasciotomies are most urgently indicated. If such equipment is not available, then clinical suspicion alone is an indication for emergency compartment decompression. The consequences of "wait and see" are potentially too devastating to justify such a policy. Procrastination leads to tissue death, not recovery!

5.7 Glossary

Anaerobic: Refers to any metabolic process which is not dependent upon oxygen. Anaerobic organisms have a metabolism which can continue in tissues deprived of oxygen.

Broad Spectrum: Refers to antibiotics which are active against a wide variety of different organisms.

Endosteal: Adjective from endosteum, which means the interior surface of a hollow bone – the wall of the medullary cavity.

Energy Transfer: When tissues are traumatised, the damage is due to energy that is transferred to the tissues. This is most commonly due to the transfer of kinetic energy from a moving object (car, missile, falling object, etc.). The greater the amount of energy transferred to the tissue, the more extensive the damage.

Fascio-cutaneous: A term describing tissue flaps which include the skin, the subcutaneous tissues and the deep fascia as a single layer.

Fasciotomy: Cutting the fascial wall of a muscle compartment, usually to release intracompartmental pressure.

Hypovolaemia: A state where the circulating blood volume is reduced. This can lead to shock.

Hypoxia: A state where the arterial blood oxygen level is pathologically reduced.

Ischaemia: Absence of blood flow.

Multifragmentary: A fracture complex that has more than three fragments is multifragmentary.

Osseo-fascial Muscle Compartment: An anatomical space, bounded on all sides by either bone or deep fascial envelope, which contains one or more muscle bellies. The relative inelasticity of its walls means that if the muscle belly swells, the pressure in the osseo-fascial envelope can build up to levels which cut off the flow of blood to the muscle tissue, resulting in its death.

Osteopoenic: An abnormal reduction in bone mass. This may be generalised, as in some bone diseases, or localised as a response to inflammation, infection, disuse, etc.

Osteosyntesis: A phrase coined by Lambotte to indicate the surgical joining together of bone fragments, usually by internal fixation. Now also used to cover external fixation.

Periosteal: Adjective from periosteum, which is the membrane covering the exterior surface of a bone. The periosteum plays an active part in the blood supply to cortical bone, and in bone remodelling.

Polytrauma: Multiple injury. Usually, a person with an Injury Severity Score of 16 or more is regarded as being multiply injured.

Prophylactic: Preventative.

Segmental: If the shaft of a bone is broken at 2 levels, leaving a separate shaft segment between the two fracture sites, if is called a "segmental" fracture complex.

Systemic: Usually refers to a route for drug or fluid administration other than via the gastro-intestinal tract, by injection.

Toxins: Poisonous chemicals. Some pathogenic organisms release powerful toxins when they multiply.

5.8 References

Gustillo R, Anderson L (1976) Prevention of infection in the treatment of one thousand and twenty-six open fractures of long bones. J Bone and Joint Surg 58 A: 453–465

Müller ME, Nazarian S, Koch P, Schatzker J (1990) The comprehensive AO classification of fractures of long bones. Springer, Berlin Heidelberg New York

Müller ME, Allgöwer M, Schneider R, Willenegger H (1991) Manual of internal fixation, 3rd edn. Springer, Berlin Heidelberg New York

Rojczyk M (1981) Keimbesiedlung und Keimverhalten bei offenen Frakturen. Unfallheilkunde 84: 458

Tscherne H, Gotzen L (1984) Fractures with soft tissue injuries. Springer, Berlin Heidelberg New York

6 AO/ASIF Instrumentation

By R. Texhammar
With Contributions by J. Disegi (6.1.1, 6.1.2),
F. Baumgart (6.1.3), and A. Murphy (6.22)

Since 1958 the AO/ASIF group has worked together closely with biologists, biomechanics and engineers to develop a uniform integrated instrumentation providing what is necessary to solve most problems encountered in the fixation of fresh fractures, pseudarthroses, osteotomies, and arthrodeses. The AO Technical Commission continuously reevaluates existing instruments and implants, supervises new developments, and ensures compatibility and high quality. Imitations of AO/ASIF instruments and implants, which are sold by nearly all the major manufacturers of surgical instruments, have contributed greatly to the spread of the AO method. However, it is important to remember that the AO/ASIF and SYNTHES are not connected with the manufacture of these products and, hence, can assume no responsibility for their quality.

All of the original AO instruments and implants can be identified by their engraved symbols, either the current registred trademark on AO/ASIF instruments and implants or the old AO symbol, which was used until 1969.

6.1 Materials Used for AO/ASIF Instruments and Implants

6.1.1 Metals Used for AO/ASIF Implants

By J. A. Disegi

6.1.1.1 316L Stainless Steel

AO/ASIF stainless steel implants are produced from implant-quality 316L stainless steel, which typically contains 62.5% iron, 17.6% chromium, 14.5% nickel, 2.8% molybdenum, and minor alloy additions. A low carbon content is specified to ensure that the material will be free from susceptibility to intergranular corrosion.

AO implant-quality 316L stainless steel meets the metallurgical requirements established by the American Society for Testing and Materials (ASTM) and the International Organization for

Standardization (ISO). The major implant-industry standards include ASTM F 138 Grade 2 (bar and wire), ASTM F 139 Grade 2 (sheet and strip), and ISO 5832–1 Composition D. AO implant-quality material must also meet stringent AO/ASIF internal specifications for composition limits, microstructure uniformity, and mechanical properties. All implant-quality material received from approved suppliers is recertified by the AO producers to provide an extra measure of quality assurance that metallurgical requirements have been met.

Certain implants, such as cerclage wire or pelvic-reconstruction plates, are produced from AO implant-quality 316L stainless steel in the annealed, or softest, condition. This is needed for applications which demand maximum contourability. The majority of AO 316L stainless steel implants are produced from cold-worked, or strengthened, material. Some small-diameter implants such as Kirschner wires, Steinmann pins and Schanz screws may be highly cold-worked to resist permanent bending deformation. AO implant-quality 316L stainless steel is completely nonmagnetic, regardless of condition. Magnetic resonance imaging may be safely used to visualize hard and soft tissue adjacent to AO stainless steel implants.

Surface treatment known as electropolishing is used for AO stainless steel implants. Electropolishing consists of applying an electric current to an implant immersed in a specially formulated chemical solution under specified conditions of time and voltage. This treatment decreases the surface roughness of the implant and provides a good combination of low surface friction and excellent corrosion resistance. For certain applications, some AO implants may be shot-peened before electropolishing. The implant surface is subjected to high-velocity impaction by metallic particles under well-defined conditions. Shot-peening produces a roughened surface with increased residual compressive stress for enhanced fatigue life.

AO/ASIF Technical Commission consists of general and orthopaedic surgeons, material experts, engineers, and manufacturing specialists, to provide broad-based expertise in implant design and development. AO instruments and implants are designed and manufactured to maintain optimum performance. For this reason, 316L stainless steel implants produced by other manufacturers should not be mixed with AO 316L stainless steel implants. The in vivo performance of a mixed implant system may be compromised as a result of composition differences, strength variations, and design or workmanship factors.

6.1.1.2 Pure Titanium

Implants made from commercially pure titanium have been successfully used in clinical practice by the AO group since 1966. AO/ASIF pure titanium does not contain major alloying elements, and the metal has a documented history of outstanding biocompatibility. Clinical experience demonstrates that tissue adjacent to pure titanium implants is well vascularized with less tendency toward capsule formation. These biologically favourable conditions may help to reduce the spread of bacteria and increase the resistance to infection.

AO/ASIF pure titanium is produced by advanced processing methods that significantly increase the strength of the material. Various combinations of strength and ductility are provided to meet the demands of each specific implant application.

All AO/ASIF pure titanium implants have a special anodized surface finish that increases the thickness of the protective oxide film. The titanium implants are immersed in a chemical solution and a known electrical voltage is applied for a specified time. The specific colour produced depends on the oxide film's thickness. This is controlled in the anodizing process. Visible-light diffraction within the oxide film creates a distinct colour.

No pigments or organic colouring agents are present in the anodized titanium oxide film. The standard AO anodizing treatment produces the golden appearance that is a distinguishing feature of AO titanium implants. The titanium anodizing process is capable of producing a variety of colours, depending on the thickness of the oxide film.

Multiple steam sterilization cycles do not significantly change the appearance of anodized titanium implants. However, fingerprint contamination from skin contact should be avoided in handling the implants between autoclave cycles. Implant areas that are touched by hand may show evidence of darkening or grey discoloration after steam autoclaving. Gloved handling of titanium implants prevents the discoloration of isolated areas during steam autoclaving.

Improved biocompatibility, proven functional performance, and excellent corrosion resistance are important advantages of AO/ASIF pure titanium implants. Additional clinical benefits include the absence of allergic reactions to metal and the option to leave the implant in situ.

6.1.1.3 Titanium Alloys

New biocompatible titanium alloys such as Ti-6Al-7Nb and other advanced compositions are being evaluated by the AO group for future implant applications. These titanium alloys offer outstanding corrosion resistance, excellent biocompatibility, and higher strength capability than pure titanium. Titanium alloy implants may be ceramic shot-peened, and either chemically passivated in nitric acid or anodized as a final surface treatment.

The simultaneous use of two different systems increases the risk of mistakes due to mixing, of improper use and failure of implants and instruments, and of loss of time: broken drills and taps, poor fit, damaged or broken screws and plates, failure of internal fixation, etc. Problems inevitably increase in number, severity, and frequency when systems are mixed, and involve liability of both surgeon and theatre staff. For a detailed survey of this problem, see Murphy (1987).

6.1.3.5 Administrative Hospital Staff

Nonmedical hospital staff bears responsibility for the administration, planning, purchase, storage, and care of appropriate and reliable equipment. All these may also have an effect on the risk to the patient.

6.1.3.6 Final Remark

Every member of the patient-care team has a duty to avoid risk to the patient.

6.1.4 References

Annual book of ASTM standards, vol 13.01, Medical devices
DIN 17443, Stähle für chirurgische Implantate, German standard for implant stainless steel
Disegi J (1989) Mixing titanium and stainless steel implants. Personal communication
Harrington Research Centre. Fracture management implant characterization study, carried out by the Harrington Research Centre, founded by AESCULAP Instrument Coorporation
ISO (1980) ISO Standard 5832 – implants for surgery – metallic materials – part 1: wrought stainless steel
Müller ME, Allgöwer M, Schneider R, Willenegger H (1991) Manual of internal fixation. Springer, Berlin Heidelberg New York
Murphy EK (1987) OR nursing law – interchanging different product components; instilling eye drops before patient signs consent. AORN J 47/1:
Perren SM, Geret V, Tepic S, Rahn B (1986) Quantatative evaluation of biocompatibility of vanadium-free titanium alloys. Biological and biomechanical performance of biomaterials. Elsevier, Amsterdam
Pohler O (1988) Unpublished investigation. Personal communication
Pohler O, Straumann F (1975) Characteristics of the stainless steel AO/ASIF implants. AO Bull
Radford WJP et al. (1989) Unacceptable variation in the core diameter of some AO type cancellous screws. J Roy Soc Med
Rüedi T (1975) Titan und Stahl in der Knochenchirurgie. Hefte Unfallheilk 3
Séquin F, Texhammar R (1981) AO/ASIF instrumentation. Springer, Berlin Heidelberg New York
Texhammar R (1986) Checklist. A guide to care and maintenance of the AO/ASIF instrumentation. SYNTHES

6.2 Classification of AO/ASIF Instrumentation

The comprehensive system of AO/ASIF instruments and implants has been organized into standard sets, which contain the minimum that the AO group consider necessary for certain procedures. Instruments and implants not contained in a set are called supplementary instruments and implants.

Standard sets should be *complete at all times*, so that a crucial instrument or implant will not be missing during surgery. The number of implants may be decreased in accordance with their rate of use; however, *all lengths and types should be represented*. For the storage of the instruments and implants there is a choice between three different types of containers:

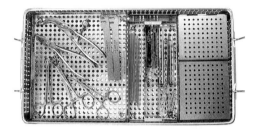

Sterilization trays in different sizes with the possibility of dividing the tray into compartments for a better overview of the contents. These trays are made entirely of stainless steel and can be obtained with graphic outlines of the contained items. Holding pegs for instruments are available. Lids of stainless steel may be used to protect the contents. The trays can be stacked on their handles, with or without lids. Advantages: durability, flexibility, easy overview.

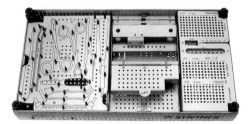

Graphic cases in different sizes made of anodized aluminium. The original brown cases with beige graphic outlines have been changed to grey cases with burgundy graphic outlines. The contents are held securely in place with pegs, brackets, and lids. Corner posts allow stacking with or without lids. Advantages: easy overview and inventory control.

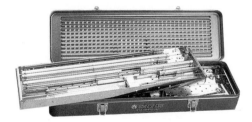

The old style *aluminium cases* in a variety of coulors, with different insert trays made of stainless steel for the storage of (especially) implants. This case is less frequently used nowadays due to its limited interior space. It has the advantage, however, of being rather small and easy to identify because of its colour.

6.3 Instruments for Fixation with Large Screws and Plates

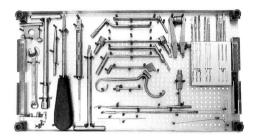

The instruments necessary for the implantation of 4.5 and 6.5 mm screws and plates are called standard instruments and contained in the basic instrument set, either in a graphic case or in a sterilizing tray. Old style aluminium cases may still be in use. Several supplementary instruments are available , which can be used in conjunction with the standard instruments.

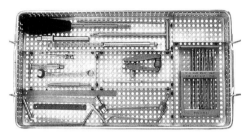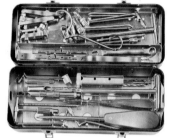

6.3.1 Standard Instruments

Drill Bit Design

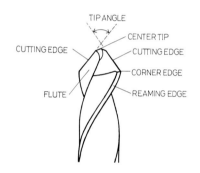

The drill bits are designed to provide optimal cutting with as little thermal damage to bone as possible. Their effectiveness depends upon their wear- and corrosion-resistant material and the design of the cutting edges.

A sharp centre tip ensures a safe first bite on the bone. The cutting edges perform the actual cutting, and their sharpness and symmetry are crucial to good function. The reaming edges clear the drill hole of bone debris and have no cutting function. Bone debris is collected in the flutes and transported away from the drilled hole. The length of flutes has recently been shortened to approximately ten times the diameter to increase the strength of the drill bit.

Table 1. Drill bit data

Standard drill bit diameter (mm)	Total length (mm)	Effective length (mm)	Double drill sleeve length[a]	Available drill bit lenght (mm)
3.2	145	120	40 mm	80
4.5	145	120	50 mm	70
2.5	110	85	30 mm	55
3.5	110	85	35 mm	50
2.7	100	75	30 mm	45
2.0	100	75	22 mm	53
1.5	85	60	18 mm	42
1.1	60	35	14 mm	21

[a] Measured from the sleeve end of the size corresponding to the respective drill bit.

Instrumentation and Techniques

As drill bits are always used in sleeves, only that portion of the drill bit projecting beyond the sleeve is available to penetrate bone (Table 1).

There are anatomical sites, for example the proximal tibia and femur, pelvis, or oblique holes in the metaphysis, where a hole deeper than that which can be made with the standard drill bit is necessary. For such instances drill bits of increased lengths are available.

Standard drill bits are two-fluted and have a quick coupling end to fit the small air drill. Bits with a triangular end to be used with a Jacobs chuck adaptor are also available.

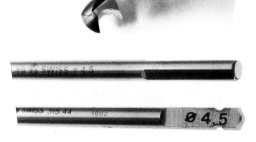

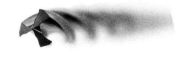

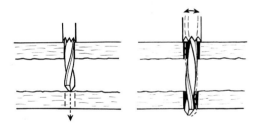

Three-fluted drill bits are best used when drilling at oblique angles. Using three cutting edges reduces the likelihood of the drill skidding off the bone, as it provides better centring of the drill bit. Cannulated drill bits of different diameters are available to be used when drilling over a previously placed Kirschner wire (see Sect. 6.6).

Calibrated, three-fluted drill bits are also available. They are used for drilling in areas where measuring with a depth gauge may be difficult, e. g. pelvic surgery. The calibration is in 5 mm increments (see Sect. 6.10).

Drill bits should always be used with a drill guide of corresponding size. Correct coaxial drilling is thereby ensured without damaging the soft tissue. Too large a sleeve may result in too large a hole. The drill bit must be stationary (not rotating) when introduced into the sleeve.

Irrigation during drilling prevents frictional heat. Ringer's lactate solution is recommended.

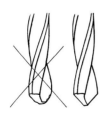

Damage to the drill bit is most frequently caused by contact with metal and unnecessary bending forces during drilling. It is essential to inspect drill bits carefully after each use and replace those which show any damage.

In the standard instrument set the drill bits have the length necessary for screws contained in the basic screw set.

Drill Bit, 3.2 mm

This bit of 145 mm/120 mm (total length/effective length) is used to prepare the thread hole for 4.5 mm cortex screws, 6.5 mm cancellous bone screws, and malleolar screws.

Fixation with Large Screws and Plates

Drill Bit, 4.5 mm

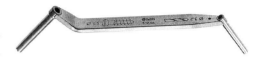

This bit of 145 mm/120 mm (total length/effective length) is used to drill the gliding hole when a 4.5 mm cortex screw is used as a lag screw to produce interfragmentary compression. If a 6.5 mm cancellous bone screw is to be inserted through hard (dense) cortical bone at its point of entry, it is necessary to enlarge the near cortex to 4.5 mm to accept the 4.5 mm shaft of the screw without splitting the bone.

Drill Bit, 2.0 mm

This bit of 100 mm/75 mm (total length/effective length) is used to pre-drill for Kirschner wires and guide wires in hard bone.

Double Drill Sleeve, 4.5 mm/3.2 mm

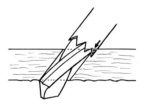

This drill sleeve can be used for several functions, thereby replacing five previous instruments. The 4.5 mm diameter sleeve is used with taps and drill bits of that size. The other end accommodates the 3.2 mm drill bit. This end also acts as the insert drill sleeve. The 4.5 mm outer diameter centres the sleeve perfectly in the gliding hole. It is long enough to reach the far cortex to drill a coaxial 3.2 mm thread hole in the far fragment for lag screw fixation of the femur and the tibia. The serrated ends of both sleeves allow precise placement and prevent slipping if pushed onto the surface of the bone. This is possible to accomplish also through plate holes.

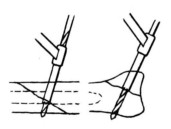

A hole in the handle accepts Kirschner wires up to 1.6 mm diameter. A 4.5 mm cortex screw can be inserted parallel to a previously placed Kirschner wire by sliding the handle over the wire and drilling parallel to it.
The angled handle allows combination with the pointed drill guide.

Insert Drill Sleeve, 4.5 mm/3.2 mm

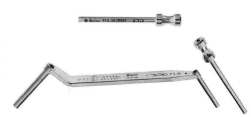

This drill sleeve is only necessary for the insertion of long 4.5 mm cortex lag screws, i. e. in the lesser trochanter, arthrodeses, pelvic fractures etc. The 60 mm long sleeve portion will reach the inner far cortex in large bones for accurate drilling of the thread hole, where the double drill sleeve end, 3.2 mm is too short.

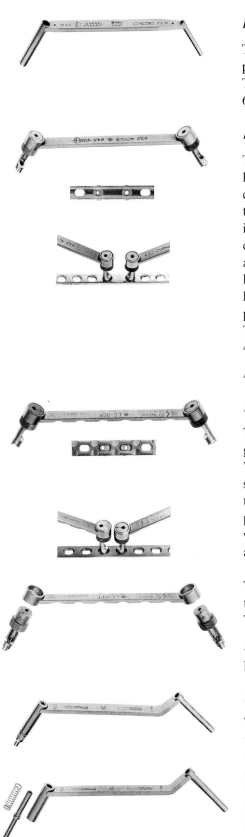

Double Drill Sleeve, 6.5 mm/3.2 mm

This drill sleeve is used to guide the 3.2 mm drill bit when preparing the thread hole for the 6.5 mm cancellous bone screw. The other end serves as the tissue protecting sleeve for the 6.5 mm tap.

DCP Drill Guide, 4.5 mm

This drill guide has a neutral (green) drill guide at one end and a load (yellow) guide at the other. The tip of each guide fits precisely in the DCP hole. The neutral, green guide accurately centres the 3.2 mm drill bit in the DCP hole to pre-drill for a screw in neutral position. The yellow guide places the screw in an eccentric load position in the DCP hole for compression, when the arrow points toward the fracture. Compression of 1 mm in the long axis of the bone is then achieved (see also p. 85). The handle can be moved around the guides into an optimal holding position.
The instrument is disassembled for cleaning. The measurement 4.5 mm in this instance refers to the screw size used.

Note: The DCP drill guide should only be used with DC plates.

LC-DCP Drill Guide, 4.5 mm

This drill guide also has a neutral (green) and a load (yellow) guide. The tip of each guide fits exactly in the LC-DCP hole. With this guide the 3.2 mm drill hole is prepared in a neutral position in the LC-DCP hole, if the arrow of the green guide points toward the fracture. The eccentric position for compression is prepared with the yellow guide, also with the arrow pointing toward the fracture. Compression of 1 mm in the long axis is then achieved. See also p. 88.

The movable handle has grooves on the undersurface similar to those of the LC-DCP. The drill guide is taken apart for cleaning. The "4.5 mm" nomenclature refers to the screw size used.

Note: The LC-DCP drill guide should only be used with LC-DC plates.

LC-DCP Universal Drill Guide, 4.5 mm

This drill guide is, as the name indicates, a guide for universal use. It was designed to be used with the LC-DCP, but may be used with any large plate. It has two sleeves combined on a handle. One sleeve has a 4.5 mm inner diameter to accommodate the 4.5 mm drill bit and tap. The other side has a sleeve consisting of three components and a spring. These components are preloaded by the spring in such way that the inner sleeve protrudes at the tip. The sleeve has an internal diameter of 3.2 mm to accept the 3.2 mm drill bit. Without applying pressure the

sleeve can be placed in any desired position in the plate hole. An eccentric position for the load screw is achieved by placing the sleeve in the far end of the plate hole, away from the fracture. This will lead to 1 mm displacement of the fragment. Placed in the near end, a buttress position of the screw is possible. By applying pressure on the outer sleeve, its rounded tip is pushed against the inclined cylinder of the plate hole and the neutral position reached, i.e. at the intersection of the horiontal and vertical cylindrical profiles of the plate hole. The neutral screw hole can then be drilled. Because of the round end of the guide, which corresponds to the undersurface of the screw head, an exact fit between the plate hole and the screw head can be established. This is important because it prevents the occurrence of undesirable torque between the bone segments. It is also possible to place a screw at an angle and still maintain a congruent fit. The degree of inclination is limited to angles that provide exact fit. See also p. 89.

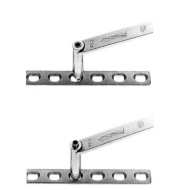

Large Countersink, 4.5 mm

This countersink is used to cut a recess for the 4.5 mm cortex screw head, when inserted as a separate lag screw. The 4.5 mm tip centres the instrument in the pre-drilled gliding hole. By turning the handle clockwise until the full diameter starts to cut, a seat for the spherical screw head is prepared. The pressure of the screw head is distributed over a larger area on the bone, thereby reducing the concentration of stress. The head also protrudes less.

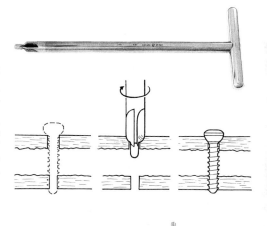

T Handle

The T handle with the quick coupling chuck is used with the 4.5 and 6.5 mm taps. In an emergency it can be used with the large hexagonal screwdriver shaft as a substitute for the regular screwdriver. The outer sleeve is pushed forward to allow coupling.

Depth Gauge, 4.5–6.5 mm

The depth gauge measures the drilling depth for the 4.5 and 6.5 mm diameter screws up to 110 mm. The hook has to engage the opposite cortex before the sleeve is pushed onto the bone or plate and the reading made. It is calibrated such that the height of the large screw head is taken into account, and can therefore only be used for the size of screws marked on the depth gauge. A new generation of depth gauges with a locking sleeve has been developed to avoid interchanging of the outer sleeves. The depth gauge is disassembled for cleaning.

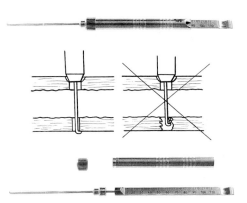

Note: Measure after countersinking, or through the plate hole, *before* tapping.

Instrumentation and Techniques

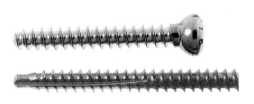

Taps – Design

A cortical bone tap is a sharp instrument designed to cut threads in bone of the same size as the screw's to facilitate insertion. The tap is sharp and has an efficient mechanism for clearing bone debris into three flutes. These flutes extend from the tip through the first ten threads, ensuring that debris does not accumulate and jam the tap. The thread lengths of standard taps correspond to the most commonly used screw lengths. If longer screws are inserted, a tap with increased length has to be used (Table 2).

Table 2. Cortex screw tap data

Taps for standard cortex screw (mm)	Total length with quick coupling (mm)	Thread length (mm)
4.5	125	70
3.5	110	50
2.7	100	33
2.0	53	24
1.5	50	20

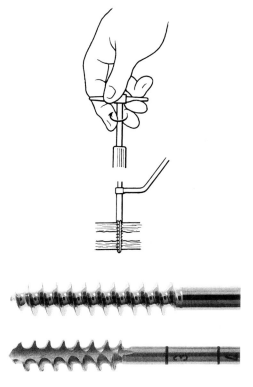

The long tip and conical run in of the cutting threads facilitate the tapping procedure. The entire far cortex must be tapped. The tip of the tap should therefore protrude completely before returning the tap.

Tapping should be done manually to avoid stripping of the threads or damage to the soft tissue. Two turns forward and a half turn in reverse, to clear the threads of debris, is recommended. Taps should always be used with a sleeve to prevent damage to the soft tissue.

The tap must be cleared of the bone debris between each tapping procedure. The sharp hook or a Kirschner wire can be used.

The tap for cancellous bone screws is designed with a short and wide thread of slightly smaller diameter than the screw). It is normally used to cut the thread in the near cortex only since cancellous bone screws can cut the thread themselves in the soft and spongy cancellous bone.

Note: Power tapping is *not* recommended. It is easy to damage the tap, the bone and especially the soft tissues if power tapping is performed.

Tap for 4.5 mm Cortex Screw

This tap is used to cut the thread in the bone before inserting a 4.5 mm cortex screw, and can also be used for malleolar screws. It is used for both plate fixation screws and lag screws, since it has a long thread and a short flute. It combines the function of the former long- and short-threaded 4.5 mm taps. Threads cut in the near cortex are protected from damage as the tap is ad-

Fixation with Large Screws and Plates

vanced through the bone. In the lag screw technique the thread is cut only in the far cortex. The full diameter of the long, unfluted threaded portion will centre the tap in the gliding hole. This allows placing the tip of the tap correctly in the thread hole, before tapping of the far cortex begins. The double drill sleeve end 4.5 mm is used to protect the surrounding soft tissue.

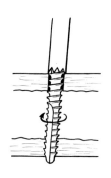

The tap has a quick coupling end and is used with the T handle. The effective cutting length of the taps in the standard set corresponds to the screw lengths in the basic screw set. Longer taps are necessary if longer screws are used.

Tap for 6.5 mm Cancellous Bone Screws

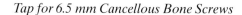

This tap is used to cut the thread, usually only in the near cortex at the point of entry, for 6.5 mm cancellous bone screws. In young patients the cancellous bone may be quite dense, making tapping of the entire screw length necessary.

The double drill sleeve end 6.5 mm is used to protect surrounding soft tissue. The tap has a quick coupling end and is used with the T handle.

In straight plates 6.5 mm tapping can only be done through the slightly larger end holes and has to be done with great care to avoid damaging the tap.

Note: Never use a power drill with the 6.5 mm cancellous bone tap.

Large Hexagonal Screwdriver

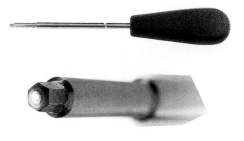

This screwdriver has a hexagonal tip which fits snuggly into the head sockets of the 4.5 and 6.5 mm screws, allowing easy insertion and removal. It must engage the full depth of the hexagonal socket of the screw head before it is turned. The shaft has a groove, which is necessary to take the large screw holding sleeve. This screwdriver has a shaft 7 mm in diameter and has replaced the previous screwdriver with a 8 mm diameter shaft. The latter can not be used with the large screw holding sleeve.

The two ring markings on the shaft indicate the insertion depth of locking bolts used for universal nails.

Note: Never use a screwdriver with a damaged tip.

Large Screw Holding Sleeve

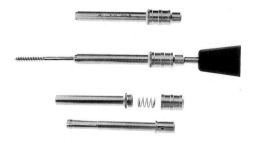

This is a self retaining, screw holding sleeve which facilitates insertion of screws in areas with reduced visibility. It must be used when removing screws with a smooth shaft, since traction may be needed to reverse the screw. It has to be disassembled carefully for cleaning.

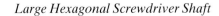

Large Hexagonal Screwdriver Shaft

This screwdriver shaft has a quick coupling end and can be used with the small air drill for the insertion and removal of 4.5 and 6.5 mm screws. However, both the final tightening after insertion and the initial loosening prior to removal have to be done manually. In emergency cases it can be used with the T handle. The 8 mm shaft diameter does not accept the large screw holding sleeve.

Articulated Tension Device, 20 mm Span

This device is designed to work in both compression and distraction modes. It is used in conjunction with plates whenever larger fracture or osteotomy gaps must be closed (and/or when the bone is soft, e.g. in porotic proximal femur where the effect of self-compression is expected to be too small).

For compression, the device is opened fully and the hook engaged in the last plate hole. The foot plate is then fixed to the bone, usually with a short cortex screw in the near cortex. While tightening the bolt using the combination wrench, the approximate compression applied is indicated by coloured rings.

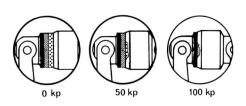

0 kp   50 kp   100 kp

▨ Yellow ring = 0–50 kp
▨ Green ring = 50–100 kp
▮ Red ring = over 100 kp

For distraction, the device is closed and the hook reversed to fit the small notch at the end of the DC plate. The foot plate is fixed to the bone with a single cortex screw. By opening the bolt of the device using the combination wrench the fracture can be distracted.

Note: The screw used in the foot plate should be discarded, as the stresses developed may cause it to bend.

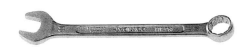

Combination Wrench, 11 mm

This wrench is used with the tension device as described above. It is also used with several other instruments that have bolts or connections with an 11 mm width across the flats of the nut.

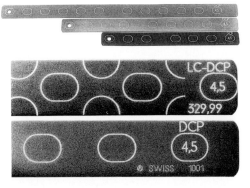

Bending Templates, 120, 155, and 210 mm

These templates, made of anodized aluminium, are moulded to conform to the shape of the bone. The templates then serve as a model when contouring a plate.
The markings correspond to the plate holes and enable exact planning of the plate placement. Newly designed templates can be used with DCP on one side and with LC-DCP on the other side. The templates are reusable.

Fixation with Large Screws and Plates

Sharp Hook

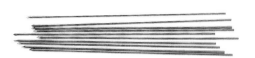

The sharp hook is used to check and reduce bone fragments. It can also be used to free the tap of bone debris or the screw head of ingrown tissue before removal.

Kirschner Wires, 2.0 mm Diameter

Kirschner wires, 150 mm long, can be used for temporary fixation or for marking different angles. They can be inserted with a power drill equipped with Jacobs chuck adaptor. In hard bone it is recommended to pre-drill with the 2.0 mm drill bit.

6.3.2 Supplementary Instruments

Pointed Drill Guide

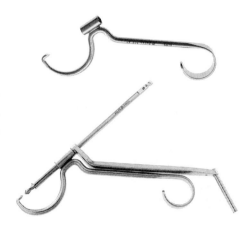

This drill guide can be used together with the 4.5 mm end of the 4.5 mm/3.2 mm double drill sleeve. It will guide the 4.5 mm drill bit for the gliding hole to align with a thread hole that has been prepared before reduction.

Drill Guide with Stop, 4.5/3.2 mm

The drill guide with a stop is used with drill bit 3.2 mm and limits the drilling depth by adjusting the sleeve length. This is especially useful in pelvic and spinal surgery.

Socket Wrench

The socket wrench for nuts of 11 mm width can be used to tighten the articulated tension device. Because of its universal joint, its strength is limited and it should not be used to apply strong forces.

Screwdriver with T Handle

This screwdriver can be used to release seized screws from the 4.5 and 6.5 mm group with a large hexagonal socket. It provides even greater turning power than a regular screwdriver.

Screwdriver with Universal Joint

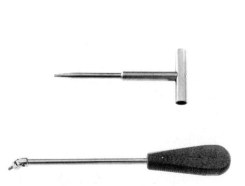

This screwdriver has a hexagonal tip which fits the large hexagonal socket of 4.5 and 6.5 mm screws. It may be advantageous to use in areas with obscured vision, e. g. pelvic or spinal surgery. The joint, however, does not allow the generation of strong torque.

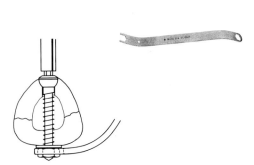

Large Hexagonal Allen Key

This Allen key fits screws with a 3.5 mm hexagonal socket. It may serve as a reserve.

Wrench, 8 mm

This wrench can be used to hold an 8 mm nut, needed in an emergency for a 4.5 mm cortex screw with stripped threads. The nut, mounted in the 8 mm wrench, is held against the opposite surface of the bone while a slightly longer than measured cortex screw is inserted.

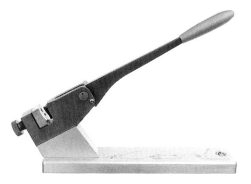

Bending Press

The bending press is used to contour large plates into convex or concave shapes. It is stable and requires little force for bending. Before using the bending press, the handle is placed in the neutral position and the jaws adjusted to the plate thickness. The anvil has two positions; for concave bending the plate is placed at the front for convex bending it is placed at the back. With the handle in the neutral position, the knurled knob is turned until the plate is held firmly between the anvil and the upper jaw.
Bending is made between holes in small increments without applying too much force until the desired shape is reached. A bending template serves as a model. While holding the plate with the press, twisting can be performed with a bending iron.
The bending press has to be disassembled for cleaning. Moving parts need lubrication. See Sect. 6.22.5.9.

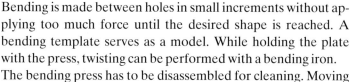

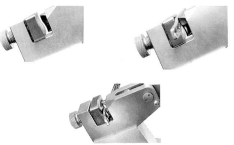

Bending Pliers

The bending pliers have three interchangeable anvils: a large size for broad plates, a medium size for 4.5 mm DCP and LC-DCP, and a small anvil for small fragment plates or mandibular plates. The upper jaw can be rotated to fit the plate cross-section – convex, concave or flat.
The pliers are adjusted to the plate thickness and to the grip of the surgeon by turning the knob at the end of the handle. Bending is performed between the holes and in small increments. Twisting is possible by placing the plate obliquely in the jaws but requires care and experience.
Complete disassembly is necessary for cleaning and lubrication. See Sect. 6.22.5.9.

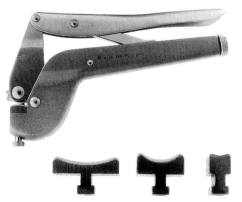

Fixation with Large Screws and Plates

69 ∎

Bending (Twisting) Irons

Bending irons are used solely to twist the plates. The two slots accept different plate thicknesses. In the newly designed irons, marked LC-DCP and DCP, the slots have rounded edges to avoid indentation and possible weakening of plates. The irons should not be used for bending, since this would cause the plate to bend at the holes and weaken it.

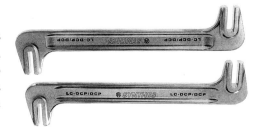

Small Air Drill

This drill with a double air hose connector and quick coupling chuck accepts all AO/ASIF drill bits and other instruments with quick coupling ends. For instruments with triangular ends, a Jacobs chuck adaptor can be fitted.
See Sect. 6.21.3

Instruments for Removal of Damaged Screws

See Sect. 6.19.

6.3.3 Obsolete Instruments

The instruments described below either are no longer manufactured or have been replaced by an improved version. However, they will still serve their function if undamaged.

Malleolar Countersink, 3.2 mm

This countersink was used with the T handle to cut the recess for the malleolar screw head. Since malleolar screws are rarely used in areas where countersinking is necessary, the instrument is obsolete. It had a 3.2 mm tip to fit the pre-drilled 3.2 mm hole for this screw.

Tap Sleeve, 6.5 mm

This tap sleeve has been replaced by double drill sleeve, 6.5 mm/3.2mm

Straight Drill Sleeve, 4.5 mm/3.2 mm

This drill sleeve was used as an insert drill sleeve for lag screw fixation. The double drill sleeve 4.5 mm/3.2 mm and the insert drill sleeve 4.5 mm/3.2 mm now serve this function.

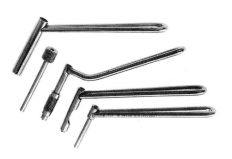

Tap Sleeve, 4.5 mm

This tap sleeve was used as the drill sleeve for the 4.5 mm drill bit and as a tap sleeve for the 4.5 mm tap. The double drill sleeve 4.5 mm/3.2 mm is the replacement.

Instrumentation and Techniques

Tap Sleeve, 3.5 mm

This tap sleeve was used as a drill sleeve for the 3.2 mm drill bit. It has been replaced by the double drill sleeve 4.5 mm/3.2 mm.

Drill Sleeve for Plates, 3.2 mm

This drill sleeve was used as a drill sleeve for plates with round holes. The double drill sleeve (3.2 mm) now serves this function.

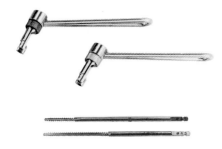

DCP Drill Guides, 4.5 mm

These drill guides, either neutral (green) or eccentric (yellow), each with a separate handle, have been replaced by the 4.5 mm DCP drill guide combined on one handle.

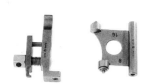

Taps with Short and Long Thread, 4.5 mm

These taps have been replaced by the long threaded 4.5 mm tap with a short flute.

Tension Device, 8 mm Span

This tension device has been replaced by the articulated tension device, which provides a longer span for compression.

Drill Sleeve for the Tension Device, 8 mm Span

This was the drill sleeve for the tension device, 8 mm.

6.4 AO/ASIF Screws for Large Bone Fractures

Screws are the basic elements for achieving interfragmentary compression. They can be used as lag screws either individually or through plates to bring two fragments together under compression. Screws are also used for the fixation of plates to bone. Screw sizes are named according to the outside diameter of their threaded portion. The correct screw type, diameter and length must be selected to correspond to the size, type and quality of bone.

There are basically two types of screws: cortex screws and cancellous bone screws. Cortex screws are designed to be used in hard cortical bone, mainly in the diaphysis of long bones, but they may also be used in the pelvis, for example. They are not self-cutting; the thread has to be cut prior to insertion.[1] The cortex screw may be fully threaded or partially threaded. Malleolar screws with cortex thread, a shaft and a trocar tip have limited use in the metaphyseal area, e. g. distal humerus, the trocanteric area, and sometimes in the ankle, where the bone is rather dense.

---

[1] A self-tapping 4.5 mm cortex screw is presently being included.

Cancellous bone screws find their application in the metaphyseal and epiphyseal regions, where the bone is softer and spongy, and the cortex thin. The screws may be fully or partially threaded, solid or cannulated.

Large AO/ASIF standard screws exist with 6.5 and 4.5 mm thread diameters, in various lengths. Measurements include both the tip and the head. The screws are available in both stainless steel and pure titanium. They may be obtained in standard lengths in either a graphic case or in a screw rack for sterilization trays. Other lengths can be obtained separately.

A screw forceps is used to remove the screws from the rack.

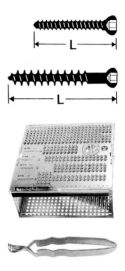

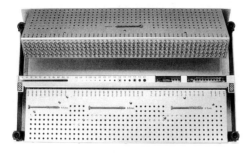

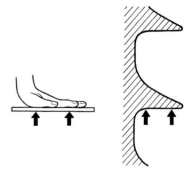

Cannulated screws, in diameters 7.0 mm, 4.5 mm, and 3.5 mm, are discussed in Sect. 6.6.

The large AO/ASIF screws have the following characteristics in common:

1. Spherical Screw Head. The 8 mm diameter head has a hemispherical undersurface. This ensures optimal annular contact between the screw and the plate hole, even if it is inserted at an angle. The hexagonal socket, 3.5 mm in width, enables easy insertion and removal with a hexagonal screwdriver of the corresponding size, without the need to apply axial pressure. It is essential that the socket be free of ingrown tissue before removal and that the screwdriver fully engage the socket. A damaged screwdriver would destroy the socket and make screw removal extremely difficult.

2. AO/ASIF Screw Thread. The design of the screw thread is the factor ultimately determining the screw's holding power in the material in which it is used. Because the strength of the bone is ten times less than that of metal, AO/ASIF screws have an asymmetrical buttress thread profile. The flat, broad pressure bearing area gives excellent hold in bone. In hard cortical bone a shallow thread and finer pitch ensure a large contact area and the best hold. In soft cancellous bone a deep thread and coarse pitch is necessary to enhance the holding power.

Another prerequisite for optimal holding power is that the thread hole be prepared to the size of the core (stem) of the screw and that the threads cut in the bone correspond exactly to the profile of the screw thread. Tapping is always necessary in

Instrumentation and Techniques

cortical bone, while in general it is not in cancellous bone, except in hard juvenile bone.

3. Core Diameter. The core is the solid stem of the screw from which the threads protrude. It should not be confused with the shaft of the screw. The 4.5 mm cortex screw , the 6.5 mm cancellous bone screw, and the malleolar screw made of stainless steel all have the same core diameter of 3.0 mm. The core diameter of the large titanium screws, however, differs, i. e. 3.1 mm for the 4.5 mm screw, and 3.2 mm for the 6.5 mm screws. The core size determines the size of the drill bit used for the pilot hole. The same size drill bit (3.2 mm) is used to pre-drill the thread hole for all the large screws.

4. Shaft Diameter. The 4.5 mm shaft screw and the 6.5 mm cancellous bone screw each have an unthreaded shaft of diameter 4.5 mm. Pre-drilling of 4.5 mm in the near cortex is therefore necessary at any entry point in hard cortical bone to avoid splitting. The shaft of malleolar screws has the same diameter as the core, so that pre-drilling of 3.2 mm is sufficient.

6.4.1 Large Standard Screws

4.5 mm Cortex Screws in Stainless Steel and Pure Titanium

These screws are usually used as lag screws or for plate fixation in the diaphyses of large bones. They are also used as fixation screws for the tension device or the pelvic reduction forceps. The 4.5 mm cortex screw is a fully threaded non-self-tapping screw. Pretapping of cortical bone is necessary before insertion of the screw. The thread and the polished surface allow easy removal of the screw, even though hard cortical bone will have grown between the threads during healing.
The 4.5 mm cortex screw has a smooth tip. It is important for the holding power of the screw that the threads engage the entire far cortex. The tip of the screw and one or two threads should therefore protrude on the opposite side of the bone. In hard cortical bone the 4.5 mm cortex screw has a holding strength of approximately 2500 N (250 kg).
Measurement of the screw length is rounded up rather than down to ensure optimal holding power. The 4.5 mm cortex screws are available in lengths from 14 mm to 110 mm in stainless steel, and from 14 mm to 140 mm in titanium.

Important dimensions:
- Head diameter: 8.0   mm
- Hexagonal socket width: 3.5   mm
- Core diameter: 3.0   mm (titanium 3.1 mm)
- Thread diameter: 4.5   mm
- Pitch: 1.75 mm
- Drill bit for gliding hole: 4.5   mm diameter
- Drill bit for thread hole: 3.2   mm diameter
- Tap diameter: 4.5   mm

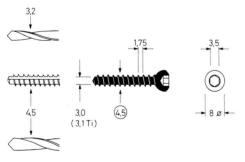

4.5 mm Shaft Screw in Pure Titanium

This screw is a recently developed cortex shaft screw to be used with the LC-DCP. It was used in stainlesss steel for some time as the locking screw in the universal nails, until the present stronger locking bolt was introduced.

It is used as a lag screw through a plate or as a free lag screw in the diaphysis. A cortex shaft screw used as a lag screw produces a more effective compression than a fully threaded cortex screw, because the shaft does not accidentally engage in the plate hole or in the gliding hole. The screw can also be inserted eccentrically in a LC-DCP hole as a load screw for axial compression. The shaft portion is five times stiffer and 3.4 times stronger in bending than the threaded portion. It therefore contributes to the improved axial compression and supplements the self-compressing effect of the plates.

The thread is of the same design as that of the fully threaded cortex screw. Pretapping is necessary before insertion of the screw. The tip and one or two threads should protrude on the opposite side of the bone to ensure optimal purchase.

The 4.5 mm shaft screws are available in lengths from 22 mm to 110 mm. The threaded portion of the screw increases from 13 mm to 26 mm in proportion to the overall screw length. Pretapping of the far cortex prior to insertion is necessary.

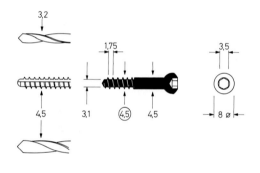

Important dimensions:
- Head diameter: 8.0 mm
- Hexagonal socket width: 3.5 mm
- Shaft diameter: 4.5 mm
- Core diameter: 3.1 mm
- Thread diameter: 4.5 mm
- Pitch: 1.75 mm
- Drill bit for gliding hole: 4.5 mm diameter
- Drill bit for thread hole: 3.2 mm diameter
- Tap: 4.5 mm

6.5 mm Cancellous Bone Screws in Stainless Steel and Pure Titanium

These screws are used only in the metaphyseal and epiphyseal areas, with fine trabecular bone and relatively thin cortex. Three different types of screws exist: one with a 16 mm thread length, another with a 32 mm thread length, and the third fully threaded. The screws with shafts are designed as lag screws; the fully threaded screw is mainly used as a plate fixation screw when the end holes of a plate are located over cancellous bone. The deep and wide threads of the cancellous bone screw ensure good purchase in the compressed cancellous trabeculae. Tapping is only necessary in the near cortex to allow introduction of the screw. The holding power in the fine trabecular bone is increased when the screw itself creates its thread by pressing bone aside. Engaging the far cortex increases the holding power of

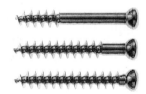

Instrumentation and Techniques

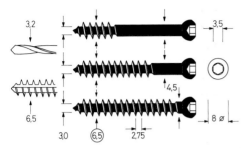

the screw, but is only necessary in porotic bone. However, the tip is pointed and care must be taken not to damage any structures on the opposite side of the bone if it is left protruding too far.

The 6.5 mm cancellous bone screws are available in 5 mm increments in lengths from 25 mm to 110 mm in stainless steel, and from 25 mm to 150 mm in pure titanium

Important dimensions:

– Head diameter:	8.0 mm
– Hexagonal socket:	3.5 mm
– Shaft diameter:	4.5 mm
– Core diameter:	3.0 mm (titanium 3.2 mm)
– Thread diameter:	6.5 mm
– Thread lengths:	16 and 32 mm, fully threaded
– Pitch:	2.75 mm
– Drill bit for thread hole:	3.2 mm diameter
– Drill bit for shaft in hard bone:	4.5 mm diameter
– Tap:	6.5 mm

Malleolar Screw, 4.5 mm

This screw was designed as a lag screw to be used in medial malleolar fractures, but due to its rather large diameter and large screw head the smaller cancellous bone screws have taken its place in this area. The malleolar screw may find its application in fractures in the metaphysis, for example in the distal humerus or in the lesser trochanter. It may also be used in some pelvic fixations.

The malleolar screw has a smooth shaft and is partially threaded. The trephine tip allows insertion without tapping, and in osteoporotic bone sometimes even without pre-drilling the cancellous bone. Because of the cortex screw thread profile it has, however, a rather poor hold.

The malleolar screw is available in lengths from 25 mm to 70 mm. The threaded portion is as the same length as the unthreaded shaft.

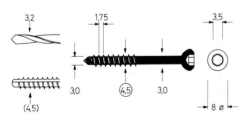

Important dimensions:

– Head diameter:	8.0 mm
– Hexagonal socket:	3.5 mm
– Shaft diameter:	3.0 mm
– Core diameter:	3.0 mm
– Thread diameter:	4.5 mm
– Pitch:	1.75 mm
– Drill bit for thread hole:	3.2 mm diameter
– Tap (rare):	4.5 mm diameter

Washer, 13 mm

This washer has a flat side, which rests on the bone, and a countersunk side which accepts the screw head. It prevents the screw head from breaking through the thin cortex in the metaphysis and epiphysis by spreading the load over a larger area.

6.4.2 Supplementary Implants

Nut for 4.5 mm Cortex Screw

This nut is an 11 mm flat stainless steel nut with a thread matching that of the 4.5 mm cortex screw and which can be used in the event of emergency if the hole for the screw has been stripped. It is held in position with the 8 mm wrench. See above.

Spiked Washer, 13.5 mm

This washer is made of polyacetate with a stainless steel reinforcement for X-ray contrast. It is used for reattachment of avulsed ligaments together with either a 6.5 mm cancellous bone screw or a 4.5 mm cortex screw. Due to structural changes in the molecules of the material, it can only be sterilized in autoclaves at a maximum of 140°C (270°F) a few times. Eight hours are required for cooling and rehardening following sterilization. Sterilization in EtO (ethylene oxide) is also possible, followed by a full-cycle aeration. It is therefore recommended to have a few in stock, separately packaged and presterilized.

6.4.3 Obsolete Implants

Epiphyseal screws had an extra high head to prevent ingrowth of bone when used in juvenile bone. Since removal still proved difficult and the fixation of slipped epiphysis was possible with large cancellous bone screws and a washer, this implant no longer exists.

6.4.4 Fixation Techniques with Large Screws

Screws are used either as lag screws to achieve interfragmentary compression or as plate fixation screws. The lag screw technique should always be used if a screw is to be inserted across a fracture, even through a plate.

Principle of lag screw technique: The screw has no purchase in the near fragment; the thread grips the far fragment only. This can be achieved with screws that have a shaft or with fully threaded screws. It is the technique of application that determines whether a screw functions as a lag screw. The technique for each individual screw will be discussed below.

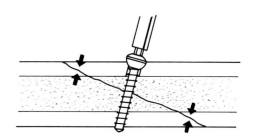

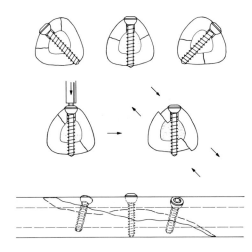

Positioning of (Cortex) Screws as Lag Screws

Maximal interfragmentary compression is achieved when the screw is placed in the middle of the fragment and directed at a right angle to the fracture plane. Any other position would cause shearing as the screw is tightened, risking displacement of the fragments. Maximal axial stability is provided by a screw placed at a right angle to the long axis of the bone. This position, however, also tends to cause displacement of fragments. Therefore, in lag screw fixation of a fracture it is best to have at least one screw at a right angle to the long axis, usually the central one, and one or two perpendicular to the fracture plane.

In diaphyseal bone lag screw fixation alone presents an exception. Only in torsional fractures resulting in a long spiral at least twice the diameter of the bone can lag screw fixation alone give sufficient stability. If comminution or other factors predisposing to redisplacement are present, interfragmentary lag screw fixation must be protected by a plate.

4.5 mm Cortex Screw Used as a Lag Screw

The fully threaded cortex screw is used as a lag screw mainly in diaphyseal bone where the cortex is thick.

To permit the screw to glide freely through the near fragment, a so-called gliding or clearance hole is drilled which is equal in size to the thread diameter. In the far fragment a coaxial thread hole is drilled which is slightly larger than the core diameter. The thread hole is then tapped with a tap which corresponds exactly in diameter and thread profile to the screw.

Standard Technique "Outside In"

Step by step procedure:
- The fracture is reduced and held with reduction forceps or Kirschner wires.
- The gliding hole is drilled in the near cortex with the 4.5 mm drill bit in the 4.5 mm end of the double drill sleeve (Fig. 1).
- The double drill sleeve is turned around and the 3.2 mm sleeve inserted into the gliding hole. It is pushed through the gliding hole until it abuts the opposite cortex.
- The thread hole is drilled in a coaxial direction in the far fragment with the 3.2 mm drill bit (Fig. 2).
- A recess is cut in the near cortical surface with the large countersink, 4.5 mm (Fig. 3).

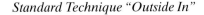

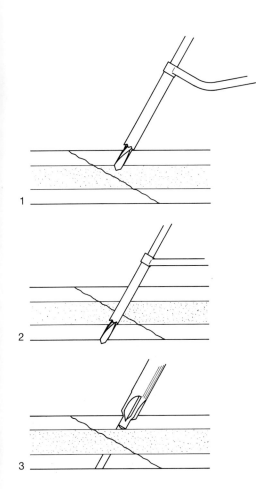

- The screw length is measured with the large depth gauge, 4.5 mm – 6.5 mm (Fig. 4).
- The thread hole in the far fragment is tapped with the tap for 4.5 mm cortex screws in the 4.5 mm end of the double drill sleeve. Two turns clockwise and one-half turn counterclockwise to free the threads of bone debris (Fig. 5).
- The 4.5 mm cortex screw is inserted with the large hexagonal screwdriver. Ensure that the screw securely engages the far cortex (Fig. 6).

Variation: If the far fragment ends in a long narrow spike, where it is essential to place the screw in its centre, then either the gliding hole or the thread hole can be drilled prior to reduction. This ensures that the screw can be positioned exactly.

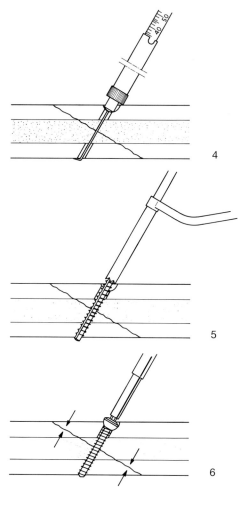

Gliding Hole First Technique "Inside Out"

Step by step procedure:
- The gliding hole is drilled from the medullary aspect in the near fragment with the 4.5 mm drill bit in the 4.5 mm end of the double drill sleeve, keeping in mind the position of the screw in the far fragment (Fig. 1).
- The fracture is reduced and temporary fixation applied.
- The thread hole is drilled in the opposite fragment, using a 3.2 mm drill bit in the 3.2 mm end of the double drill guide inserted into the 4.5 mm hole (Fig. 2). It is then countersunk, measured and tapped as described above, before inserting the screw.

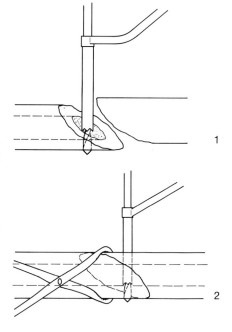

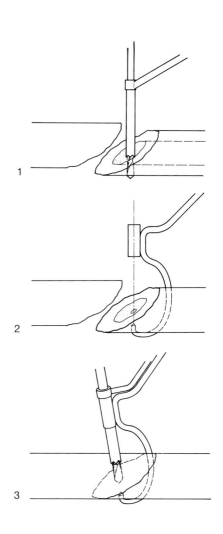

1

2

3

Thread Hole First Technique "Inside Out"

Step by step procedure:
- The thread hole is drilled in the centre of the medullary surface of the far bony spike under direct vision, using the 3.2 mm drill bit and the 3.2 mm end of the double drill sleeve (Fig. 1).
- The pointed drill guide is hooked into the thread hole and held absolutely centred (Fig. 2).
- The fracture is reduced and temporary fixation applied.
- The 4.5 mm end of the double drill sleeve is pushed into the cylindrical sleeve of the pointed drill guide until it abuts the bone. The handles of the 4.5 mm drill guide and the pointed drill guide are squeezed together to grip the bone and steady the direction.
- The gliding hole is drilled in the near cortex with the 4.5 mm drill bit passed through the pointed drill guide assembly, without changing the guide's position (Fig. 3).
- The countersink, the depth gauge, and the tap are then used as described for the standard technique.

*Note:*This technique demands that care is taken not to damage the periosteum when passing the pointed drill guide around the bone. It is also necessary to hold the tip of the guide absolutely centred; coaxial drilling of the gliding hole is impossible otherwise.

The 4.5 mm Cortex Screw Used as a Plate Fixation Screw

Large plates used for fractures in the diaphysis are fixed with 4.5 mm cortex screws. For plate fixation the threads of the cortex screw engage both cortices, or exceptionally only the near cortex. The appropriate drill guide must be used.

Step by step procedure:
- The fracture is reduced and the plate fixed provisionally to the bone.
- The thread hole is drilled with the 3.2 mm drill bit in the correct drill guide through the plate hole and through both cortices.
- The screw length is measured through the plate hole with the depth gauge, 4.5–6.5 mm.
- Both cortices are tapped with the tap for 4.5 mm cortex screws in the double drill sleeve, 4.5 mm/3.2 mm.
- The screw is inserted with the large hexagonal screwdriver.

The Malleolar Screw as a Lag Screw

The malleolar screw is primarily used for lag screw fixation in the metaphysis. Its shaft allows gliding and the 4.5 mm cortex thread should have purchase only in the far fragment.

Step by step procedure:
– The fracture is reduced and temporarily fixed.
– The thread hole is drilled with the 3.2 mm drill bit in the 3.2 mm end of the double drill sleeve, 4.5 mm/3.2 mm.
– The screw length is measured with the depth gauge, 4.5–6.5 mm
– If necessary, the bone is tapped with the tap for 4.5 mm cortex screws in the double drill sleeve end, 4.5 mm.
– The screw is inserted with the large hexagonal screwdriver.

6.4.5 AO/ASIF Instruments for Insertion and Removal of Large Screws

Instruments for the insertion of 4.5 mm cortex screws as lag screws

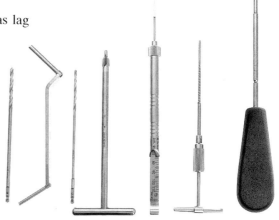

Instruments for the insertion of 6.5 mm cancellous bone screws   Instruments for large screw removal

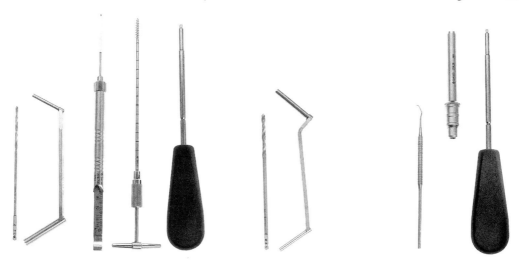

6.5 Plates for Large Bone Fractures

The large AO/ASIF plates have been designed for the fixation of certain fractures in large bones, i.e. humerus, pelvis, femur and tibia. They are also referred to as large plates because they are fixed to the bone by means of the large screws described in Sect. 6.4.

Each plate has a name, which either describes the design of the plate (e.g. semitubular plate), the part of the bone on which it is used (e.g. lateral tibial head plate) or a very special feature of the plate (e.g. Limited Contact-Dynamic Compression Plate or LC-DCP). Plates can also be referred to by the function they fulfil in a particular fixation, e.g. a tension band plate, neutralization or protection plate, compression plate (see Sect. 6.5.4). These functions, however, can be performed by different plates.

There are three main groups of large plates: the straight plates, the special plates and the angled blade plates. Of these, the straight plates are used mainly in the diaphysis, the special plates in the metaphyseal and epiphyseal areas and the angled blade plates in the proximal and distal femur. In this section only straight and special plates are discussed. Angled blade plates are described in Sect. 6.8.

Most plates and screws are available both in stainless steel and in commercially pure AO titanium. High quality stainless steel has been the standard material for implants for a long time. It offers good mechanical strength, together with excellent ductility. This steel is available in different degrees of strength, which allows the choice of a material corresponding to the function of the implant. Although highly purified and of an optimized chemical composition, stainless steel may still show local corrosion and eventually pitting corrosion, which may eventually cause a tissue reaction.

The attractive biological characteristics of commercially pure AO titanium (p.Ti), when cold worked to high strength, has therefore made this an implant material of choice, especially for patients suffering from metal allergy. Due to its mechanical properties, the handling of pure titanium plates, for example, contouring, feels somewhat different from that of stainless steel plates. Whatever material is chosen for plates, though, it is recommended that the same material be used for screws. See also Sect. 6.1.1

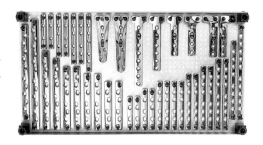

6.5.1 Standard Plates

The standard plates may be obtained in either a graphic case or a sterilizing tray. The old aluminium cases can also be used for storage.

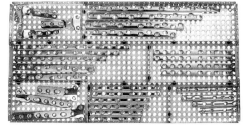

6.5.1.1 Straight Plates

DCP, 4.5 mm

The term DCP stands for dynamic compression plate. The term DCP plate is therefore incorrect. It is nevertheless used since DCP is a registered term rather than the descriptive expression. The DCP was developed to improve the former plating techniques with round hole plates. Over the years the DCP has been used for successful fixations of many fractures, especially in the long bones. The special geometry of the plate hole allows for self-compression and a congruent fit between screw head and plate hole at different angles of inclination. The plate can thus fulfil different plate functions, e. g. compression plating, tension band plating, neutralization (protection) plating, and buttress plating. See Sect. 4.2

Plate Hole and the "Spherical Gliding" Principle

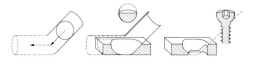

The plate hole can best be described as a part of an inclined and horizontal cylinder in which a sphere can be moved downwardly and horizontally to the intersection of the two cylinders. The cylinders represent the plate hole and the sphere the screw head. Axial compression between fragments can be achived by using this feature of the plate holes.

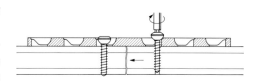

A screw placed at the inclined plane, i.e eccentrically (load position), will move the underlying bone horizontally in relation to the plate until the screw head reaches the intersection of the two cylinders. At this point the screw has optimal contact with the hole, ensuring maximal stability. The horizontal "cylinder" prevents jamming as well as undesired distraction. A 4.5 mm cortex screw can be placed in three different positions in the plate hole: eccentric (or load) position, neutral position, and buttress position.

All holes in the DCP embody the spherical gliding principle.

The DCP Drill Guide, Neutral and Load

A special drill guide is necessary for the correct placement of the screws. The two ends connected on a handle fit exactly in the plate holes.

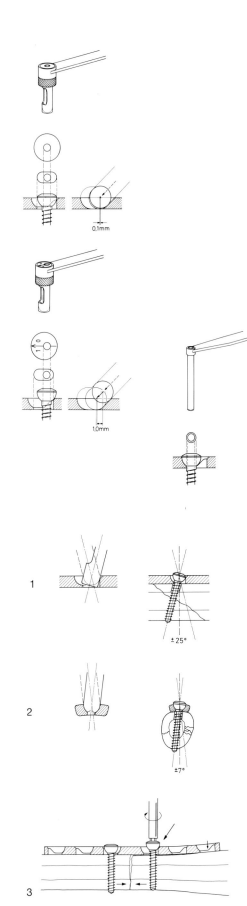

The *neutral, green* end of the DCP drill guide is used when drilling for a screw in the neutral position, that is, at the intersection of the two cylinders. A minimal movement of 0.1 mm in fact occurs when this guide is used. The neutral DCP drill guide is the one most frequently used.

The *load, yellow* DCP drill guide allows eccentric drilling, placing the screw in a load position. The little arrow on the top must point toward the fracture, because when the screw is driven home, it is displaced 1.0 mm horizontally. This guide is used only to achieve axial compression once the fracture has been anatomically reduced and fixed with at least one screw in the opposite fragment.

The buttress position of a screw is obtained by using the 3.2 mm side of the double drill sleeve. The sleeve is placed snugly at the inner limit of the plate hole near the fracture. This position is needed when the plate is being used to prevent collapse of a fracture reduction, i.e in comminuted or metaphyseal fractures.

Advantages of the DCP Design

The DCP holes offer several advantages:
– Inclined insertion of the screw with hemispherical screw head is possible up to an angle of 25° longitudinally (Fig. 1), 7° sideways (Fig. 2).
– Placement of a screw in neutral position without the danger of distraction of fragments.
– Insertion of a load screw into the hole positioned most favourably for a given fracture. All holes permit compression (Fig. 3).

- Symmetrical spherical gliding holes: the basic principle of spherical gliding of the screw head in the plate hole is preserved, but augmented. Both ends of each plate hole offer the gliding possibility, which means more versatility in use. The holes allow 1.0 mm displacement of the fragment if a load screw is inserted.

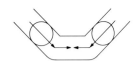

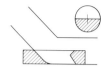 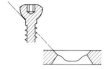

- Undercut plate holes: undercut at each end of the plate hole allows 40° tilting of screws both ways along the long axis of the plate. Lag screw fixation of short oblique fractures is thereby possible. Screws can be tilted ±7° in the transverse plane. Furthermore, the undercuts reduce the contact area between plate and bone even more.
- The end holes of the plate allow use of the articulated tension device if further compression is necessary, i.e. in fractures of the femur with a wide gap.

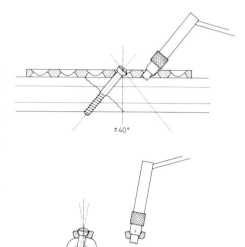

Before applying a LC-DCP, the plate must be contoured or prebent and the fracture anatomically reduced.

The LC-DCP, 4.5 mm, is fixed to the bone with 4.5 mm cortex screws and 4.5 mm shaft screws, or in the end holes with 6.5 mm cancellous bone screws. The 4.5 mm screws can be inserted in three different positions: neutral, load, and buttress. For this pupose special drill guides have to be used, either the LC-DCP drill guide, 4.5 mm, or the universal drill guide, 4.5 mm.

LC-DCP Drill Guides

The LC-DCP drill guide, 4.5 mm, is similar to the DCP drill guide, 4.5 mm, in that it has a neutral (green) and a load (yellow) guide combined on a handle. The inserts will only fit this special handle, which has been designed with the same undercuts as the plate to distinguish it from the DCP drill guide handle. The green neutral guide places the screw in a neutral position if the arrow points toward the fracture. Turned 180°, the arrow pointing away from the fracture, a buttress position is obtained. The yellow load guide places the screw in an eccentric position for compression, when the arrow points toward the fracture. The displacement is 1.0 mm.

Because of the spherical end of the guides, they have a congruent fit in the plate hole, also when tilted 40° in the longitudinal and ±7° in the transverse plane.

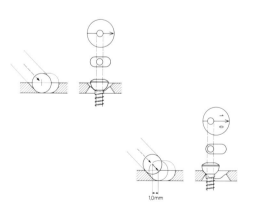

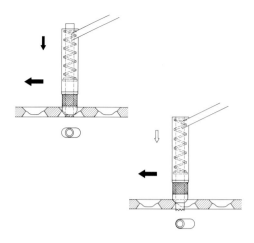

The LC-DCP universal drill guide, 4.5 mm, has two different sleeves combined on a handle. One sleeve has an inner diameter of 4.5 mm and is used with the 4.5 mm drill bit and the tap for 4.5 mm cortex screws. The other end consists of an outer sleeve, which has an end that corresponds exactly to the hemispherical undersurface of the screw head, and an inner sleeve with diameters 4.5 mm/3.2 mm used with the 3.2 mm drill bit. The two sleeves are preloaded by a spring in such a way that the inner sleeve protrudes at the tip. By applying pressure the inner sleeve is pushed back into the outer sleeve. When the sleeve is placed in the plate hole and pressure is applied, the rounded end of the outer sleeve follows the inclined "cylinder" of the plate hole to neutral position. The load position for a screw is obtained by placing the protruding inner sleeve in the far end (away from the fracture) of the plate hole. Similarly, the buttress position is obtained when this sleeve is placed in the end of the plate hole nearer the fracture.

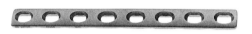

Narrow LC-DCP, 4.5 mm in Pure Titanium

This plate has been specially designed for use on the tibia, but it can be used sometimes on the radius or ulna in a large patient. The plate can function as a neutralization, tension band or buttress plate, as desired. It is fixed with 4.5 mm titanium cortex screws and, if located over cancellous bone, with 6.5 mm titanium cancellous bone screws. The 4.5 mm titanium shaft screws are used as load screws for axial compression and as lag screws for interfragmentary compression. The narrow 4.5 mm LC-DCP is available with 2 to 16 holes.

Important dimensions:
- Profile: see figure
- Thickness: 4.6 mm
- Width: 13.5 mm
- Hole spacing: 18   mm
- Hole length: 8.5 mm

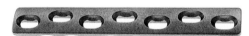

Broad LC-DCP, 4.5 mm in Pure Titanium

This plate is designed for use on the femur and for pseudarthroses of the humerus. Any desired plate function can be achieved with it. The broad LC-DCP, 4.5 mm is available with 6 to 18 holes, which are staggered to prevent fissuring of the bone.

Important dimensions:
- Profile: see figure
- Thickness: 6.0 mm
- Width: 17.5 mm
- Hole spacing: 18   mm
- Hole length: 8.5 mm

Semitubular Plates

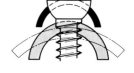

As their name implies, semitubular plates are designed in the shape of a half tube. They are only 1 mm thick and have low rigidity. The plate should be used only in areas where they are subject to tensile forces. Good rotational stability can be achieved by means of the edges that dig into the bone. The oval plate holes allow some axial compression if the 4.5 mm cortex screws are inserted eccentrically on each side of the fracture.

A slight disadvantage of the plate hole is the deep penetration of the unthreaded neck of the screw into the cortex, which entails some risk of cortical splitting. Enlarging the cortex to 4.5 mm would prevent such splitting.

In the past the semitubular plate found its application in forearm fractures. Today it may occasionally be used as a tension band plate in open book injuries of the pelvis and as a second plate in comminuted fractures in the metaphysis of long bones. Sometimes it is used also for special orthopaedic procedures.

The semitubular plates can be used with the tension device.

Semitubular plates are available with 2 to 12 holes.

Important dimensions:
- Profile: see figure
- Thickness: 1 mm
- Width: 11 mm
- Hole spacing: 16 and 26 mm

Reconstruction Plates, 4.5 mm

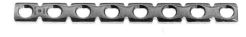

Reconstruction plates have been specially designed such that they can be bent and twisted in two dimensions. They are therefore suitable in areas where exact and complex contouring is necessary, e. g. the pelvis. The notches alongside the plate make it possible to bend it into a curve on the flat, using special bending irons for reconstruction plates. It should be noted that the already low strength of the plate is further diminished by three-dimensional bending. Bending angles greater than 15° at any one site must be avoided.

The oval plate holes permit self-compression and accept both 4.5 mm cortex screws and 6.5 mm cancellous bone screws. The plates are available with 3 to 16 holes.

Important dimensions:
- Profile: see figure
- Thickness: 2.8 mm
- Width: 12   mm
- Hole spacing: 16   mm

6.5.1.2 Special Plates

The special plates are shaped to conform to specific anatomical locations in the metaphysis and the epiphysis. In general they are applied according to the same principles as the straight plates, i.e. as compression plates, neutralization plates or buttress plates.

T Plates

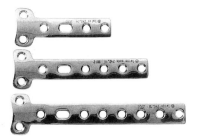

T plates are designed to be used as buttress plates, especially on the medial aspect of the tibial plateau. They are also applied in proximal humerus fractures, for axial compression of a large head fragment. The tension device is then used to exert compression.

The head of the plate accommodates 6.5 mm cancellous bone screws. The elongated hole is for loose temporary fixation with a cortex screw. Longitudinal adjustment and tightening with the tension device is then possible before fixation of the shaft. Angled lag screws can also be inserted through the elongated hole.

T plates are available with 3, 4, 5, 6 and 8 holes in the shaft and 68, 84, 100, 116 and 148 mm in length.

Important dimensions:
- Thickness: 2.0 mm
- Width shaft: 17   mm

T and L Buttress Plates

T and L buttress plates are designed as buttress plates for the lateral aspect of the tibial plateau. They differ from the ordinary T plates only in their double bend, which contours to the lateral side of the tibial plateau. The L buttress plates have an offset head, one for the left and one for the right leg, to enable more lateral buttressing without disturbing the fibula.

T buttress plates are available with 4, 5 and 6 holes in the shaft and in lengths of 81, 96 and 112 mm, respectively The L buttress plates have 4 holes only and are 81 mm long.

Important dimensions:
- Thickness: 2.0 mm
- Width shaft T buttress plate: 17   mm
- Width shaft L buttress plate: 16   mm

6.5.2 Supplementary Plates

Lateral Tibial Head Buttress Plates

Lateral tibial head buttress plates are also designed as buttress plates for fractures of the lateral tibial plateau with proximal diaphyseal involvment. The plate has an expanded and shaped upper portion or head. This is thinner than the shaft of the plate, which has the same form as the narrow DCP, 4.5 mm. The shaft is thicker than in the plates mentioned in 6.5.1.2 and is preferable when proximal tibial fractures extend down into the diaphyseal zone.

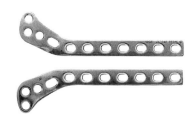

The DCP holes in the shaft accept 4.5 mm cortex screws; the round holes in the slightly thinner head accommodate 6.5 mm cancellous bone screws. The plate can be used with the tension device.

Lateral tibial head buttress plates are available with 5, 7 and 9 holes in the shaft, for both the left and the right tibia.

Important dimensions:
- Profile: see figure
- Shaft thickness: 3.8 mm
- Width: 14   mm
- Hole spacing: 16   mm

Condylar Buttress Plates

Condylar buttress plates are used for the fixation of comminuted fractures (C3) in the distal femur if a right angled condylar plate cannot be used. The shaft is similar in size to that of the broad DCP, and the DCP holes are staggered. The tension device can be hooked in the notch at the end of the plate. The head portion with its round holes accepts the 6.5 mm cancellous bone screws.

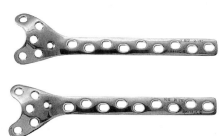

The plate is available with 7, 9, 11, 13 and 15 holes for both the left and the right tibia.

Important dimensions:
- Profile: see figure
- Shaft thickness: 5 mm
- Width: 16 mm
- Hole spacing: 16 mm

Cobra Head Plates

Cobra head plates are used for arthrodesis of the hip. The head portion of the plate has round holes and is fixed with 4.5 mm cortex screws. This plate also has a shaft similar to that of the broad DCP with staggered DCP holes since it is applied to the femur. A notch at the end of the shaft accepts the tension device, which is always used with this plate to exert enough axial compression for the fusion.

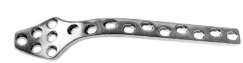

Instrumentation and Techniques

For the technique of application, see the *Manual of Internal Fixation* (Müller et al. 1979, pp. 388–389).

Long drill bits and taps are needed for the insertion of long screws.

The cobra head plate is available with 8, 9, 10 and 11 holes in the shaft.

Important dimensions:
- Profile: see figure
- Shaft thickness: 6 mm
- Width of shaft: 16 mm

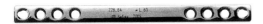

Narrow Lengthening Plates, 8 Holes

Narrow lengthening plates are used in special lengthening procedures with the lengthening apparatus (see Sect. 6.13.4). The plate has a middle section, without holes, in different lengths. Depending on the achieved lengthening a corresponding plate is chosen. The holes are of round hole design accepting 4.5 mm cortex screws; 6.5 mm cancellous bone screws can be inserted in the end holes, which also have notches for the tension device used for distraction. The plate has 4 holes on each side and can be used for lengthenings of 30, 40, 50, 60, 70 and 80 mm.

Important dimensions:
- Profile: see figure
- Thickness: 3.6 mm
- Width: 12   mm
- Hole spacing: 12   mm

Broad Lengthening Plates, 8 and 10 Holes

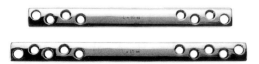

Broad lengthening plates are used for stabilisation of a lengthened femur. The plates therefore have staggered holes, 4 on each side, but their use is otherwise similar to that of the narrow lengthening plate. They may be applied when lengthenings of 30, 40, 50 and 60 mm have been achieved.

Important dimensions:
- Profile: see figure
- Thickness: 4.5 mm
- Width: 16   mm
- Hole spacing: 12   mm

Broad Lengthening Plates, 10 Holes

These broad lengthening plates have 5 holes on each side instead of 4, but design and use are otherwise the same as that of the previously mentioned plates. Lengthenings of 50, 60, 70, 80, 90, 100, 110 and 120 mm can be stabilised with these plates.

Plates for Large Bone Fractures

Titanium screws are used with titanium plates.

Prerequisites:
- Lag screw fixation separately, and if possible through the plate.
- Exact contouring of the plate. See Sect. 6.5.6.

Plate length: depends on fracture site and configuration. Two to four screws in each main fragment.

Step by step procedure:
- Reduction of the fracture and lag screw fixation with either 4.5 mm or 3.5 mm cortex screws (Fig. 1).
- Using a template as model, the plate is carefully contoured and provisionally fixed to the bone with reduction forceps.
- The first plate screw is inserted in one of the main fragments without crossing the fracture. The drill bit, 3.2 mm, in the LC-DCP drill guide, 4.5 mm, is used to drill the thread hole (Fig. 2).
- The screw length is measured using the depth gauge (Fig. 3).
- The thread hole is tapped with the tap for 4.5 mm cortex screws in the 4.5 mm end of the double drill guide (Fig. 4).
- The 4.5 mm titanium cortex screw is inserted with the large hexagonal screwdriver (Fig. 5).
- If any of the subsequent screws are crossing the fracture, they should be inserted as lag screws: The LC-DCP universal drill guide, 4.5 mm, is pressed into the plate hole in the desired direction and the thread hole drilled with the 3.2 mm drill bit in both cortices (Fig. 6).
- The length is measured (Fig. 7).
- The tap for 4.5 mm cortex screws in the 4.5 mm end of the universal drill guide is used to tap both fragments (Fig. 8).
- Without changing direction the near cortex is overdrilled with the 4.5 mm drill bit in the 4.5 mm end of the LC-DCP universal drill guide (Fig. 9).
- The chosen 4.5 mm titanium shaft screw is inserted with the large hexagonal screwdriver (Fig. 10).
- Interfragmentary compression has been achieved.
- The remaining screws, not crossing the fracture, can be inserted as regular plate screws using the neutral LC-DCP drill guide, 4.5 mm (Fig. 11).
- Final tightening of all screws (Fig. 12).

Note: Not all plate holes need to be occupied by screws. A short screw can be inserted if the fracture location so requires.

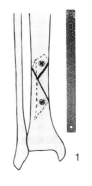

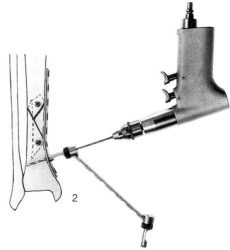

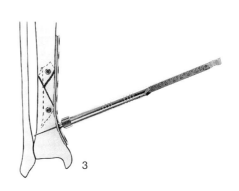

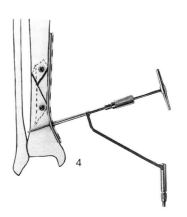

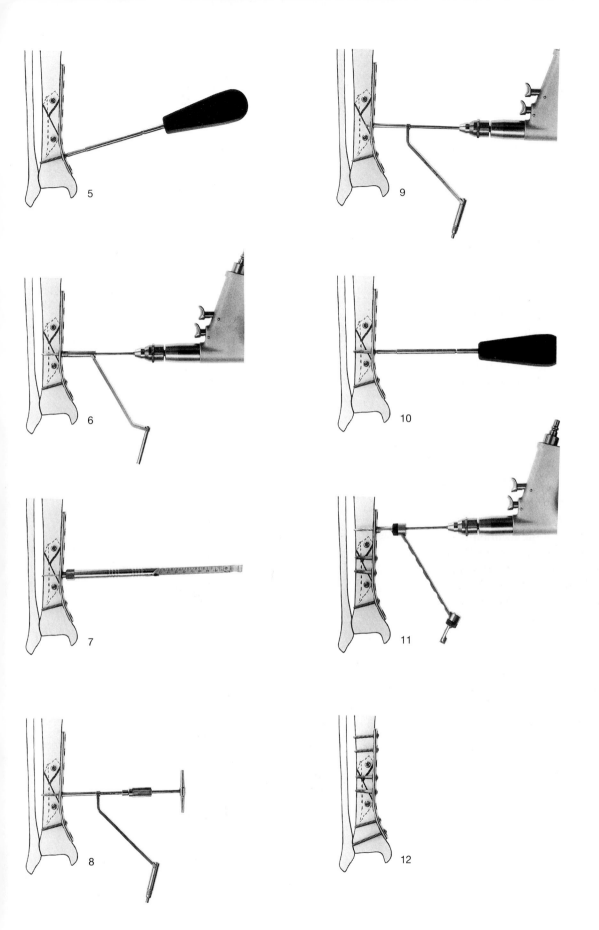

LC-DCP, 4.5 mm, Applied as a Buttress Plate

Like the DCP, the LC-DCP can be used as a buttress or as a bridging plate to prevent fracture zone collapse. All screws should be inserted in the buttress position to avoid compression.

Prerequisites:
– Careful contouring of the plate. See Sect. 6.5.6.
– All screws in buttress position.

Plate length: depends on the localization of the fracture.

Step by step procedure:
– The fracture is reduced and the contoured plate fixed to the bone with reduction forceps.
– The first screw is inserted near the fracture using the green neutral LC-DCP drill guide with the arrow pointing *away* from the fracture. The thread hole is drilled with the 3.2 mm drill bit.
– The screw length is measured and the hole tapped with the tap for 4.5 mm cortex screws and the double drill sleeve, 4.5 mm.
– The 4.5 mm titanium cortex screw is inserted with the large hexagonal screwdriver and tightened firmly.
– The procedure is repeated in the opposite fragment. Using the neutral LC-DCP drill guide with the arrow pointing *away* from the fracture, the thread hole is drilled, measured, and tapped, and the 4.5 mm titanium cortex screw inserted.
– If required, a lag screw can be inserted through the plate. Depending on the location it may be a cortex or a cancellous bone screw.
– The remaining screws are inserted in the buttress position using the technique described for the first screw.
– Final tightening of all screws.

6.5.3.3 Application of Semitubular Plates

Semitubular Plate as a Tension Band Plate

The semitubular plate can be used for the fixation of transverse fractures in, for example, the forearm, where the plate would be subject to tension only. The oval holes allow insertion of screws in a slightly eccentric position. If the fracture is perfectly reduced, axial compression can be exerted through this self-compressing effect.
If a cancellous bone screw is used in this plate it is inserted first.

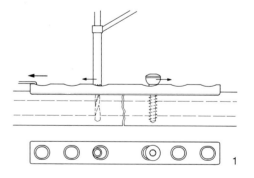

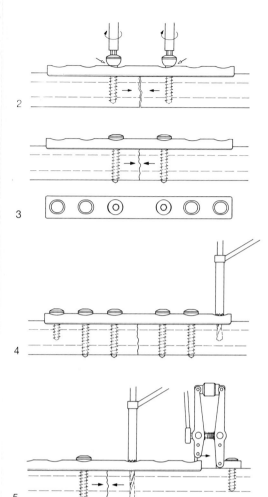

2

3

4

5

Step by step procedure:
- Reduction and careful contouring and overbending of the plate.
- In the plate hole nearest the fracture on one side a hole is drilled with the 3.2 mm drill bit in the 3.2 mm end of the double drill sleeve, in an eccentric position, away from the fracture.
- The screw length is measured.
- The hole is tapped with the 4.5 mm tap in the 4.5 mm end of the double drill sleeve.
- The 4.5 mm cortex screw is inserted until the screw head abuts the plate.
- After pulling the plate toward the opposite fragment, the second screw hole is drilled through the plate hole nearest the fracture in this fragment. This is also in eccentric position. The reduction must be maintained (Fig. 1).
- The length is measured.
- Tapping for 4.5 mm cortex screw.
- Insertion of the second cortex screw (Fig. 2).
- Final tightening of the first screw. A certain amount of axial compression is achieved (Fig. 3).
- Insertion of the remaining screws, alternating from one side to the other: drilling 3.2 mm, measuring and tapping 4.5 mm (Fig. 4).

Note: The articulated tension device can also be used with the semitubular plates. It is used as described for DCP, 4.5 mm (Fig. 5).

6.5.3.4 Application of 4.5 mm Reconstruction Plates

4.5 mm Reconstruction Plate as a Self-compressing Plate

The 4.5 mm reconstruction plate is mainly used for the fixation of pelvic fractures in large individuals.
By means of the oval shaped holes, axial compression can be exerted by inserting the screws eccentrically on each side of the fracture. Depending on the bone quality, 4.5 mm cortex screws or fully threaded 6.5 mm cancellous bone screws are used.
The plate should be contoured carefully by using the special bending irons. The plate holes may otherwise be distorted and cannot accept the screws. Bending angles greater than 15° at any one site must be avoided. See Sect. 6.10.1.

Step by step procedure:
- The fracture is reduced and the plate carefully contoured and applied to the bone with reduction forceps.
- The first screw hole is drilled in the plate hole nearest the fracture with the 3.2 mm drill bit in the 3.2 mm end of the double drill sleeve.

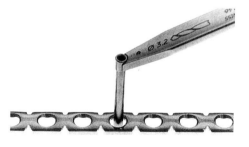

Plates for Large Bone Fractures

Note: In the US some of the large plates have modified plate holes to accommodate the 7.0 mm cannulated screw. See the SYNTHES USA catalogue.

6.6.1.1 Instruments

Threaded Guide Wire, 2.0 mm Diameter, 230 mm

The guide wire has a threaded spade point tip to facilitate insertion. It is inserted after reduction at the site where the screw is to be placed. The use of a drill sleeve prevents creeping of the wire on the bone surface. The 8 mm long threaded tip should be well anchored in the subchondral bone to ensure correct measurement of the screw length with the measuring device. The correct position is confirmed with an image intensifier.
For easy identification some of the wires are coloured blue. The guide wire must be checked for damage and bends before insertion, or else it will bind and be pushed forward with the drill bit, causing damage.

Drill Bit, 2.0 mm Diameter

The drill bit, 100 mm/75 mm, is used to pre-drill a dense cortex before insertion of the threaded guide wire or a Kirschner wire used for reduction.

Cannulated Drill Bit, 4.5 mm Diameter, Three-Fluted

The 4.5 mm, three-fluted cannulated drill bit, 230 mm/210 mm, has a cannulation of 2.1 mm to fit over the threaded guide wire, 2.0 mm. The three cutting edges facilitate cutting at angles and prevent skidding. It is calibrated to allow direct reading of the drilled depth, except when drilling through the percutaneous sleeve assembly. The drill bit has a triangular end which fits into a Jacobs chuck. Because of the cannulation the drill bit is weaker than a solid one. Bending or excessive axial force must be avoided during drilling to prevent breakage. It should always be used with a drill sleeve of the same diameter.

Percutaneus Sleeve Assembly

– The *protection sleeve*, 11.0 mm/8.0 mm, 88 mm long, with handle is used as the outermost component in the percutaneous sleeve assembly. All steps can be performed through this sleeve, including measuring, tapping and inserting screws.

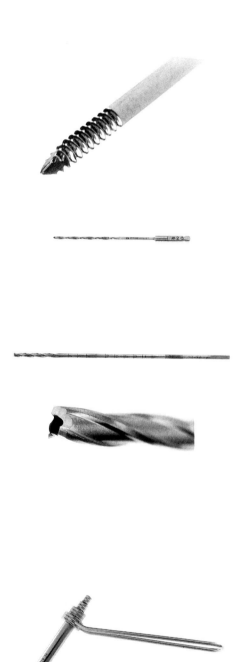

Instrumentation and Techniques

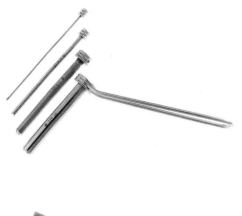

- The *drill sleeve*, 8.0 mm/4.5 mm in diameter, 99 mm long, is used within the sleeve mentioned above while drilling.
- The *drill sleeve*, 4.5 mm/2.0 mm in diameter, 108 mm long, is used inside the two instruments just described to reduce the risk of deflection when inserting the threaded guide wire, 2.0 mm.
- The *trocar*, 2.0 mm in diameter, 118 mm long, is the innermost part of the percutaneous sleeve assembly and is used to facilitate passage of the assembly through soft tissue down to the bone.

Parallel Drill Guide, 4.5 mm Diameter

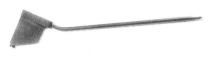

With the drill guide additional, parallel threaded guide wires can be placed for parallel screws in percutaneous or open procedures. These may be inserted at distances of 10, 14, or 18 mm. If washers are to be used with the screws the 14 or 18 mm marked holes should be used to allow enough space for the washers.

Parallel Wire Guide, 2.0 mm Diameter

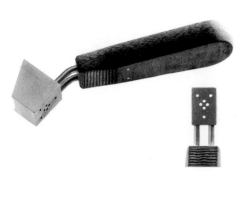

With the wire guide, it is possible to place threaded guide wires in parallel at 130° in open fixation of femoral neck fractures so that multiple screws can be placed accurately. The centre holes are used for preliminary fixation and the threaded guide wires for the cannulated screws are inserted through the outer holes. The head has spikes to help secure the instrument on the bone surface during use.

Double Drill Sleeve, 4.5 mm/3.2 mm

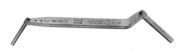

The drill sleeve is used with the cannulated drill bit.

Cannulated Screw Measuring Device, 7.0 mm

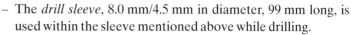

The cannulated screw measuring device is used to determine the screw length by sliding it over the guide wire. The length measured is 8 mm shorter (length of the threaded tip) than the overall length of the guide wire within the bone. The screw is thus prevented from penetrating the far cortex, and the threaded portion of the guide wire remains anchored during drilling, tapping, and screw insertion, provided the measured depth is not exceeded. The pencil-like measuring device formerly used has been replaced by this device, which can be used also in percutaneous procedures through the protection sleeve, 11 mm/8 mm. Some devices are made of anodised aluminium and coloured

Cannulated Screw System

blue. Care must be taken when cleaning these devices. See Sect. 6.22.4.2

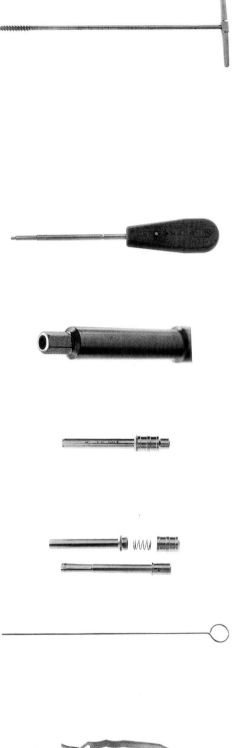

Cannulated Tap for the 7.0 mm Cannulated Screw

The cannulated tap is used to cut the thread in the near cortex (or the entire length of the nonthreaded part of the guide wire in dense bone) prior to insertion of the screw. The calibration helps confirm the tapping depth. The percutaneous protection sleeve, 11 mm/8 mm, or the tap sleeve for the 6.5 mm cancellous bone tap can be used for soft tissue protection.

Note: The calibration is designed to be read at the bone surface and *not* at the outer end of the drill sleeve.

Large Cannulated Hexagonal Screwdriver

The large cannulated hexagonal screwdriver, 3.5 mm in width across flats, is used to insert the 7.0 mm cannulated screws over the guide wire. Because of its cannulation, excessive force should not be applied with this screwdriver since it is not as strong as a solid one. The ordinary, large hexagonal screwdriver should be used for final tightening and to remove the screws. The screwdriver is fully cannulated and the shaft has a groove to accept the large holding sleeve.

Large Holding Sleeve

The large holding sleeve is a self-retaining screw-holding sleeve, which can be used with those large hexagonal screwdrivers equipped with a grooved shaft. The holding sleeve grips the screw head during insertion in areas with reduced visibiliy, or when removing screws with a smooth shaft, allowing traction to be applied. The sleeve must be carefully disassembled for cleaning. See also Sect. 6.22.4.

Cleaning Stylet, 2.0 mm Diameter

The stylet is used for cleaning all cannulated instruments, also intraoperatively to prevent accumulation of debris and therefore binding of the instruments around the guide wire.

Screw Forceps

The screw forceps is self-retaining and used to remove screws from the screw rack.

6.6.1.2 Supplementary Instruments

Cleaning Brush, 2.1 mm

The brush is made of autoclavable nylon on a steel shaft. It is used to clean 2.1 mm cannulated instruments.

6.6.1.3 Implants

The 7.0 mm Cannulated Screw

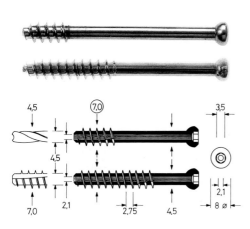

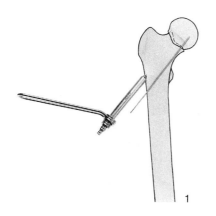

Important dimensions:
– Screw head diameter: 8.0 mm
– Screw head height: 4.5 mm
– Hexagonal socket width: 3.5 mm
– Shaft diameter: 4.5 mm
– Core diameter: 4.5 mm
– Thread diameter: 7.0 mm
– Pitch: 2.75 mm
– Cannulation: 2.1 mm

The screws are available with a 16 mm long thread in lengths of 30 mm–130 mm and with a 32 mm long thread in 45 mm–130 mm in 5 mm increments. Fully threaded screws are also available as supplementary implants if desired. The screw also has reverse-cutting flutes for easy removal.

Washer, 13 mm

The washer is used with the screw to prevent the screw head from sinking into the thin cortex in the metaphysis or the epiphysis. The flat surface is placed onto the bone; the countersink receives the screwhead.

6.6.1.4 Technique of Insertion of 7.0 mm Cannulated Screws

In, for example, a femoral neck fracture three screws are usually inserted. Image intensification is strongly recommended.

Percutaneous Insertion of Screws, Closed Procedure

– The fracture is reduced, and a regular, 230 mm long Kirschner wire or threaded guide wire is inserted along the anterior aspect of the femoral neck to determine the anteversion. The telescoping wire guide may be used. Image intensification is used for confirming correct placement.
– Through a stab incision and by blunt dissection the percutaneous sleeve assembly is pushed onto the lateral cortex and positioned parallel to the anteversion wire in the coronal plane (Fig. 1).

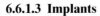

1

117 ■

- The 2.0 mm trocar is removed and the 2.0 mm threaded guide wire inserted to the appropriate depth. To prevent slippage the 4.5 mm/2.0 mm sleeve may be tapped with a hammer to seat its teeth in the bone. The drill should be run at maximum speed to minimise deflection while gradually advancing the wire (Fig. 2). The correct position in antero-posterior (AP) and lateral views is verified with the image intensifier.
- Proper screw length is determined with the cannulated screw measuring device, used through the 11.0 mm/8.0 mm protection sleeve (Fig. 3). The length measured is 8 mm short of the threaded portion of the wire to prevent penetration of the far cortex (see also p. 115).
- The 8.0 mm/4.5 mm drill sleeve is reinserted and the cannulated drill bit, 4.5 mm, used to drill over the threaded guide wire under image intensifier control. Depending upon the bone quality, only the near cortex may be drilled. In dense bone the entire unthreaded length of the guide wire is drilled (Fig. 4). The drill is removed slowly and pulled back straight, taking care not to pull out the wire. The drill should not be run in reverse as this risks unthreading the guide wire, should there be any binding between wire and drill.
- The 8.0 mm/4.5 mm sleeve is removed and the near cortex tapped through the 11.0 mm/8.0 mm protection sleeve. In dense bone virtually the entire length over the unthreaded part of the guide wire is tapped (Fig. 5).
- The large cannulated hexagonal screwdriver, without holding sleeve, is used to insert the selected screw through the 11.0 mm/8.0 mm sleeve. If a washer is used, the protection sleeve has to be removed to place the washer over the guide wire (Fig. 6).
- A second and a third screw may be inserted using the same technique as described for the first screw. Another possibility is to use the parallel drill guide.

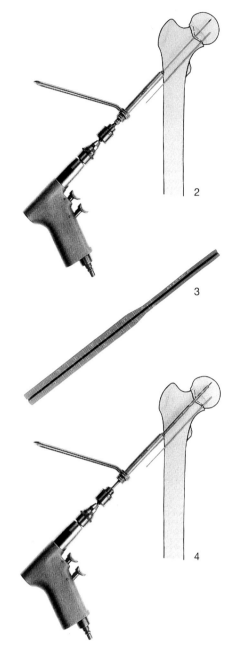

2

3

4

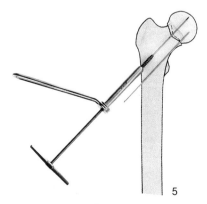

5

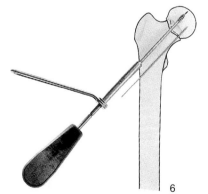

6

**Insertion of Parallel Guide Wires Percutaneously
Using the Parallel Drill Guide**

When planning where the different guide wires are to be placed, the possible distances offered by the parallel drill guide should be taken into consideration. Measured from the centre of the main hole to the centres of the others, the distance can be 10, 14, and 18 mm.

Note: To prevent loss of reduction, each screw is fully inserted before starting with the next.

- After insertion of the first guide wire as described above, the percutaneous sleeve assembly is removed.
- The parallel drill guide is prepared with the drill sleeve, 4.5 mm/2.0 mm, in its outermost 4.5 mm hole marked 0. This combination is placed over the first inserted guide wire.
- A second 4.5 mm/2.0 mm drill sleeve and 2.0 mm trocar are inserted into one of the other three holes in the parallel drill guide. After stab incision the trocar is pressed onto the near cortex.
- The trocar is removed and a threaded guide wire inserted to the appropriate depth with the small air drill. Any bending force on the first guide wire must be avoided, as this will affect the parallel alignment of the holes.
- Further guide wires can be inserted using this technique. Any previously inserted guide wire can be used in the outermost hole for parallel placement of the next wire.
- The remaining steps for insertion of the screws are performed through the protection sleeve, 11.0 mm/8.0 mm, as described above.
- The anteversion wire is removed using the small air drill (reverse trigger) once correct placement of the guide wire is confirmed.

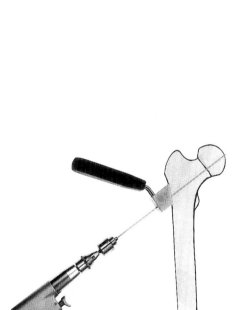

**Insertion of 7.0 mm Cannulated Screws in Femoral Neck
Fractures Using the Parallel Wire Guide, Open Procedure**

- After reduction, the anteversion of the femoral neck is determined by placing a 2.0 mm Kirschner wire or a threaded guide wire along the anterior aspect of the femoral neck. The position is confirmed with an image intensifier.
- Using the parallel wire guide, a 2.0 mm threaded guide wire is inserted as a positioning wire into the centre of the femoral head parallel to both the anteversion wire in AP and axial views. The drill should run at maximum speed to minimise deflection (Fig. 1). In dense bone pre-drilling of the cortex with the 2.0 mm drill bit is recommended.

Cannulated Screw System

Instruments for insertion of 7.0 mm cannulated screws using the parallel wire guide

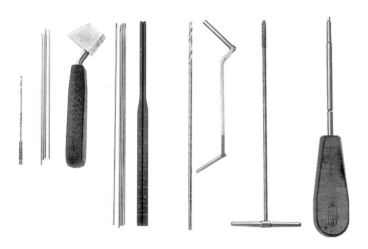

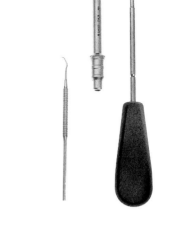

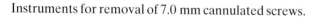

Instruments for removal of 7.0 mm cannulated screws.

The 7.0 mm cannulated screws are removed using the regular large hexagonal screwdriver and large holding sleeve. The hexagonal recess must be freed from any debris before the screwdriver is engaged. The holding sleeve is used when traction is needed, i.e. for partially threaded screws. The reverse-cutting flutes in the thread facilitate removal even in dense bone.

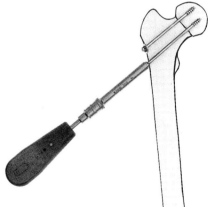

6.6.2 The 4.5 mm Cannulated Screw System

The 4.5 mm cannulated screw is used primarily in malleolar fractures, in fractures of the proximal and distal humerus, patellar fractures, and fractures of the calcaneus and talus. It may also be used for certain fractures of the pelvis, the acetabulum and of the tibial plateau.
The 4.5 mm cannulated screws and the instruments necessary for their application may be obtained in either a graphic case, a sterilising tray or in an aluminium case.

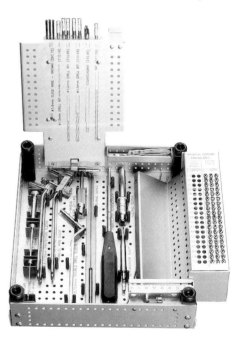

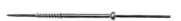

Instrumentation and Techniques

6.6.2.1 Instruments

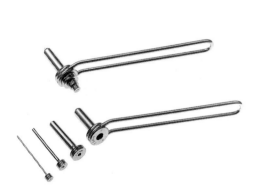

Threaded Guide Wire, 1.6 mm Diameter, 150 mm

The 1.6 mm guide wire, coloured brown for easy identification, has a spade point tip for better cutting ability and smooth insertion using the small air drill. It is inserted after reduction at the site where the screw is to be placed. The 5 mm threaded tip has to be anchored safely in the far cortex for correct measurement. The position is confirmed by image intensification. The drill guide should be used so as to avoid creeping of the wire on the bone surface. In hard juvenile bone pre-drilling with a 1.5 mm drill bit is recommended.
The guide wire must not be damaged during use.

Drill Bit, 1.5 mm

The 1.5 mm drill bit, 110 mm/85 mm, is used to pre-drill a hard cortex before inserting the threaded guide wire, 1.6 mm.

Cannulated Drill Bit, 3.2 mm, Four-Fluted

The 3.2 mm, four-fluted cannulated drill bit, 170 mm/140 mm, has a cannulation of 1.7 mm to fit over the 1.6 mm guide wire. The four cutting edges prevent skidding. The drill bit has a quick coupling end to fit into the small air drill. The drill bit is used to pre-drill for the 4.5 mm cannulated screw. Because of the cannulation the drill bit must be used with great care so as to avoid breakage. Cleaning of the cannulation with the cleaning stylet is imperative to prevent binding about the wire.

Percutaneous Sleeve Assembly

- The *protection sleeve*, 9.5 mm/7.0 mm, 39 mm long, has a handle and is used when measuring and inserting the screw in percutaneous procedures. It is also used to guide the other parts of the assembly. The sleeve allows a working depth of 31 mm.
- The *drill sleeve*, 7.0 mm/3.2 mm, 46 mm long, is used inside the protection sleeve, 9.5 mm/7.0 mm, as a drill sleeve for the 3.2 mm cannulated drill bit.
- The *drill sleeve*, 3.2 mm/1.6 mm, 52 mm long, inserted into the two sleeves described above is used a guide for the threaded guide wire to avoid the risk of wire deflection during insertion.
- The *trocar*, 1.6 mm, 59 mm long, is used within the assembly when passing it through the soft tissue down to the bone.

Adjustable Parallel Wire Guide

The adjustable parallel wire guide is used for parallel placement of additional guide wires when parallel screws are to be placed. The sleeve can be removed and placed in the desired position within the slot. It is locked by turning the knurled top.

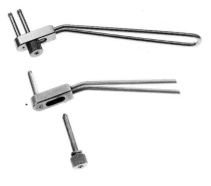

Double Drill Sleeve, 4.5 mm/3.2 mm

The double drill sleeve is used when drilling and tapping in open procedures.

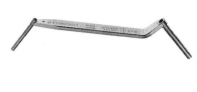

Cannulated Countersink, Tip 3.0 mm

The cannulated countersink is used to cut a recess in the bone for the 4.5 mm cannulated screw head. It has a quick coupling end to fit the T handle.

T Handle

The T handle, with quick coupling, is used as handle for the countersink and for the tap.

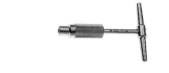

Cannulated Screw Measuring Device, 4.5 mm

The cannulated screw measuring device can be used separately in open procedures (or through the protection sleeve, 9.5 mm/7.0 mm in percutaneous applications) to measure the screw length. It is calibrated such that the threaded portion of the guide wire (5 mm) is deducted, thus preventing the screw from penetrating the far cortex. The scale at the end of the device is used to set the drilling depth if the drill guide with stop from the 3.5 mm cannulated screw set is used. Some devices are made of anodised aluminium and are brown in colour. Care must be taken when cleaning these devices. See Sect. 6.22.4.2

Cannulated Tap for 4.5 mm Cannulated Screw

The cannulated tap is used to cut the thread in dense bone when necessary. It has a quick coupling end to fit the T handle.
The double drill sleeve end, 4.5 mm, is used as a tap sleeve. The cleaning stylet must be inserted after each use to prevent debris from collecting in the cannulation.

Instrumentation and Techniques

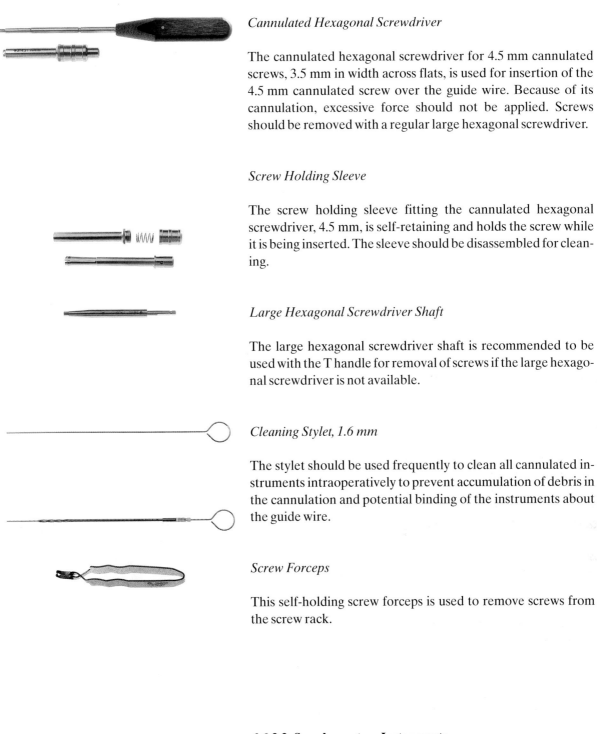

Cannulated Hexagonal Screwdriver

The cannulated hexagonal screwdriver for 4.5 mm cannulated screws, 3.5 mm in width across flats, is used for insertion of the 4.5 mm cannulated screw over the guide wire. Because of its cannulation, excessive force should not be applied. Screws should be removed with a regular large hexagonal screwdriver.

Screw Holding Sleeve

The screw holding sleeve fitting the cannulated hexagonal screwdriver, 4.5 mm, is self-retaining and holds the screw while it is being inserted. The sleeve should be disassembled for cleaning.

Large Hexagonal Screwdriver Shaft

The large hexagonal screwdriver shaft is recommended to be used with the T handle for removal of screws if the large hexagonal screwdriver is not available.

Cleaning Stylet, 1.6 mm

The stylet should be used frequently to clean all cannulated instruments intraoperatively to prevent accumulation of debris in the cannulation and potential binding of the instruments about the guide wire.

Screw Forceps

This self-holding screw forceps is used to remove screws from the screw rack.

6.6.2.2 Supplementary Instruments

Cannulated Drill Bit, 4.5 mm, Four-Fluted

The 4.5 mm, four-fluted cannulated drill bit, 170 mm/140 mm, 1.7 mm cannulation, can be used to prepare a gliding hole for the fully threaded 4.5 mm cannulated screw. It is four-fluted, and has a quick coupling end to fit the small air drill.

Cannulated Screw System

Cleaning Brush, 1.75 mm

The brush, made of autoclavable nylon and with a steel shaft, is used to clean 4.5 mm cannulated instruments.

6.6.2.3 Implants

The 4.5 mm Cannulated Screw, Partially Threaded

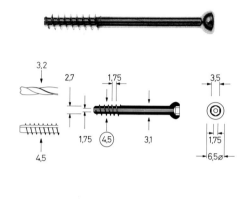

Important dimensions:
- Screw head diameter: 6.5 mm
- Screw head height: 4.0 mm
- Hexagonal socket width: 3.5 mm
- Shaft diameter: 2.7 mm
- Core diameter: 3.1 mm
- Thread diameter: 4.5 mm
- Pitch: 1.75 mm
- Cannulation: 1.75 mm

The cancellous thread finds excellent purchase in the spongy cancellous bone. The screw is self-tapping and has reverse-cutting flutes to facilitate removal of the screw. Partially threaded screws in lengths from 20 mm to 72 mm are available. The threaded portion increases stepwise from 7 mm in the 20 mm screws to 24 mm in the 72 mm screws. These screws can be obtained in a set together with the necessary instruments. The screws are compatible with the small fragment plates, because the size of the screw head has been reduced.

Fully threaded screws in lengths of 20 mm–72 mm are also available. See SYNTHES catalogue for details.

Washer, 10 mm Outer Diameter

The washer is used to prevent the screw head from cracking a thin cortex and sinking into the spongy cancellous bone. The flat side is placed on the bone, the recessed side against the screw head.

6.6.2.4 Technique of Insertion of 4.5 mm Cannulated Screws

Percutaneous Insertion of Screws

- The fracture is reduced and temporarily fixed with a Kirschner wire or with a pointed reduction forceps.
- A stab incision is made and the percutaneous sleeve assembly inserted through the soft tissue after blunt dissection down to the bone.
- The trocar is removed and a 1.6 mm threaded guide wire inserted to the appropriate depth through the drill sleeve,

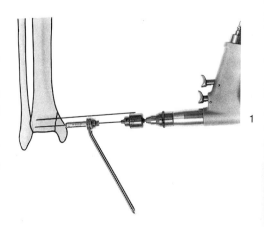
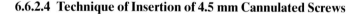

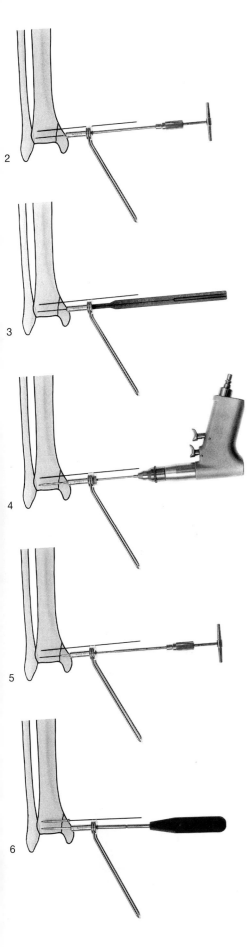

3.2 mm/1.6 mm under image intensification. The drill shoud be run at maximum speed to minimise deflection while gradually advancing the guide wire (Fig. 1).

- Additional parallel wires may be placed using the adjustable parallel wire guide as indicated below.
- In dense bone the cannulated countersink may be used through the 9.5 mm/7.0 mm sleeve to cut a recess in the bone (Fig. 2).
- The cannulated screw measuring device is used through the 9.5 mm/7.0 mm protection sleeve to measure the proper screw length (Fig. 3). The measured depth is 5 mm short of the threaded guide wire tip (the threaded portion of the wire), to prevent the screw from penetrating the far cortex.
- The 7.0 mm/3.2 mm drill sleeve is reinserted into the outer sleeve, and the 3.2 mm cannulated drill bit passed over the guide wire. The near cortex is drilled, allowing the drill to follow the guide wire. It must not be forced or directed at a different angle. In dense bone the entire length of the unthreaded part of the wire may have to be drilled (Fig. 4). The drill guide with stop, with 3.2 mm insert, from the 3.5 mm cannulated screw set can be used (see below). The correct drilling depth is confirmed with image intensification.
- In dense bone the tap for 4.5 mm cannulated screws is used to tap the thread in the bone over the guide wire. The double drill sleeve, 4.5mm, or the protection sleeve 9.5 mm/7.0 mm, is used for tissue protection (Fig. 5).
- The cannulated hexagonal screwdriver 4.5, without holding sleeve, is used to insert the selected screw through the 9.5 mm/7.0 mm protection sleeve. Because of the cannulation, excessive force should be avoided while tightening (Fig. 6).
- In osteoporotic bone a washer may be needed to prevent the screw head from cracking the cortex and sinking into the bone. The washer cannot be placed through the protection sleeve. This has to be removed to place the washer over the guide wire before inserting the screw.
- A second screw is inserted either in the place of the previously inserted Kirschner wire or over a newly placed guide wire (Fig. 7).
- After insertion of the screw, the threaded guide wire is removed using the Jacobs chuck, and the reverse trigger of the small air drill.

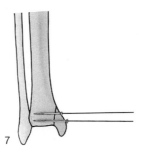

Insertion of Additional Parallel Threaded Guide Wires

– After placing the first wire as described above, the percutaneous sleeve assembly is removed. The fixed sleeve of the adjustable parallel wire guide is placed over the first wire.
– The movable sleeve is adjusted to the desired position and the
knurled nut tightened. A separate incision may be necessary.
– Without placing any bending force on the first guide wire,
which would affect the parallel alignment, a second 1.6 mm
threaded guide wire is inserted and its position confirmed
with image intensification.
– Any additional guide wires can be inserted following the
same procedure, using one of the previously inserted wires as
guide.
– To prevent loss of reduction, insert each screw over the guide
wire according to the technique described above before proceeding to the next screw.

6.6.2.5 Instruments for Insertion and Removal of 4.5 mm Cannulated Screws

Instruments for insertion of 4.5 mm cannulated screws

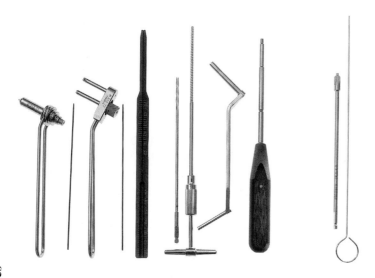

Instruments for removal of the 4.5 mm cannulated screw: When
necessary, the 4.5 mm cannulated screws are removed using the
regular, large hexagonal screwdriver. The screw head must be
cleared of all debris prior to removal.

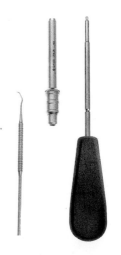

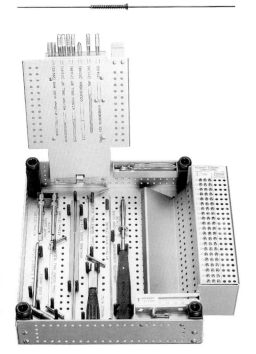

6.6.3 The 3.5 mm Cannulated Screw System

The 3.5 mm screw finds application in fractures of the carpus, metacarpals, and metatarsals. It may also be used in osteochondral fractures, epiphyseal fractures in children and for ligament fixation. The screw is compatible with the 2.7 mm stainless steel implants and some 3.5 mm implants, i.e. small T plate, cloverleaf plate.

The 3.5 mm cannulated screws and the instruments necessary for their application may be obtained in a graphic case, a sterilising tray, or an aluminium case

6.6.3.1 Instruments

Threaded Guide Wire, 1.25 mm , 150 mm

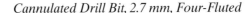

The guide wire has a self-cutting spade point tip. This wire is inserted as guide wire where the 3.5 mm cannulated screw is to be placed. Its position is confirmed with image intensification. The 5 mm threaded tip should be well anchored in the far cortex before drilling.

Cannulated Drill Bit, 2.7 mm, Four-Fluted

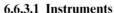

The 2.7 mm, four-fluted cannulated drill bit, 160 mm/130 mm, is used to drill the thread hole over the 1.25 mm guide wire for the 3.5 mm cannulated screw. The four cutting edges prevent skidding when cutting at angles. It has a quick coupling end and connects to the small air drill. Because of its 1.35 mm diameter cannulation the drill bit is more susceptible to breakage than solid drill bits. Excessive force and bending must be avoided. The cannulation must be free of any debris before use to prevent binding about the wire. The cleaning stylet must be inserted to clear the cannulation after each use.

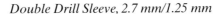

Double Drill Sleeve, 2.7 mm/1.25 mm

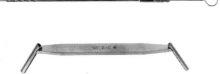

The 2.7 mm double drill sleeve is used as a drill sleeve for the 1.25 mm guide wire, and at the other end for the 2.7 mm cannulated drill bit.

Cannulated Screw System

Double Drill Sleeve, 3.5 mm/2.5 mm

The 3.5/2.5 mm double drill sleeve is used as protection sleeve for the cannulated tap and drill bit 3.5 mm.

Drill Guide with Stop, 3.5 mm/2.7 mm

The drill guide with stop, with two inserts, is used as a drill guide for drilling to a predetermined depth. The inserts have diameters of 2.7 mm and 3.5 mm. They can be screwed into the handle. To set the drilling depth the drill bit which has been selected is inserted into the corresponding size guide until its quick coupling end rests on the drill guide. It is then slid into the end of the measuring device. The knurled nut is loosened and the threaded end turned until the protruding drill bit length corresponds to the drilling depth. The nut is tightened in this position.

Cannulated Countersink, 2.4 mm Tip

The cannulated countersink has a quick coupling end to fit the handle with quick coupling. It is used to cut a recess in bone to accommodate the screw head.

Handle with Quick Coupling

The quick-coupling handle connects with the cannulated countersink and tap. Thanks to the rotating handle it rests in the palm and can be gently turned with two fingers.

Cannulated Screw Measuring Device, 3.5 mm

The cannulated screw measuring device is used to determine the screw length. It measures 5 mm short of the guide wire tip (the length of the threaded portion of the wire), preventing the screw from penetrating the far cortex. The other end can be used in combination with the drill guide with stop, 3.5 mm/2.7 mm, to set the drilling depth as described above. Some devices are made of anodised aluminium and are silver in colour. Care must be taken when cleaning these devices. See Sect. 6.22.4.2.

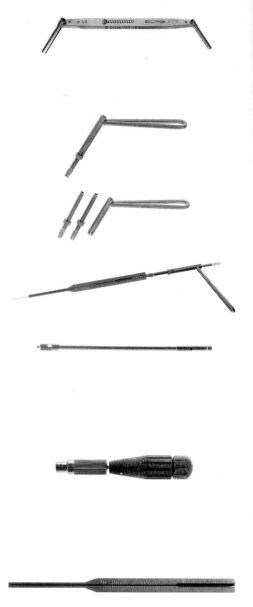

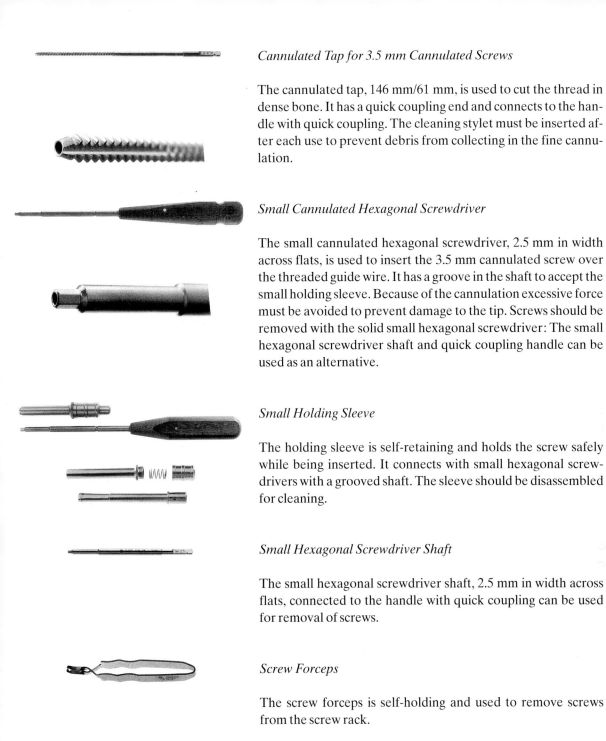

Cannulated Tap for 3.5 mm Cannulated Screws

The cannulated tap, 146 mm/61 mm, is used to cut the thread in dense bone. It has a quick coupling end and connects to the handle with quick coupling. The cleaning stylet must be inserted after each use to prevent debris from collecting in the fine cannulation.

Small Cannulated Hexagonal Screwdriver

The small cannulated hexagonal screwdriver, 2.5 mm in width across flats, is used to insert the 3.5 mm cannulated screw over the threaded guide wire. It has a groove in the shaft to accept the small holding sleeve. Because of the cannulation excessive force must be avoided to prevent damage to the tip. Screws should be removed with the solid small hexagonal screwdriver: The small hexagonal screwdriver shaft and quick coupling handle can be used as an alternative.

Small Holding Sleeve

The holding sleeve is self-retaining and holds the screw safely while being inserted. It connects with small hexagonal screwdrivers with a grooved shaft. The sleeve should be disassembled for cleaning.

Small Hexagonal Screwdriver Shaft

The small hexagonal screwdriver shaft, 2.5 mm in width across flats, connected to the handle with quick coupling can be used for removal of screws.

Screw Forceps

The screw forceps is self-holding and used to remove screws from the screw rack.

Cleaning Stylet, 1.25 mm Diameter

The stylet is used for cleaning cannulated instruments intraoperatively and after surgery.

6.6.3.2 Supplementary Instruments

Cannulated Drill Bit, 3.5 mm, Four-Fluted

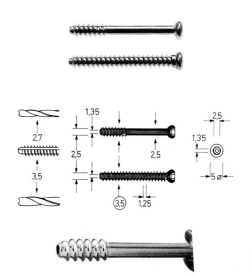

The 3.5 mm, four-fluted cannulated drill bit, 160 mm/130 mm, has a 1.35 mm cannulation to fit over the 1.25 mm guide wire. It has four cutting edges and a quick coupling end. It is used to pre-drill a gliding hole for the fully threaded 3.5 mm cannulated screw, if necessary.

Cleaning Brush, 1.35 mm Diameter

The brush is used for cleaning the cannulated instruments. It has bristles of autoclavable nylon on a steel shaft.

6.6.3.3 Implants

The 3.5 mm Cannulated Screw

Important dimensions:
- Screw head diameter: 5.0 mm
- Screw head height: 2.0 mm
- Hexagonal head recess: 2.5 mm
- Shaft diameter: 2.5 mm
- Core diameter: 2.5 mm
- Thread diameter: 3.5 mm
- Pitch: 1.25 mm
- Cannulation: 1.35 mm

The low profile of the screw head is advantageous when used for fractures near an articular surface. The tapered tip facilitates insertion; the reverse-cutting flutes aid removal.

The screws are available partially threaded in lengths from 10 mm to 50 mm in 2 mm increments. The threaded portion of the screws increases stepwise from 5 mm in the 10 mm screws to 16 mm in the 50 mm screw. Fully threaded screws are available in lengths of 10 mm to 50 mm, in 2 mm increments.

Washer, 7.0 mm

The washer is used to prevent the screw head from cracking a thin cortex and sinking into cancellous bone. The flat side is placed on the bone; the recessed side against the screw head. The holding clip holds the washers.

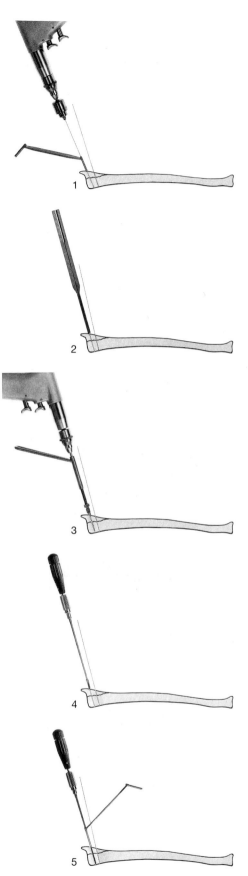

6.6.3.4 Technique of Insertion of 3.5 mm Cannulated Screws

Image intensification is essential when using this technique.

– The fracture is reduced and held with pointed reduction forceps.
– A 1.25 mm threaded guide wire is inserted at the site where screw insertion is planned, using the small air drill and the Jacobs chuck. The double drill sleeve, 1.25 mm, is used as a guide and tissue protector. A second wire is inserted parallel to the first to prevent rotation of the fragments. The reduction forceps is removed and the position of the wires confirmed with image intensification (Fig. 1).
– The length is measured with the cannulated screw measuring device (Fig. 2).
– The drilling depth is set to the desired depth using the direct measuring device and drill guide with stop. See figure.
– The assembly is placed over the threaded guide wire and the drilling performed until the quick coupling end contacts the drill guide with stop (Fig. 3).

Note: The drill bit must not be directed but rather allowed to follow the guide wire. It should be removed slowly while running the drill forward to prevent guide wire pull out. The reverse gear must not be used as this may unscrew the threaded guide wire tip.

– In dense bone the cannulated countersink is used to cut a recess in the bone. In osteoporotic bone a washer is used instead (Fig. 4).
– The cannulated tap is connected to the handle with quick coupling and used to cut the thread in the near cortex. In dense metaphyseal bone tapping over the entire nonthreaded length of the guide wire may be necessary. The double drill sleeve, 3.5 mm, is used as a tissue protector (Fig. 5).
– The 3.5 mm cannulated screw which has been selected is inserted over the guide wire with the small cannulated screwdriver (Fig. 6. Here the old style screwholding sleeve is shown).

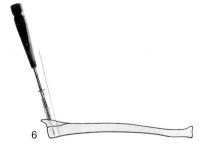

- The second screw is inserted using the same technique as described for the first screw (Fig. 7).
- The threaded guide wires are removed using Jacobs chuck and the reverse trigger of the small air drill. Used guide wires should be discarded (Fig. 8).

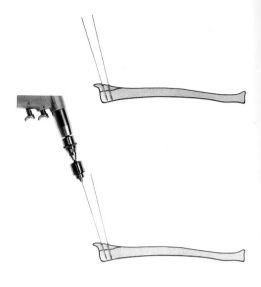

6.6.3.5 Instruments for Insertion and Removal of 3.5 mm Cannulated Screws

Instruments for insertion of 3.5 mm cannulated screws

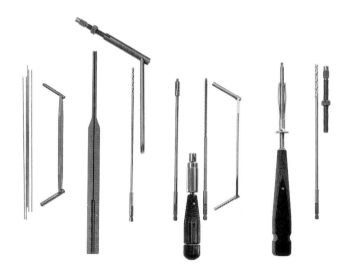

Instrumentation and Techniques

Instruments for removal of the 3.5 mm cannulated screws. If the screws are to be removed, the regular, small hexagonal screwdriver should be used. The small holding sleeve is of great advantage if traction is needed for removal, for example, of partially threaded screws. It is essential to clear the screw head socket of debris prior to removal.

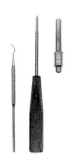

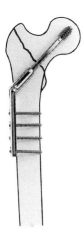

6.7 Dynamic Hip Screw and Dynamic Condylar Screw Instrument and Implant System

The dynamic hip screw (DHS) implant system has been designed primarily for the fixation of trochanteric fractures. It may also be used for certain subtrochanteric fractures as well as for selected basi-cervical femoral fractures.

The implant is based on the sliding nail principle which allows impaction of the fracture. This is made possible by the insertion of a wide diameter screw into the femoral head. A side plate, which has a barrel at a fixed angle is slid over the screw and fixed to the femoral shaft. The barrel and the screw each have two corresponding flats, which allow the smooth shaft of the screw to slide within the barrel and yet retain rotational stability. Thus, the femoral head fragment fixed with the screw can be impacted, either deliberately or from weight-bearing.

The correct placement of the implant is essential for the success. The anteversion of the femoral neck has to be determined with a guide wire as well as the site of the screw in the middle of the femoral head with a guide pin. The correct position of the guide pin must be checked with two-plane radiography. All steps necessary for the insertion of the implant are performed over the guide pin.

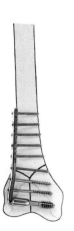

The barrel angle can be predetermined by evaluating the angle subtended between the femoral neck and shaft axes (CCD, or collum–centre–diaphysis, angle) of the uninjured side. The 135° barrel angle is the most commonly indicated.

The dynamic condylar screw (DCS) is similar to the DHS in its design and concept. The fixed angle between plate and barrel is 95° and the plate is contoured to fit the lateral surface of the distal end of the femur.

The main indications are fractures of the distal femur and intercondylar fractures. It may also be used for certain intertrochanteric fractures and very proximal subtrochanteric fractures. Preplanning the exact site of the screw is essential also for the successful application of DCS. For application in the distal femur the axis of the knee joint as well as the inclination of the patellar articular surface of the condyles have to be predetermined. Impaction or compression of the fracture is achieved by using the compression screw.

6.7.1 DHS and DCS Instruments

For the application of the DHS and the DCS special instruments are necessary. These have to be used correctly and in a special order to ensure optimal placement of the implant. DHS/DCS instruments are available in either a graphic case or in sterilising trays. Implant cases are also available. Basic instruments are necessary for the fixation of the plate to the femur with the large screws. A graphic case containing DHS instruments as well as the necessary basic instruments is obtainable.

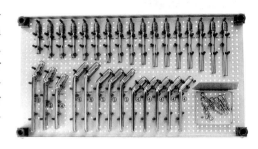

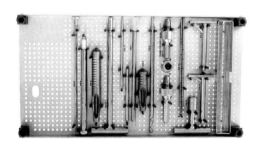

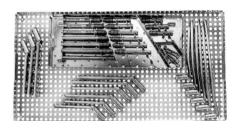

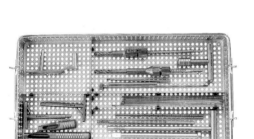

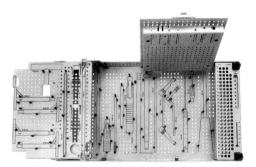

DHS/DCS Guide Pins, 2.5 mm Diameter, 230 mm Long

These pins are the special guide pins to be used when inserting DHS/DCS screws. They must be straight and absolutely undamaged when introduced. The threaded tip anchors the guide pin in the subchondral bone.

Drill Bit, 2.0 mm

This bit 100 mm/75 mm may be used to drill the hard juvenile cortex before introducing the DHS/DCS guide pin.

DHS/DCS T Handle

This handle with a quick coupling connects to the angle guides and to the DHS/DCS tap.

Instrumentation and Techniques

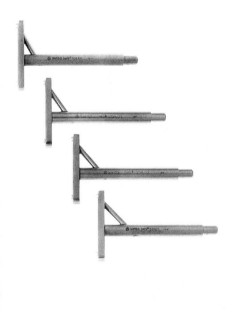

DHS Angle Guides, 135°, 140°, 145°, and 150°

These guides allow placement of the DHS/DCS guide pin at the desired angle in the femoral head. The 135° angle guide is the one most commonly used, since it corresponds most closely to the anatomical neck/shaft angle. The guide is connected to the DHS/DCS T handle and held against the bone surface while inserting the guide pin. The spikes on the foot plate prevent slipping.

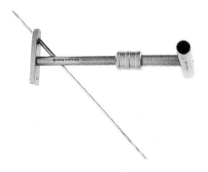

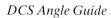

DCS Angle Guide

This guide connected to the DHS/DCS T handle aids the insertion of the guide pin at 95° in the distal femur when placed over the correct insertion point. The angle guide has spikes to prevent slipping off the bone. The new version has a redesigned bend, which fits better to the curvature of the bone than the older model.

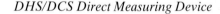

DHS/DCS Direct Measuring Device

This device is used to read off directly the inserted depth of the DHS/DCS guide pin. Other pins can not be used. Devices made of anodised aluminium must be cleaned according to the guidelines made in Sect. 6.22.4.2

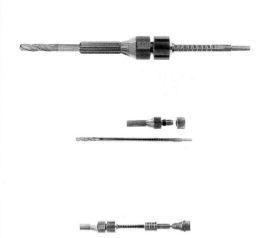

DHS Triple Reamer

This reamer prepares the seat for the screw and for plates with the 38 mm standard barrel. It consists of three elements: an 8 mm diameter drill bit for the screw, a reamer head for the barrel and the conical barrel/plate junction, and a locking nut. To assemble the three parts, the reamer head is slid onto the drill bit with the set screw aligned with the flat on the drill bit. The reamer head is pushed forward until it engages the notch with the desired depth marking. The nut is then tightened firmly.
Special quick couplings are available to connect the triple reamer with either the small air drill, or the universal air drill.
The triple reamer is cannulated allowing reaming over the guide wire. The cannulation needs special attention when cleaning the instrument. See Sect. 6.22.5.1.

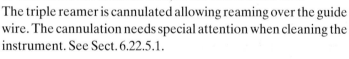

This reamer is marked DHS and should not be confused with the DCS triple reamer.

DHS Short Triple Reamer

This reamer is used in similar manner for plates with 25 mm short barrel. It consists of the same three elements as the standard reamer, but the reaming portion is shorter.

DCS Triple Reamer

This reamer is clearly marked DCS and should only be used to ream for DCS. The drill and the locking nut are the same as for the DHS triple reamer. The reamer, however, is shorter and has no conical section.

DHS/DCS Tap

This is used to tap for the 12.5 mm DHS/DCS screw in juvenile bone. Before use the short centring sleeve is slid on, and the DHS/DCS T handle connected. Tapping is done over the guide wire. The tapped length can be read on the calibrated shaft.

Centring Sleeve for DHS/DCS Tap (Short)

This sleeve is slid on the tap and pushed into the hole, which is reamed to the barrel size. The sleeve centres the tap during tapping. The window allows the tapping depth to be read. The golden coloured sleeve is made of anodised aluminium and care must be taken when it is cleaned. See Sect. 6.22.4.2

Guide Shaft

This shaft is used with the coupling screw to insert DHS/DCS screws. The ridges should interdigitate with the notches of the outer end of the screw. Some guide shafts have flats on the side that align with the flats of the lag screw, when assembled for insertion. This allows positioning the plate correctly, with the flats of lag screw before pushing the plate in place.

Coupling Screw

This screw is pushed through the guide shaft and screwed into the DHS/DCS screw for insertion. It is cannulated to allow the assembly to be slid over the guide pin.

Note: This assembly should not be used for extraction.

DHS/DCS Wrench

This wrench is necessary for the insertion and the extraction of the DHS/DCS screw. For insertion the long centring sleeve is pushed onto the wrench. The screw, assembled with the guide

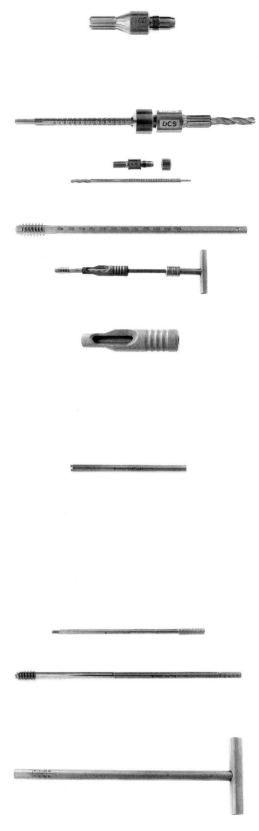

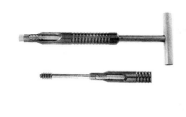

shaft and the coupling screw, is then slid into the wrench. The flat sides of the screw should match the internal flats of the wrench to allow visualisation of the screw end through the small window. To insert the screw the complete assembly is slid over the guide pin, the centring sleeve pushed into the reamed bone and the wrench turned clockwise.

To extract a DHS/DCS screw, the wrench is coupled with the long coupling screw. and positioned such that the flat sides of the wrench and those of the screw shaft match. The long coupling screw is then screwed into the screw end. By pulling and turning the wrench anticlockwise the screw can be extracted.

Centring Sleeve for DHS/DCS Wrench (Long)

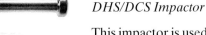

This sleeve is pushed onto the wrench to centre it in the bone when inserting the DHS/DCS screw. It is made of anodised aluminium and needs special care when it is cleaned. See Sect. 6.22.4.2.

DHS/DCS Impactor

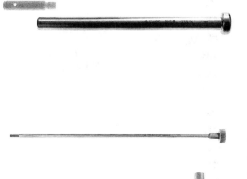

This impactor is used to finally seat the DHS and DCS plates by gentle blows with a hammer. The plastic tip must be seated correctly in the plate barrel or else it may break. The tip is interchangeable. A pin is inserted in the hole of the tip to unscrew it.

Long Coupling Screw

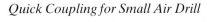

This screw is necessary for the extraction of DHS/DCS screws. It is pushed through the wrench and then screwed into the end of the DHS/DCS screw. The screw end should be free of debris before attempting connection with the long coupling screw. By pulling and turning the wrench anticlockwise, the screw can be extracted.

Quick Coupling for Small Air Drill

This is necessary to connect the DHS or DCS triple reamer to the small air drill.

Quick Coupling for the Universal Air Drill

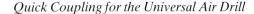

This is necessary to connect the DHS or DCS triple reamer to the universal air drill.

DHS and DCS Instrument and Implant System

 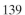

Combined DHS/DCS Wrench

This wrench has recently been developed to facilitate the insertion of a DHS/DCS screw and plate. The wrench has the same outer diameter as the screw shaft. It is coupled with a long coupling screw, which has a locking spring to prevent it falling off. The selected DHS or DCS plate is slid over the wrench, and the coupling screw tightened in the selected DHS/DCS screw, until the cams and the notches interdigitate. An open centring sleeve is placed and locked over the wrench. The assembly can then be used for insertion of both screw and plate simultaneously. A side impactor is used to finally seat the plate without having to disassemble the instruments.

Any disimpaction at the fracture site can be reduced by gentle pull on the wrench while impacting the plate.

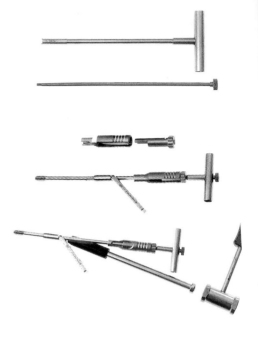

6.7.2 DHS/DCS Implants

DHS/DCS Screws

These screws are designed for insertion in both the distal and the proximal femur. The screw has a smooth shaft with two flat sides and is partially threaded. The thread is tapered at the tip and has a reverse cutting flute for easier extraction. The two flat sides of the shaft correspond to the two flats inside the plate barrel, enhancing rotational stability. The screw is cannulated and has an inside thread at the outer end for the compression screw and two notches for coupling with instruments for insertion and extraction.

The screws are available in lengths from 50 mm to 145 mm, in 5 mm increments

Important dimensions:
- Thread diameter: 12.5 mm
- Thread length: 22 mm
- Shaft diameter: 8 mm

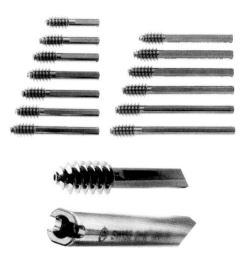

DHS/DCS Compression Screw

This can be screwed into the end of the DHS/DCS screw to achieve final impaction. It may also be used in unstable fractures to prevent disengagement of the screw from the plate barrel in non-weight-bearing patients. When using the compression screw in osteoporotic bone, great care must be taken not to strip the thread of the DHS/DCS screw within the bone.

Instrumentation and Techniques

The compression screw is left in place in a DCS, in a DHS removal is optional. It is 36 mm long and has a hexagonal socket to fit the large hexagonal screwdriver.

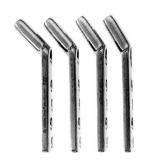

DHS Plates, Standard Barrel, 38 mm

This is the standard plate with barrel angles 135°, 140°, 145°, and 150°. Most commonly indicated is the plate with 135°. Greater barrel angles may offer biomechanical advantages in unstable cases: i.e. better gliding characteristics, reduction of bending stresses on plate/barrel junction. Correct placement of the implant becomes technically more difficult as barrel angles increase (see Regazzoni et al. 1985).

Two flats within the barrel correspond to the flat sides of the DHS/DCS screw. Thus, rotation of the screw within the barrel is prevented.

The side plate has staggered DCP holes accepting 4.5 mm screws.

The DHS plate 135° is available with 2, 4, 5, 6, 8, 10, 12, 14, or 16 holes, in lengths from 46 mm to 270 mm.

DHS plates 140° and 145° are available with 4, 5, or 6 holes in lengths from 78 mm to 110 mm.

DHS plate 150° is available with 2, 4, 5, 6, 8, 10, or 12 holes, in lengths from 46 mm to 206 mm.

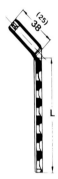

Important dimensions:
– Profile:	See figure
– Thickness:	5.8 mm
– Width:	19 mm
– Hole spacing:	16 mm
– Barrel outside diameter:	12.6 mm

DHS Plate 135°, 25 mm Barrel

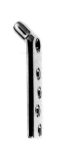

These plates are rarely indicated, but may be necessary to use in unusually small femurs. If a long impaction distance is expected and the screw might "run out of glide", the short barrel plate may be chosen. It is sometimes used in the fixation of a medial displacement osteotomy. The plate is applied in similar manner to the standard DHS, but the short reamer must be used.

The short barrel plates are available with 4, 5 or 6 holes, in lengths from 78 mm to 110 mm. The other dimensions are similar to those of the standard plate.

- The direct measuring device is slid over the guide pin and the inserted depth measured. The calibration provides a direct reading (Fig. 6).
- The anteversion Kirschner wire is removed.
- The DHS triple reamer is set at the desired reaming depth: 5–10 mm less than measured.
- A special quick coupling is used to connect the reamer to the air drill. The reamer is slid over the guide pin and reaming started. The speed should be diminished when each portion of the reamer enters the lateral cortex to avoid further damage to the bone. The reamer drills for the screw, reams for the barrel and countersinks for the plate/barrel junction.
- The reamer must "follow" the guide pin, or else it would damage it or push it forward into the acetabulum (Fig. 7).
- The reamer is carefully withdrawn leaving the guide pin in place. If the guide pin is inadvertently removed it must be repositioned. By placing a screw retrograde into the short centring sleeve the guide pin can be accurately reinserted.
- In young patients the dense cancellous bone may have to be tapped. The short centring sleeve is mounted on the tap and the T handle attached.
- When tapping, the centring sleeve is pushed into the bone to prevent "wobbling" and damage of the thread in the bone. The tapping depth (i.e. screw length) can be checked through the window of the centring sleeve (Fig. 8).
- The selected screw, 5–10 mm shorter than the guide pin depth measurement, is assembled with the guide shaft and the coupling screw.
- The long centring sleeve is pushed onto the DHS/DCS wrench and the screw assembly inserted.
- To stabilise the assembly, the centring sleeve is seated fully in the bone. By turning the wrench clockwise the screw is inserted until the zero mark aligns with the lateral cortex. The tip of the screw now lies 10 mm from the joint surface (Fig. 9). In

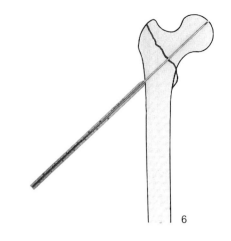

6

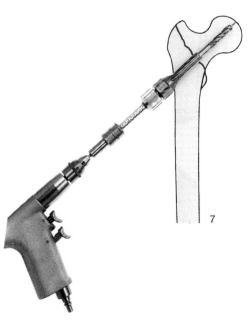

7

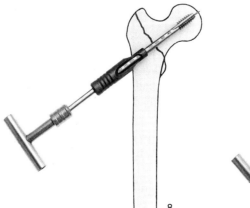

8

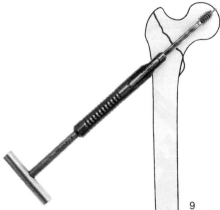

9

Instrumentation and Techniques

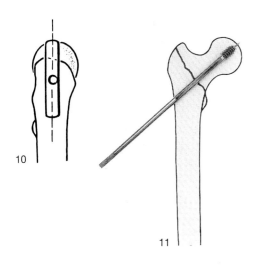

10

11

porotic bone, the screw should be inserted additional 5 mm to increase the holding power. Before removing the T handle, its handle should be aligned parallel to the long axis of the femur. This ensures proper placement of the side plate (Fig. 10).

- The T handle and the centring sleeve are removed; the guide shaft and coupling screw are left in place (Fig. 11).
- The selected DHS plate is slid onto the guide shaft assembly and pushed onto the screw (Fig. 12).
- After removal of the guide shaft assembly, and guide pin (Fig. 13), the impactor is used gently to seat the plate on the bone (Fig. 14).
- The side plate is fixed to the femur with 4.5 mm cortex screws: Drilling 3.2 mm, measuring, tapping, and insertion of the screw (Fig. 15).
- The remaining screws are inserted using the same technique (Fig. 16).

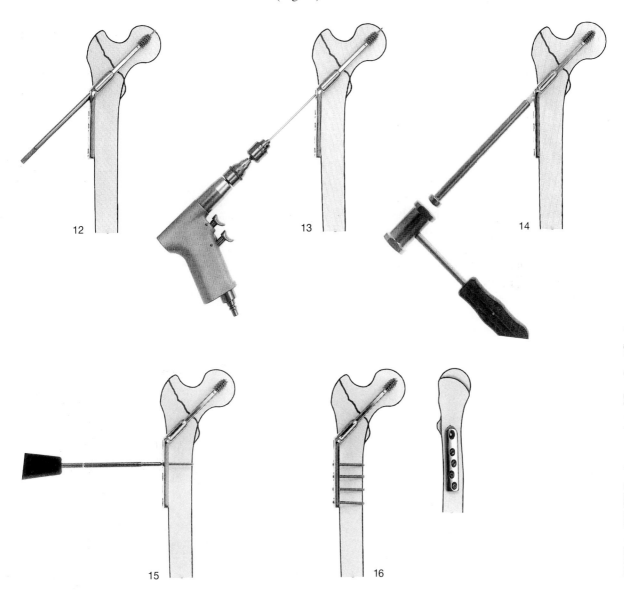

12   13   14

15   16

- For further compression of trochanteric fractures, the compression screw may be inserted into the DHS/DCS screw and tightened with great care to avoid stripping the DHS/DCS screw thread in the bone. Leaving the compression screw in is optional.

Example of measurements:
- Length measured   105 mm
- Reamer setting   95 mm
- Tapping depth   95 mm
- DHS/DCS screw length   95 mm

6.7.3.2 Application of DCS in the Distal Femur

Note: A DCS can be used only if at least 4 cm of the distal femur is intact to provide support for the implant. Also, the medial cortex of the distal femur must be intact or the medial support reconstituted with a cancellous graft to avoid failure of the implant.
The patient is positioned on a regular table in such a way that the knee can be flexed through 90°. Intraoperative radiography is essential and image intensification preferable.

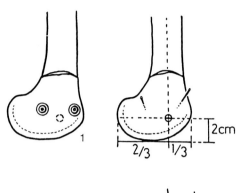

Step by step procedure:
- The fracture is reduced and temporarily fixed. Intercondylar fractures are fixed with 6.5 mm cancellous bone screws as lag screws (Fig. 1) taking care to avoid the planned site of insertion of the DCS screw (Fig. 2).
- After reconstruction of the condyles, three Kirschner wires are used to determine the correct site for the DHS/DCS screw.
- First, a Kirschner wire is inserted through the knee joint along the distal end of the condyles (*1*) to mark the plane of the tibio-femoral articulation (Fig. 3).
- A second Kirschner wire is inserted anteriorly over the condyles (*2*) to mark the plane of the patellar surface of the femoral condyles (Fig. 4).
- Thirdly, a DHS/DCS guide pin (*3*) is inserted with the air drill (Fig. 5) at the predetermined point of insertion parallel to wire (*1*) in anteroposterior view (Fig. 6), and parallel to the anterior wire (*2*) in axial view (Fig. 7).

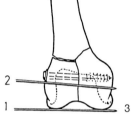

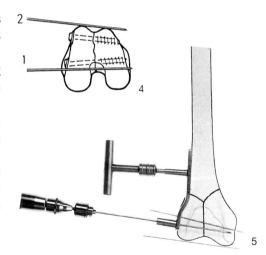

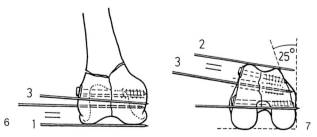

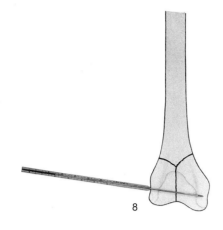

8

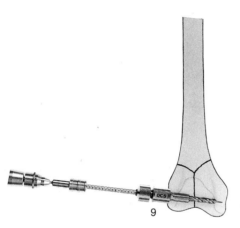

9

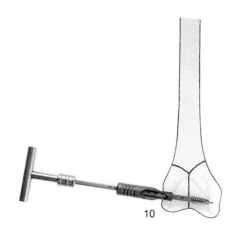

10

– The threaded end should be anchored in the medial cortical bone. This pin determines placement of the DCS implant and must be correct. Misplacement can result in varus/valgus or rotational malalignment.
– Correct placement is verified with image intensifier.
– The Kirschner wires are removed.
– The inserted depth is measured with the direct measuring device (e. g. 85 mm) (Fig. 8).
– The DCS triple reamer is assembled: The reamer head marked DCS is slid onto the drill bit, with the set screw aligned with the flat on the drill bit. When the reamer head engages the notch with the desired reaming depth (e. g. 75 mm), the nut is tightened firmly.
– The DCS triple reamer is connected to the special quick coupling and then to the air drill.
– The triple reamer is slid over the guide pin and reaming started. The speed is diminished when each portion of the reamer enters the lateral cortex. Two steps are prepared: the hole for the screw, and the seat for the plate barrel. The guide pin must not be damaged when drilling (Fig. 9).
– If the guide pin is inadvertently withdrawn when removing the triple reamer, it must be reinserted. The short centring sleeve pushed into the bone and a screw inserted in a retrograde position, makes reinsertion easy. The guide pin should remain in place until the side plate has been attached.
– In young patients with dense bone, tapping may be necessary. The short centring sleeve is mounted on the tap and the T handle connected. The centring sleeve is pushed into the bone to avoid "wobbling" when tapping. The tapping depth (i. e. reamed depth; e. g. 75 mm) is checked through the small window in the sleeve (Fig. 10).
– A DHS/DCS screw 5 mm shorter than the reamer setting (e. g. 70 mm) is chosen. The screw is connected to the guide shaft/coupling screw assembly. The notches of the screw must interdigitate with the ridges of the guide shaft.

– The long centring sleeve is pushed onto the DHS/DCS wrench and the screw assembly inserted. The screw end should be visible through the window in the wrench. While inserting the screw over the guide pin the wrench is centred in the bone with the long centring sleeve (Fig. 11). The screw is inserted until the 5 mm mark on the wrench aligns with the lateral cortex. This leaves a 5 mm gliding capacity in the barrel when the fracture is compressed.
– In osteoporotic bone the screw may be inserted to the 10 mm mark, enhancing the grip of the screw.
– The handle of the wrench should be aligned with the long axis of the femur before being removed (Fig. 12).
– The wrench and the centring sleeve are removed; the guide shaft/coupling screw are left in place at this stage.
– The barrel of the selected DCS plate is pushed over the screw assembly until the flat sides align (Fig. 13).
– After removal of the guide shaft/coupling screw, the guide pin is removed using the Jacobs chuck in the small air drill (reverse trigger) (Fig. 14).
– The plate is gently seated with the impactor. The cortex at the proximal rim of the insertion hole may have to be chiselled to seat the plate further (Fig. 15).
– The compression screw is used carefully to compress the fracture without stripping the thread in the bone. It also locks the plate to the condylar screw (Fig. 16).

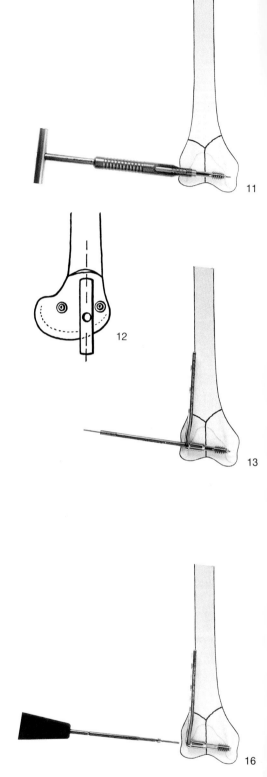

11

12

13

14

15

16

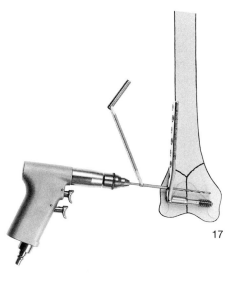

17

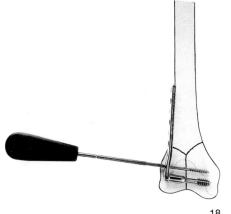

18

– Two 6.5 mm cancellous bone screws are inserted through the two distal plate holes to increase the interfragmentary compression and provide rotational stability of the implant in the distal fragment. Drilling 3.2 mm (Fig. 17), measuring, tapping, and insertion of a long threaded 6.5 mm cancellous bone screw (Fig. 18).

– For the final reduction of the condylar complex and the femoral shaft, the articulated tension device may be used. It is attached first in distraction mode for indirect reduction, and then hooked in the last plate hole for axial compression. A 4.5 mm cortex screw is used to fix the device to the bone. The bolt of the device is tightened using the open end wrench (Fig. 19).

– Before the articulated tension device is removed, at least three 4.5 mm cortex screws should have been inserted through the plate. If a screw is crossing the fracture it has to be inserted as a lag screw: Drilling 4.5 mm for the gliding hole, then 3.2 for the thread hole, measuring, tapping, and insertion of the screw (Fig. 20).

– Insertion of the remaining screws (Fig. 21).

Example of measurements:
– Length measured   85 mm
– Reamer setting   75 mm
– Tapping depth   75 mm
– DHS/DCS screw   70 mm

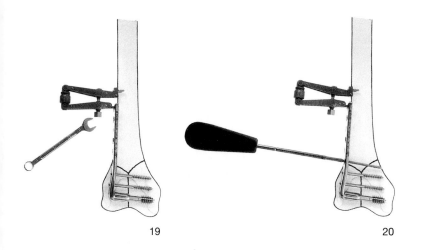

19   20   21

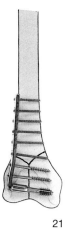

6.7.3.3 Application of DCS in the Proximal Femur

The technique of application of the DCS in the proximal femur
is similar to the technique described above for the distal femur.
The positioning of the guide pin in the femoral neck has to be
correct to ensure proper placement of the implant.

A Kirschner wire is inserted to determine the anteversion of the
femoral neck (see Fig. 1, p. 143). The condylar guide (85°) is
then used to place the DHS/DSC guide pin correctly in the
greater trochanter. The wire should also be parallel to the anteversion wire. The point of entry is at the junction of the anterior and middle third of the trochanter massive. The guide pin
should not lie less than 1 cm from the superior cortex, and its tip
approximately 2 cm short of the articular surface in the lower
part of the femoral neck.

For preparation and insertion of the DCS, see illustrations.

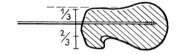

6.7.4 AO/ASIF Instruments for Application and Removal of DHS and DCS

Instruments for the application of DHS

Instruments for the application of DCS

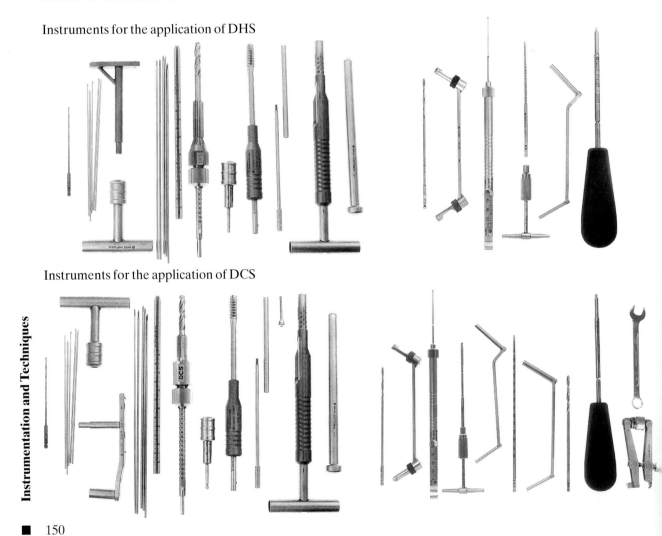

Instrumentation and Techniques

150

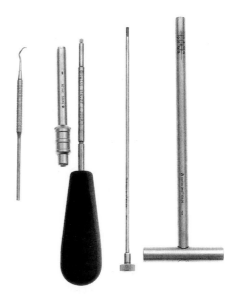

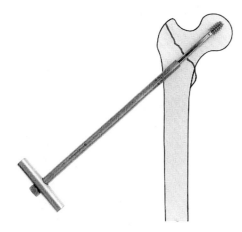

Procedure:
- After cleaning the screw head recess of debris the plate fixation screws are removed with the large hexagonal screwdriver. Likewise an eventual compression screw, and the plate are removed.
- The DHS/DCS wrench is assembled with the long coupling screw and placed on the DHS/DCS screw end with the flats aligned. The coupling screw is screwed in the DHS/DCS screw end.
- By pulling the assembly and turning anticlockwise, the DHS/DCS screw can be removed.

6.7.5 References

Regazzoni P, Rüedi T, Winquist R, Allgöver M (1985) The dynamic hip screw implant system. Springer, Berlin Heidelberg New York

DHS and DCS Instrument and Implant System

6.8 Angled Blade Plates and Instruments

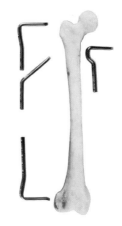

Angled blade plates were developed for the fixation of proximal and distal femoral fractures. Later osteotomy plates with different angles were introduced. All angle blade plates are of one-piece construction with a fixed angle between shaft and blade. The fixed angle increases the strength of the implant and makes it less susceptible to corrosion. A further advantage of the fixed angle is the possibility of accurate placement of the plate in osteotomies.

Angled blade plates with 95° and 130° angles are mainly used for fracture fixations. Osteotomy plates of various angles are available in sizes for both adults, adolescents, children and infants.

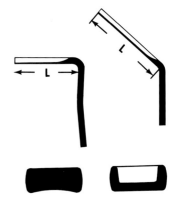

The blade of the plates for adults has a U-cross-section, which provides high strength with minimum bone displacement. Angle blade plates for small adults, adolescents, children and infants have a T-shaped blade cross-section. Although sharp at the tip, the seat of the blade must be prepared with a seating chisel with the corresponding cross-section.

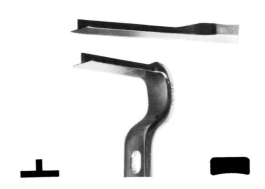

The shaft of the plate is slightly thicker than that of the straight, broad plate and can withstand higher stresses. The dynamic compression holes are arranged in an offset mode, similar to the straight broad plates. These holes accept 4.5 mm cortex screws; the round holes in some types of plates will accept 6.5 mm cancellous bone screws. For axial compression of fractures of the femur, it is often necessary to use the articulated tension device instead of the self-compressing DCP holes.

Due to its special design, the insertion of the angled blade plate requires great precision. Preoperative planning is essential to determine the exact placement of the plate. The blade must be correctly placed in both the frontal and the sagittal planes, and the shaft must line up with the axis of the femur. The anatomical landmarks must be known and guide wires inserted for orientation at the time of surgery. Misplacement of the plate may lead to varus, valgus or rotational deformities.

Instrumentation and Techniques

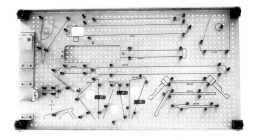

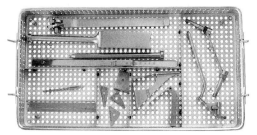

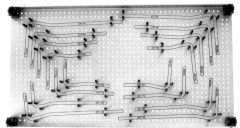

6.8.1 Angled Blade Plate Instruments

The instruments for angled blade plate application can be obtained in either a graphic case or in a sterilising tray. A graphic case for condylar plates is also available.

6.8.1.1 Standard Instruments

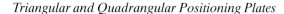

Drill Bit, 2.0 mm

This bit is used to pre-drill for the Kirschner wires necessary when planning the procedure.

Kirschner Wires, 2.0 mm Diameter, 150 mm

These wires are used to mark the different angles when planning for the insertion of angled blade plates. They are inserted with the small air drill using the Jacobs chuck.

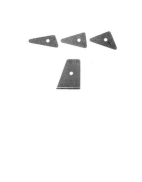

Triangular and Quadrangular Positioning Plates

These small positioning plates are used to determine the angles for inserting the Kirschner wires necessary for all angled blade plate procedures. They help indicate correct angulation of the seating chisel and to set the angle of the flap of the seating chisel guide. They are also used to determine correct osteotomy angles.

Due to their small size, vision is not obscured during insertion of the Kirschner wires. They can be held with a long forceps.

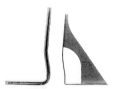

Condylar Plate Guide

This condylar plate guide is used to determine the best site and the correct angle for the condylar plate. Its side is an exact negative of the plate and the angle of 95° corresponds to that of the plate.

Angled Blade Plates and Instruments

Triple Drill Guide

The triple drill guide has a set angle of 130° and was originally designed to be used as a drill guide when preparing the seat for the 130° plate. It has a removable attachment with a ball bearing, which directs the 3.2 mm drill bit or a 3.0 mm Steinmann pin inserted along the femoral neck. The three holes accept the 4.5 mm drill bit, which is employed to open the cortex.
If slid on to the condylar guide, it can be used as a drill guide for condylar plates too.

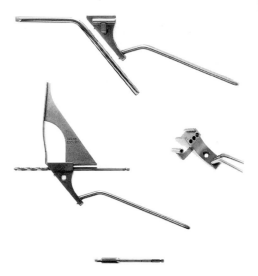

Router, 7 mm Diameter

The router is used to enlarge the three 4.5 mm holes into a slot before the seating chisel is inserted. It is both front and side cutting. It is available with both a quick coupling end to fit the small air drill and a triangular end to fit the Jacobs chuck.

Seating Chisel, 320 mm, U Profile

The seating chisel is used to cut the channel for the angled blade plates. Its U-shaped cross-section corresponds to that of the blade. The engraved millimetre scale to 110 mm indicates the depth of insertion. The tip of the chisel is ground such that it will not bite into the calcar when inserted obliquely. The sides are ground to converge slightly, which enhances the centring of the chisel in the femoral neck. Resharpening of the chisel must therefore be done by the manufacturer.
A 500-g hammer is used for insertion, the slotted hammer for extraction of the seating chisel.
The long seating chisel gives enough "driving way" for removal from dense bone.

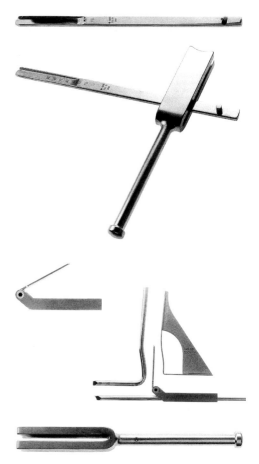

Chisel Guide

The chisel guide is slid onto the seating chisel from the front and used to control the rotation of the chisel about its long axis. The flap can be set at the same angle as the blade plate and the condylar plate guide. The locking screw is tightened with the hexagonal screwdriver. When inserting the seating chisel, the flap of the chisel guide should be in line with the long axis of the femur to avoid flexion/extension malposition.

Slotted Hammer

The slotted hammer is used to adjust and maintain the orientation of the seating chisel during insertion. It is also employed to extract the chisel. If necessary, it can be used to remove angled blade plates mounted with the inserter – extractor.

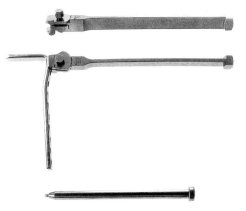

Inserter – Extractor

The inserter – extractor has a notched head into which the plate is mounted for insertion and, if necessary, for extraction. It must be placed as close as possible to the shoulder of the plate. The handle and the blade of the plate should be on horizontal line: after loosening the bolt, the notched head is moved into the correct position, the plate inserted and the bolt tightened firmly with the combination wrench.

Impactor

The impactor is used to finally seat the plate in close contact with the bone. Its tip fits into the depression near the shoulder of the plate.

DCP Hip Drill Guide, 4.5 mm

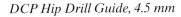

The drill guide, neutral (green) and load (load), is used with the 3.2 mm drill bit to drill for the 4.5 mm cortex screws necessary for the fixation of the angled blade plate.
Its 60 mm length allows the handle to extend beyond the muscles in the hip region.

6.8.1.2 Supplementary Instruments

Seating Chisel, 260 mm, T Profile

The seating chisel is used to prepare the seat for angled blade plates for small adults, adolescents and children. The T cross-section corresponds to that of the plates. It is used with the chisel guide for control of the rotation. The chisel has a blade length with a full T profile of 80 mm.

Small Seating Chisel, 260 mm, T Profile

The small seating chisel is used to prepare the track for the blade of the infant hip plate. It has a T-shaped cross-section that corresponds to that of infant hip plates. The shaft accepts the chisel guide, which is necessary to control rotation during insertion of the seating chisel. The blade length with full T profile of this chisel is 30 mm.

Inserter – Extractor

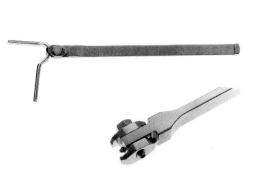

The inserter – extractor with adjustable head can be set in two positions for insertion of angled blade plates, for small adults and adolescents (marked A) and for children.
Once mounted, the plate is locked in place by tightening the bolt with the combination wrench.

Small Inserter – Extractor

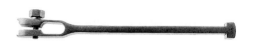

The small inserter – extractor can hold both the infant hip plate and the bifurcated plate for insertion. The bolt is carefully tightened with the combination wrench. Since infant bone is quite soft, the insertion of the infant hip plate may be possible without hammering the inserter.

6.8.1.3 Obsolete Instruments

Large triangular and quadrangular positioning plates have been replaced by the small positioning plates, since the large ones often obscured the field of vision.

The drill guide for round hole plates has been replaced by the double drill sleeve, 4.5 mm/3.2 mm, which is now used when the two round holes in the condylar plates are fixed with large cancellous bone screws.

6.8.2 Angled Blade Plates

Condylar Plate, 95°, U Profile

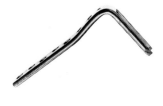

The condylar plate was primarily designed for the distal femur in adults. The 95° angle was chosen to maintain the physiological angle between the femoral shaft and the knee joint, when the plate is inserted parallel to the knee joint. The condylar plate has found increasing use also in proximal femur fractures. Then, the plate has to be inserted through the anterior half of the greater trochanter into the centre of the neck, and parallel to the neck axis in the coronal plane. The best position of the plate is just below the point of the trabecular intersection. Guide wires are used to determine the different planes. X-ray or image intensification is used only to verify the definitive insertion of the seating chisel.

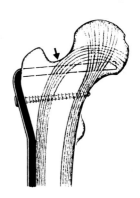

Condylar plates are available with 50, 60, 70, and 80 mm blade lengths. The shaft has 5, 7, 9 or 12 holes. The two round holes nearest the blade accept the 6.5 mm cancellous bone screws. The rest are DCP holes for 4.5 mm cortex screws; the last one has a notch for the tension device.

Important dimensions:
– Thickness: 5.6 mm
– Width: 16   mm
– Hole spacing: 16   mm
– U profile blade: 6.5–16 mm

Instrumentation and Techniques

■ 156

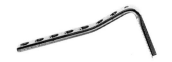

Condylar Plate, 95°, T Profile

The condylar plate is to be used in small adults for fractures of the distal and proximal femur as for intertrochanteric osteotomies, where the U profile would be too wide and might cause breakage of the neck. Four different blade lengths are available: 40, 50, 60, and 70 mm. The shaft is slightly smaller than that of the regular plate, but has DCP dynamic compression holes accepting 4.5 mm cortex screws. The two holes nearest the blade are round and accept 6.5 mm cancellous screws. The plates are available with 5, 7 and 9 holes and blade lengths of 40, 50, 60, and 70 mm. A seating chisel with the same T profile is necessary to prepare the seat of the blade. The inserter – extractor for large plates is used for insertion of the plate.

The preplanning of surgery and the insertion and fixation of the implant are otherwise similar to that of the large condylar plate.

Important dimensions:
- Thickness: 5.3 mm
- Width: 14   mm
- Hole spacing: 16   mm
- T profile blade: 5–11.7 mm

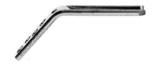

Angled Blade Plates, 130°, U Profile

The angled blade plates were developed for intertrochanteric and for certain subtrochanteric fractures; their use, however, has declined since the introduction of the DHS. When used, the preplanning of the procedure is as essential as when using the condylar plate.

The anteversion of the femoral neck must be predetermined and marked with a Kirschner wire.

The correct entry point for the 130° plate is approximately 3 cm distal to the rough line of the greater trochanter. When inserted, the plate should be in the centre of the femoral neck and about 6–8 mm above the calcar. The tip of the plate will then be at the intersection of the tension and compression trabeculae, where the plate has the best purchase.

The 130° plate is available with 4, 6, 9 and 12 DCP holes, the last with a notch for the tension device. The indentation at the junction between blade and shaft is for impaction of the plate.

Different blade lengths also are available: 50, 60, 70, 80, 90, 100, and 110 mm.

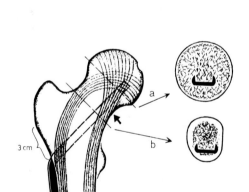

Important dimensions:
- Thickness: 5.6 mm
- Width: 16   mm
- Hole spacing: 16   mm
- U profile blade: 6.5–16   mm

Angled Blade Plates, 130°, T Profile

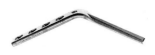

The angled blade plates are used in small adults for fixation of fracture of femoral neck and pertrochanteric fractures.

The T profile of the blade and the slightly smaller shaft fits the small bone better. The insertion is similar to that of the large angled blade plate, 130°. The seating chisel must have the same T profile as the blade. The inserter – extractor for the large angle blade plates can be used.

They are available with 4, 6 and 9 holes and with blade lengths of 50, 60, 70, and 80 mm.

Important dimensions:
- Thickness: 5.3 mm
- Width: 14 mm
- Hole spacing: 16 mm
- T profile blade: 5–14 mm

Osteotomy Plates for Adults, U Profile

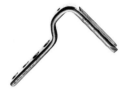

The osteotomy plates for adults are available with different angles between blade and shaft. Standard plates have angles of 90°, 100°, 110°, 120° and 130°, but any other desired angle can be obtained on special request. See SYNTHES catalogue.

The 90° and 100° plates have an offset to accommodate the greater trochanter in intertrochanteric osteotomies. Depending on the blade length (L), the depth of the offset (T) is either 10, 15, or 20 mm. The hole in the bend is for impaction of the plate and for fixation of the calcar with a 4.5 mm cortex screw. The blade lengths are 40, 50, and 60 mm.

The angled blade plates with an angle of 110° or more are used for repositioning osteotomies in pseudarthroses or nonunions of the femoral neck. The blade length varies from 65 to 110 mm. The shaft of all osteotomy plates has 4 DCP holes with a notch for the tension device in the end holes.

Osteotomies are carefully planned and carried out only after all anatomical landmarks and angles have been identified and marked with Kirschner wires. The seating chisel and sometimes the blade of the plate are inserted before the osteotomy is carried out, using the same techniques and instruments as for the regular angled blade plates.

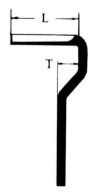

Important dimensions:
- Profile: See figure
- Thickness: 5.6 mm
- Width: 16 mm
- Hole spacing: 16 mm
- U profile blade: 6.5–16 mm
- Overall height: 94 mm

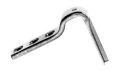

Osteotomy Plates for Small Adults and Adolescents, 90° T Profile

The osteotomy plates are used for intertrochanteric osteotomies in small adults and adolescents, where the U profile would be too wide and could cause breakage of the neck. The plates have an offset (T) with a depth of either 10 or 15 mm to accommodate the trochanter. The blade (L) with T profile is available in lengths of 40, 50, or 60 mm. For the preparation of the seat of the blade, a seating chisel with the same T profile is needed.

The shafts of the plates have 3 DCP holes for 4.5 mm cortex screws, the last with a notch for the tension device. The indentation in the offset is for impaction of the plate.

As in all procedures with angled blade plates, preplanning is essential for the successful insertion of the implant. Anatomical landmarks are identified and Kirschner wires inserted for orientation. The seating chisel and sometimes the blade of the plate are inserted before the osteotomy is carried out.

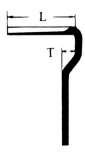

Important dimensions:
- Profile: See figure
- Thickness: 4.5 mm
- Width: 14 mm
- Hole spacing: 16 mm
- T profile blade: 5–11.7 mm
- Overall height: 78 mm

Osteotomy Plates for Children, T Profile

These plates conform to the small diameter of the femoral neck of children up to 10 years and are used for derotation and varus osteotomies. The plates are available with three different angles: 80°, 90°, and 100°; two blade lengths 35 and 45 mm; and an offset of 8 mm.

The shaft of the plates has 3 DCP holes for 4.5 mm cortex screws. The small indentation in the offset is for careful impaction of the plate.

A seating chisel with corresponding T profile has to be used and a special inserter – extractor.

The intervention is carefully planned and Kirschner wires inserted as landmarks. The seating chisel and sometimes the blade of the plate are inserted before the osteotomy is carried out.

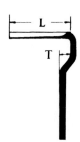

Important dimensions:
- Profile: See figure
- Thickness: 3.5 mm
- Width: 11.3 mm
- Hole spacing: 16 mm
- T profile blade: 4.5–11.2 mm
- Overall height: 74 mm

Angled Blade Plates and Instruments

Infant Hip Plates, 90° T Profile

These plates are used for derotation and varus osteotomies in infants and in children up to 5 years. The plates are available in two different blade lengths: 25 and 32 mm with offsets of 7 and 12 mm. The shaft has 3 DCP holes for 3.5 mm cortex screws.
A seating chisel with T profile of corresponding size is needed to prepare the seat of the blade.

Important dimensions:
- Thickness: 2 mm
- Width: 11 mm
- Hole spacing: 10 mm
- T profile blade: 2–8 mm
- Overall height: 46 mm

Bifurcated Osteotomy Plate, 115°

The bifurcated plate is used for proximal femoral osteotomies in small infants. The forked blade is designed to be inserted into the medulla of the femoral neck. The shaft has 2 oval holes for 3.5 mm cortex screws. The blade lengths are 30 and 35 mm. A special inserter – extractor is used for the insertion.

Important dimensions:
- Thickness: 1.1 mm
- Width: 11   mm
- Hole spacing: 20   mm

6.8.3 Technique of Application

The application of the different angled blade plates both proximally and distally requires great care and needs meticulous planning. The fixed angle between the blade and the shaft does not allow for mistakes in the application.
The insertion techniques will be described in general terms in the following.
Depending on the fracture pattern, the techniques may have to be modified.

Instrumentation and Techniques

6.8.3.1 Application of the Condylar Plate in the Proximal Femur

Before starting the application in the proximal femur, the following has to be determined:
– The length of the blade
– The length of the plate shaft
– The entry point for the blade
– The position of the plate

This is best done by using a reversed X-ray to normal scale of the contralateral side. It must be taken with the femur internally rotated to obtain the true length of the femoral neck. The transparent template of the condylar plate is placed on the reversed film along the femoral shaft. The tip of the blade should lie in the inferior half of the femoral head just below the intersection of the tension and compression trabeculae where the blade has its best purchase (see p. 156). In the femoral neck the blade passes about 10 mm below the superior cortex in the centre of the neck. (See AO/ASIF preoperative planner).
The blade length can now be determined. The shaft length will depend on the fracture pattern. The entry point in relation to the rough line (innominate tubercule) of the greater trochanter is noted.

Step by step procedure for the example of a subtrochanteric femur fracture:
– Any wedge fragment is fixed with a 4.5 mm cortex screw as a lag screw.
– A Kirschner wire, 2.0 mm in diameter, is placed below the anterior ridge which runs along the front of the intertrochanteric area, onto the anterior surface of the femoral neck, and driven into the head. It marks the plane of anteversion of the neck (Fig. 1).
– Taking the predetermined entry point in the anterior half of the greater trochanter into consideration, the condylar plate guide is placed along the lateral cortex of the femoral shaft. A second Kirschner wire is inserted (after pre-drilling with a 2.0 mm drill bit in dense bone) parallel to the upper edge of the plate guide into the apex of the greater trochanter. It should also be parallel to the anteversion Kirschner wire in the coronal plane. This wire indicates the direction of the blade of the plate (Fig. 2).
– The first Kirschner wire can now be removed.
– The level of the entry in the anterior half of the lateral eminence of the greater trochanter is marked with a chisel.
– The slot is prepared in the cortex with the 16 mm chisel, approximately 17 mm wide and 10 mm high.

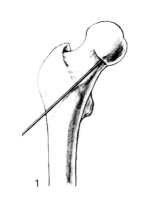

1

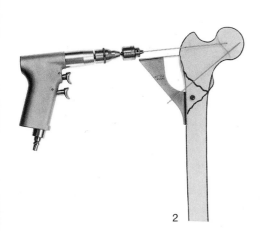

2

- In dense bone it is necessary to drill for the channel with the 4.5 mm drill bit in the double drill sleeve end, 4.5 mm (Fig. 3). The triple drill guide attached to the condylar plate guide can also serve as a drill guide. The slot is formed with the router (Fig. 4).
- The distal rim is bevelled to receive the shoulder of the plate (Fig. 5).
- The chisel guide is set at an 85° angle (using the plate itself or the condylar plate guide) and mounted on the seating chisel (Fig. 6).
- The seating chisel is hammered into the bone parallel to the Kirschner wire in both planes. The slotted hammer is used to control rotation about its long axis. The flap of the chisel guide should lie in line with the long axis of the femur throughout the insertion. The chisel is inserted to the predetermined depth (Fig. 7).

Note: The chisel should not be driven forcefully, since this may shatter the bone. Removing the chisel and drilling with the 4.5 mm drill bit may be necessary.
- The chisel is hammered back out with the slotted hammer.
- Insertion of the condylar plate: The plate is fixed in the inserter – extractor with its handle on a horizontal line with the

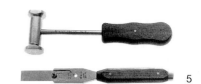

5

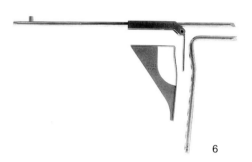

6

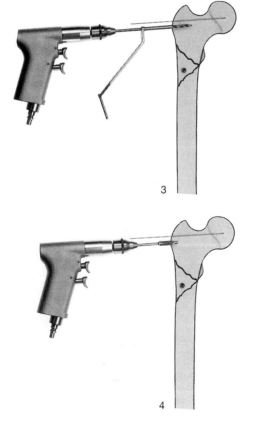

3

4

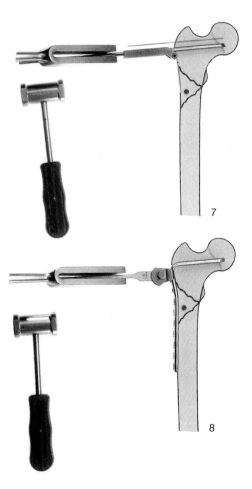

7

8

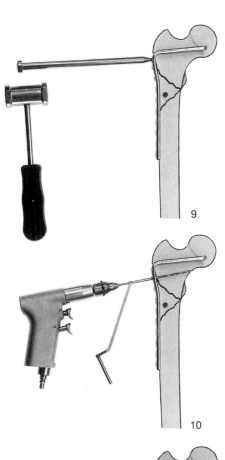

9

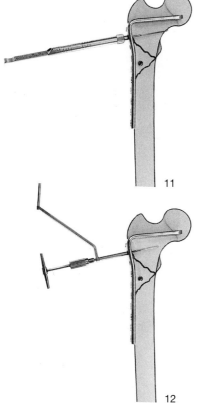

10

blade. The bolt is tightened with the open end wrench. It is pushed into the pre-cut channel and inserted with light hammer blows (Fig. 8).

– The inserter – extractor is removed and the impactor used to seat the plate against the lateral cortex (Fig. 9).
– To triangulate the fixation, a 4.5 mm cortex screw is inserted through the first plate hole into the calcar.
– With the 3.2 mm drill bit and the double drill sleeve end, 3.2 mm, the thread hole is drilled (Fig. 10).
– The length is determined with the large depth gauge (Fig. 11).
– Tapping with the 4.5 mm tap and sleeve (Fig. 12).
– Insertion of the 4.5 mm cortex screw (Fig. 13). (In intertrochanteric fractures it is inserted as a lag screw.)
– If suitable, a second screw is inserted through the next hole in similar manner.
– If necessary, axial compression is achieved with the articulated tension device: the opened device is hooked into the last plate hole and a thread hole drilled through its footplate using the 3.2 mm drill bit in the double drill sleeve end, 3.2 mm. Tapping for 4.5 mm cortex screw and insertion of a short screw (Fig. 14).

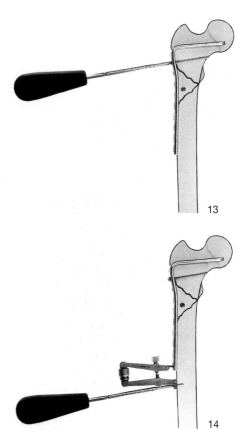

11

13

12

14

Angled Blade Plates and Instruments

- The bolt of the device is tightened with the open end wrench until the desired compression is obtained (Fig. 15).
- The remaining 4.5 mm cortex screws are inserted in the plate. Any screw crossing the fracture is inserted as a lag screw (Fig. 16). The rest are inserted after drilling 3.2 mm, measuring, and tapping as described above (Fig. 17).
- The articulated tension device is removed and the last plate hole fixed with a cortex screw (Fig. 18 a, b).

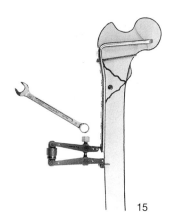

15

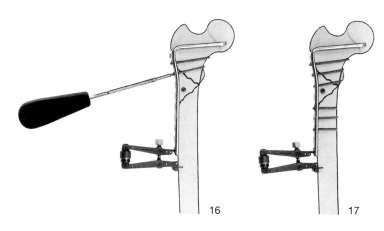

16   17

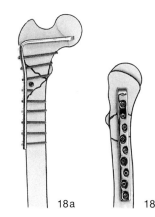

18a   18b

6.8.3.2 Application of the Condylar Plate in the Distal Femur

Before the condylar plate can be inserted in the distal femur, the following has to be determined through careful preoperative planning:
- The length of the blade
- The plate length
- The point of entry
- The position of the plate

AP and lateral X-rays of the normal side are taken and used reversed to plan the different steps of application. (See the AO/ASIF preoperative planner.)

Anatomical features to consider:
- When the distal femur is viewed laterally, the anterior part of the condyle is the continuation of the femoral shaft. Therefore, the point of entry must be in the middle of the anterior half of the condylar mass so as to have the plate lined up with the femoral shaft. The entry point is in the extension of the long axis about 1.5 cm to 2 cm above the knee joint. The slot is made at this distance parallel to an imaginary line marking the longest diameter of the elliptically shaped lateral femoral condyle.

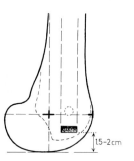

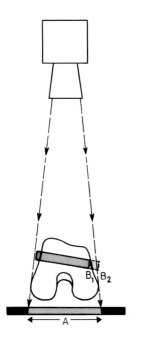

– When viewed from below the femur has a trapezoidal shape. The lateral side of the anterior part has an inclination of approximately 10°, the medial side of approximately 25°. The length of the blade (B1) must therefore be shorter than the AP (A) view suggests. The anterior surface is inclined towards the medial side. This corresponds to the inclination of the patellofemoral joint. The blade must be inserted with the same inclination.
– In the horizontal plane the blade should be parallel to the knee joint and about 1.5–2 cm from the distal end.

Step by step procedure for the example of a Y fracture:
– Fixation of the condylar fragments with two 6.5 mm cancellous bone screws as lag screws avoiding the planned insertion site of the blade (p. 81).
– The knee is bent 90° and the knee joint axis marked with a first Kirschner wire (1).
– The second Kirschner wire (2) is inserted anteriorly over the patellofemoral surface of the condyles to mark the inclination.
– The entry slot for the plate is marked and a third Kirschner wire inserted distal to the slot. This third wire (3) must be parallel to the first wire (1) in the AP view and to the second wire (2) in the axial view. Wires 1 and 2 can be removed. The third wire is the definitive guide for the direction of insertion of the seating chisel. The position can be checked with the condylar plate guide (Fig. 1).
– The entry slot is prepared with a 16 mm chisel: approx. 17 mm wide, 10 mm high and 10 mm deep. In hard juvenile bone the channel has to be pre-drilled with the 4.5 mm drill bit in the double drill sleeve end, 4.5 mm (Fig. 2). The proximal rim is bevelled with the chisel (Fig. 3).

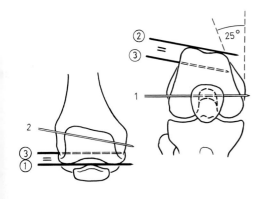

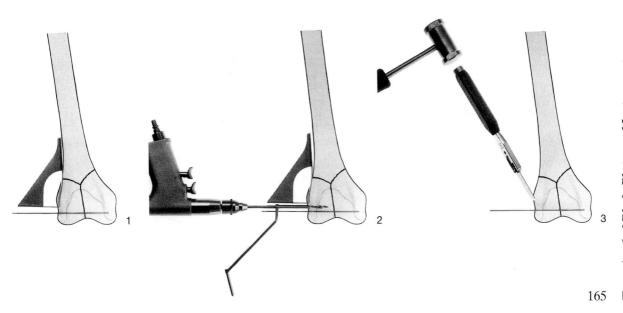

- The chisel guide is set at 85° (using the plate itself or the condylar plate guide) and mounted on the seating chisel (Fig. 4).
- The seating chisel is hammered in parallel to the definitive Kirschner wire in both planes. The flap of the chisel guide must be in line with the femoral shaft axis. The rotation is controlled with the slotted hammer (Fig. 5).
- After reaching the desired depth the chisel guide is taken off and the seating chisel removed with the slotted hammer.
- The selected plate is fixed in the inserter – extractor with the blade on a horizontal line with the handle. The bolt is tightened with the open end wrench.
- The plate is pushed into the prepared channel and inserted with light hammer blows. Rotation about its axis is controlled with the slotted hammer (Fig. 6).
- After removal of the inserter – extractor, final seating of the plate using the impactor (Fig. 7).
- The plate is fixed to the distal fragment with two 6.5 mm cancellous bone screws. In Y fractures these screws should be inserted as lag screws.
- The 3.2 mm drill bit in the double drill sleeve end, 3.2 mm, is used to drill through the round plate hole nearest the blade (Fig. 8). In hard juvenile bone the near cortex may have to be drilled with the 4.5 mm drill bit to accept the screwshaft without cracking.
- The length is measured (Fig. 9).
- The hole is tapped using the 6.5 mm tap and the double drill sleeve end, 6.5 mm (Fig. 10).

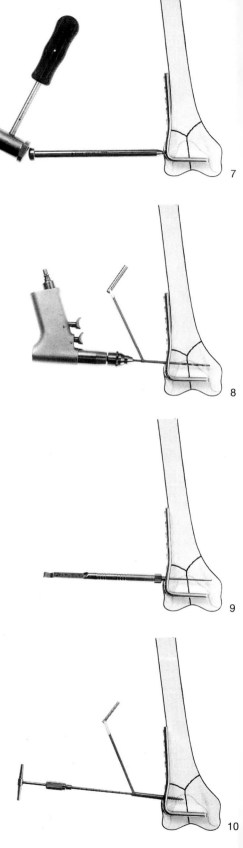

7

8

9

10

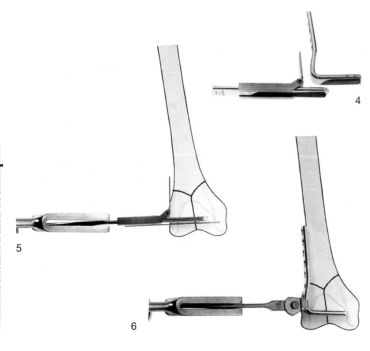

4

5

6

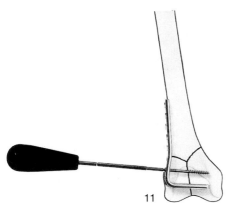

11

- The appropriate 6.5 mm cancellous bone screw is inserted (Fig. 11).
- These steps are repeated in the second round plate hole.
- If axial compression is desired the articulated tension device is used: The opened device is hooked into the last plate hole and fixed to the bone with a short cortex screw. By tightening the the bolt of the device the necessary compression can be obtained (Fig. 12).
- Fixation of the plate by inserting 4.5 mm cortex screws one by one: Drill bit 3.2 mm and the DCP drill guide 4.5 mm are used to drill the thread hole (Fig. 13). Measuring, tapping and insertion of the screws (Fig. 14).
- Removal of the articulated tension device.
- Insertion of the remaining 4.5 mm cortex screws (Fig. 15 a, b).

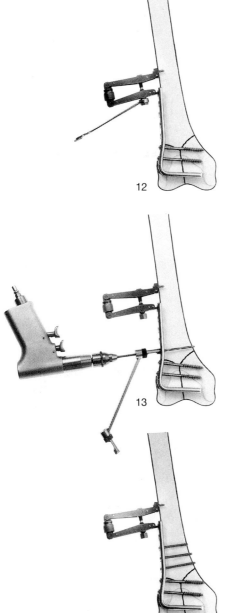

12

13

14

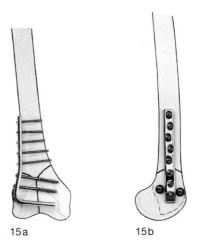

15a   15b

6.8.3.3 Application of the 130° Angled Blade Plate in the Proximal Femur

The use of the 130° angled blade plate has decreased since the DHS was introduced, but is still used in intertrochanteric fractures, especially if the DHS system is not available.

Preoperative planning is necessary to obtain the following important information:
- The position of the plate
- The point of entry
- The length of the blade
- The length of the plate

An X-ray of the uninjured side is used in reverse for the planning. This is taken with the femur internally rotated 15° – 20° to obtain the true length of the femoral neck. Using the transparent template of the 130° plate (see the AO/ASIF preoperative planner), the position of the plate is determined. The tip of the blade should lie in the centre of the femoral neck just below the

Angled Blade Plates and Instruments

intersection of the tension and compression trabeculae about 8–10 mm above the calcar (see p. 157). This is where the plate has the best purchase. The length of the blade is noted.

With the shaft lined up against the femur the entry point can be determined. It is approx. 3 cm distal to the rough line (innominate tubercle) of the greater trochanter.

The fracture pattern determines the length of the plate and the steps of insertion. Four or six hole plates are most commonly used.

Step by step procedure for the example of a subcapital fracture:

– After reduction the first Kirschner wire is inserted to determine the anteversion of the femoral neck axis. It is placed below the anterior ridge running along the front of the intertrochanteric area and driven into the head (Fig. 1).

– Variation: using the triple drill guide with the attached side guide, a 3.2 mm drill bit or a 3.0 mm Kirschner wire is inserted instead of the first Kirschner wire in the same position about 8–10 mm above the calcar.

– A second Kirschner wire is driven into the greater trochanter (pre-drilling with 2.0 mm drill bit in dense bone) parallel to the first wire in the coronal plane and parallel to the upper edge of the 50° triangular positioning plate placed on the femur along the lateral cortex (Fig. 2). This wire indicates the direction of plate insertion. The first wire is removed.

– The triple drill guide placed on the lateral cortex can be used for the preparation of the slot. This should be midway between the anterior and posterior surfaces of the femoral shaft. A 4.5 mm drill bit is used to drill for the channel (Fig. 3). Leaving this drill bit in place, a second 4.5 mm drill bit is used to drill the two remaining holes. Removal of the triple drill guide and drills.

– The router mounted in the small air drill is used to combine the three holes into a slot (Fig. 4).

– The distal rim is bevelled with a 16 mm chisel to avoid shattering of the cortex (Fig. 5).

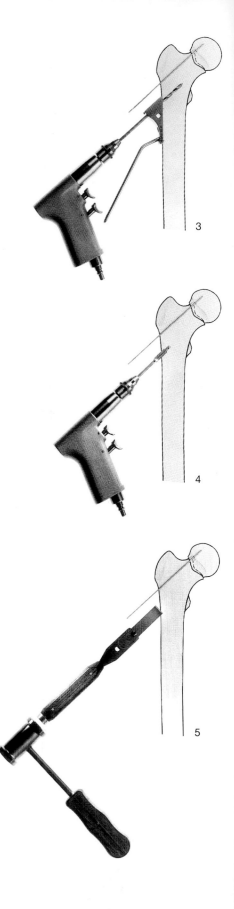

3

4

5

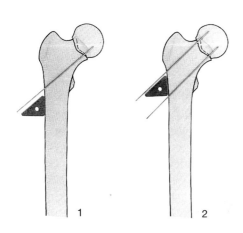

1

2

Instrumentation and Techniques

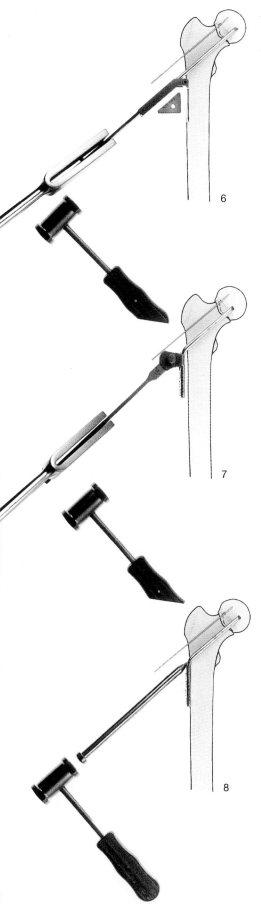

– The chisel guide is set at 50° using the plate itself or the triangular plate guide. It is mounted on the seating chisel.
– The seating chisel is inserted parallel to the Kirschner wire in both planes. The flap of the chisel guide must remain in line with the long axis of the femur. The slotted hammer is used to maintain and, if necessary, to correct the rotational alignment of the seating chisel (Fig. 6).
– When the desired insertion depth is reached, the chisel guide is removed and the slotted hammer used to remove the seating chisel.
– The selected plate is tightened in the inserter – extractor as close to the shoulder as possible. The handle must be on a horizontal line with the blade (Fig. 7).
– The plate is pushed into the prepared channel by hand and then inserted with light hammer blows. Removal of the inserter – extractor.
– The impactor is used to finally seat the plate. If correctly planned, the plate should be aligned with the femoral shaft (Fig. 8).
– Fixation of the plate with 4.5 mm cortex screws. Drill bit, 3.2 mm, in the DCP drill guide, 4.5 mm (Fig. 9).
– The length is measured (Fig. 10).

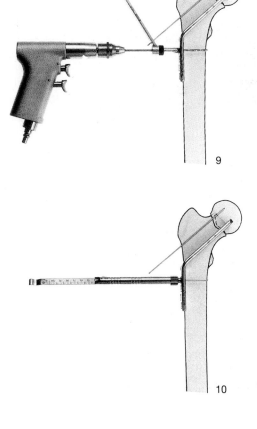

Angled Blade Plates and Instruments

- Tapping with the 4.5 mm tap in the double drill sleeve end, 4.5 mm (Fig. 11).
- Insertion of the 4.5 mm cortex screw (Fig. 12).
- The remaining screws are inserted using the same technique (Fig. 13).
- Removal of the Kirschner wire. Final tightening of the screws (Fig. 14 a, b).

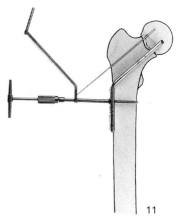

11

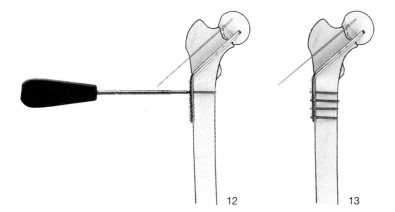

12   13   14a

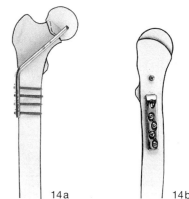

14b

6.8.3.4 Application of the Osteotomy Plates

Intertrochanteric osteotomies are performed to correct a varus, valgus, extension, flexion, or rotational deformity of the femoral neck (or combination deformities). Repositioning osteotomies are occasionally indicated for fresh fractures of the femoral neck, but most frequently for subcapital pseudarthrosis with a viable head.

Owing to the fixed angle of the AO/ASIF angled blade plates, it is possible to perform highly accurate osteotomies by carefully planning the procedure in advance.

Prior to surgery it it necessary to quantify all the components of deformity and calculate the necessary angles of correction. The basis of these calculations is the preoperative drawing made from radiographs of the unaffected side. (See AO/ASIF preoperative planner.)

As in the fixation of fractures it is necessary to identify the following before the insertion of the osteotomy plate:
- The point of insertion
- The direction of blade insertion
- The displacement angles
- The type of osteotomy plate

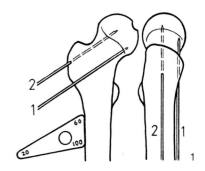

Instrumentation and Techniques

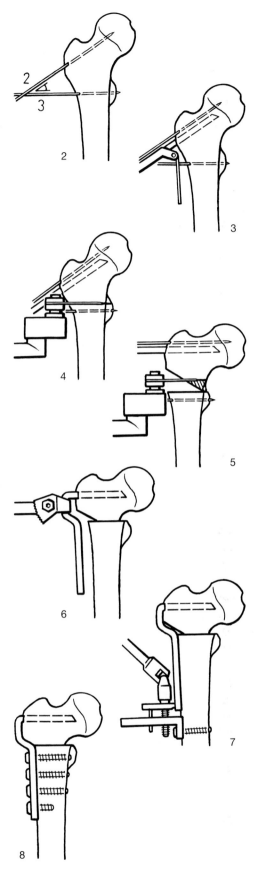

Step by step procedure for the example of a varus inter-trochanteric osteotomy:

– A first Kirschner wire (1) is inserted along the front of the femoral neck into the femoral head to indicate the anteversion of the neck.

– A second Kirschner wire (2) is inserted into the greater trochanter parallel to the upper edge of the triangular guide plate (e.g. 60°). This wire is also parallel to the front of the femoral neck axis as marked by the first wire and establishes the blade direction (Fig. 1).

– The first wire can be removed.

– About 5 mm distal to the site of the planned osteotomy, a 2.0 mm hole is drilled perpendicular to the femoral shaft axis, and a third Kirschner wire (Fig. 2) is inserted at the same anteversion angle as the second Kirschner wire.

– In derotation osteotomies, two additional Kirschner wires may be inserted to mark the necessary angles of correction.

– About 20 mm above the site of the planned osteotomy, and in the anterior half of the greater trochanter aligned with the long axis of the femur, the entry slot for the blade is prepared with a chisel.

– The seating chisel is inserted approx. 40–50 mm with the hammer in the same direction as the second Kirschner wire indicates. The flap of the chisel guide is in line with femoral shaft; the rotation controlled with the slotted hammer (Fig. 3).

– The chisel is then withdrawn 10–20 mm to facilitate later removal.

– The osteotomy is performed with the oscillating bone saw at the planned site (Fig. 4).

– Using the seating chisel as a handle, the proximal fragment is tipped into varus.

– Starting from the middle of the osteotomy, another cut is made into the proximal fragment parallel to the seating chisel. The 30° excised wedge is removed (Fig. 5).

– The seating chisel is extracted with the slotted hammer. Care must be taken not to dislocate the proximal fragment. A second slotted hammer is useful to hold the fragment.

– The selected osteotomy plate is fixed in the inserter – extractor at the shoulder. The blade and the handle are on one line.

– The plate is pushed into the pre-cut channel by hand (Fig. 6). It is further inserted with light hammer blows and, finally, after removal of the inserter-extractor, with the impactor.

– The plate is held against the shaft with a reduction forceps.

– The tension device is hooked into the last plate hole and fixed with a short cortex screw. Tightening the screw will produce the desired compression (Fig. 7).

– The plate is fixed with 4.5 mm cortex screws: drill bit, 3.2 mm, and DCP drill guide, 4.5 mm, large depth gauge, tap for 4.5 mm cortex screw, and insertion of the screw.

– The tension device is removed and the last screw inserted (Fig. 8).

6.8.4 AO/ASIF Instruments for Application and Removal of Angled Blade Plates

Instruments for the application of condylar plates in adults

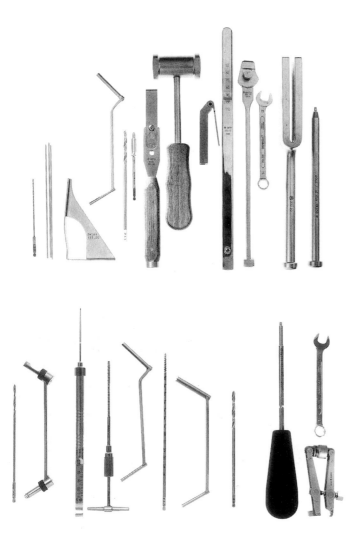

Instruments for the application of 130° angled blade plates in adults

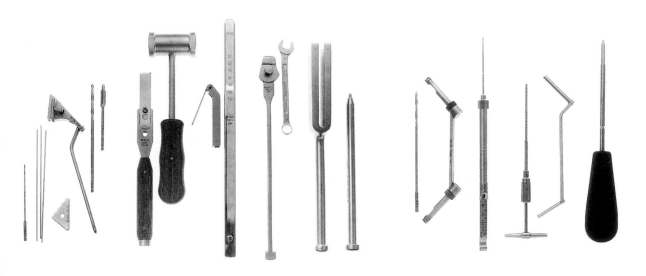

Instruments for the application of osteotomy plates in adults

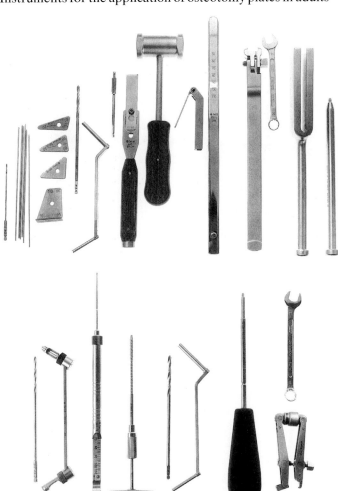

173 ■

Instruments for the application of condylar plates in small adults and adolescents

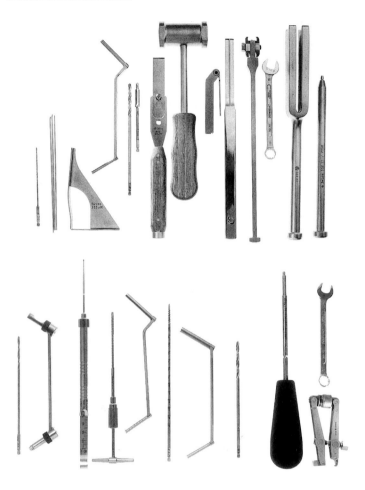

Instruments for the application of 130° angled blade plates in small adults

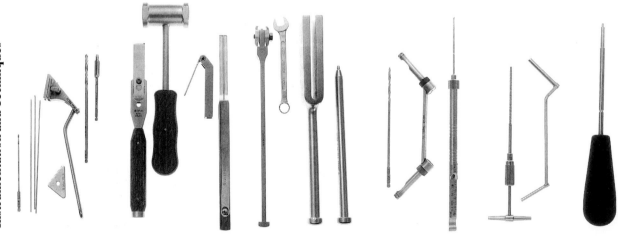

Instruments for the application of osteotomy plates in small adults, adolecents and children

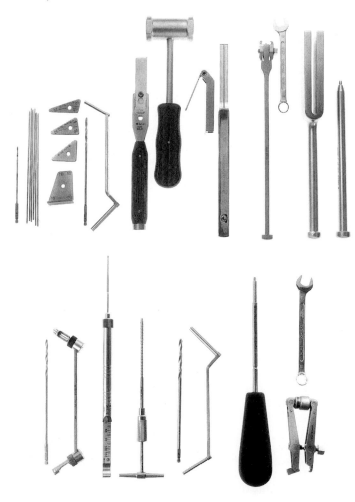

Instruments for the application of osteotomy plates in infants

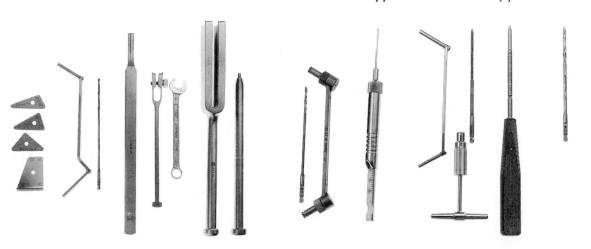

175 ■

Instruments for the removal of angled blade plates in adults

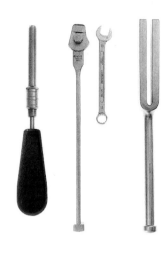

Instruments for the removal of angled blade plates and osteotomy plates in small adults, adolescents and children

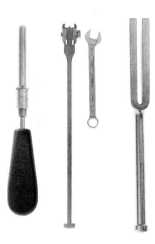

Instruments for the removal of osteotomy plates in infants

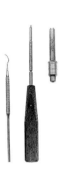

Procedure

After removal of the screws, the appropriate inserter – extractor is fixed at the shoulder of the plate, the handle in line with the blade. The slotted hammer is used to hammer out the plate.

6.9 Small Fragment Instruments and Implants

6.9.1 Small Fragment Instruments

The instruments used for reduction, temporary fixation of small fragments, and insertion of small fragment implants, are similar in principle to those used for large fragments, but of dimensions that correspond to the bone size. The general characteristics of instruments described in Sect. 6.3.1 apply also to those mentioned below. In this section the specific use of each instrument will be discussed.

Small fragment instruments and implants can be obtained in either a graphic case or in a sterilising tray

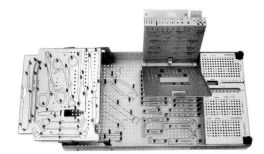
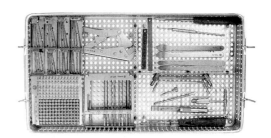

6.9.1.1 Standard Instruments

On drill bit and tap design, see Sect. 6.2

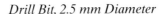

Drill Bit, 2.5 mm Diameter

This bit, 110 mm/85 mm (total and effective lengths), two-fluted, is used to prepare the thread hole for the 3.5 mm cortex screw and the 4.0 mm cancellous bone screws. It is gold/brown-coloured for easy identification. To simplify the insertion technique, it is now the drill bit of choice for all small fragment screws. The quick coupling end fits the small air drill. The drill bit should always be used with a drill guide or sleeve of corresponding size.

Drill Bit, 3.5 mm Diameter

This bit, 110 mm/85 mm (total and effective lengths), is used for the gliding or clearance hole when the 3.5 mm cortex screw is inserted as a lag screw. It has a quick coupling end to fit the small air drill. A drill sleeve of the same size should be used to protect the soft tissue.

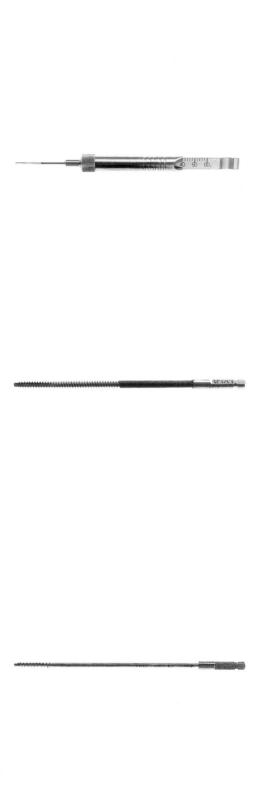

Small Countersink, 3.5 mm/4.0 mm

This is used to cut a recess in thick cortex to accommodate the screw head and to distribute its pressure evenly. It is used when small fragment screws are inserted as single screws. The 2.0 mm diameter tip centres the countersink in the pre-drilled thread hole. It is used with the T handle, never with power.

Countersinks manufactured now have five cutting edges instead of four. This increases the cutting capability and reduces the rattling.

Depth Gauge, 3.5 mm – 4.0 mm

This gauge measures the drilled depth for small fragment screws up to 60 mm. The hook has to engage the opposite cortex securely before the sleeve is pushed onto the bone, or plate, and the measurement read. If the drill hole is at an angle the longest diameter must be measured.

Depth gauges of recent design have a locking screw to avoid interchanging the sleeve with that of a different sized depth gauge. The old-style depth gauge measuring up to 50 mm may still be used.

Note: Always measure before tapping.

Tap for 3.5 mm Cortex Screws

This tap is gold/brown-coloured and is used to pre-cut the thread in the bone before the cortex screw can be inserted. The 50 mm long thread has the same 1.25 mm pitch as the screw thread, but only the first two conically increasing threads are cutting. Bone debris is deposited in the flutes, which now extend from the tip through the first ten threads. The long thread protects the already cut thread as the tap is advanced. Using the T handle, it is turned clockwise twice and anticlockwise once to clear the thread of bone debris. It is not recommended to tap with a machine, since the tap advances with too high a speed, and the sensation of completion of tapping the far cortex is lost. This may result in overpenetration and damage to the soft tissue on the far side of the bone. The tap should always be used with a protecting sleeve.

Tap for 4.0 mm Cancellous Bone Screws

This tap has been redesigned for easier identification. It now resembles the large 6.5 mm tap with short thread and a shaft. The short threaded part with 1.75 mm pitch is long enough to cut the near cortex before inserting a 4.0 mm cancellous bone screw. If tapping the opposite cortex is necessary, care must be taken not to destroy the already tapped bone. The rather narrow shaft of the tap makes this easier. It is used with the T handle and a protecting sleeve.

The previous, long threaded tap for 4.0 mm screws may still be used.

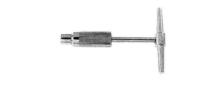

T Handle

This handle with quick coupling is used with the countersink and the taps. With this handle more force can be exerted when tapping hard bone than with a straight handle.

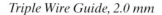

Triple Wire Guide, 2.0 mm

This wire guide can be used as a guide when Kirschner wires are inserted. The three holes on one side allow parallel placement of wires, especially in the tension band wiring technique.

Double Drill Sleeve, 3.5 mm/2.5 mm

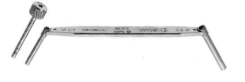

This piece has a sleeve at each side of a handle. One sleeve has an inside diameter of 3.5 mm to accept the 3.5 mm drill bit and tap. The sleeve on the other end has an inside diameter of 2.5 mm and an outside diameter of 3.5 mm. This is used with the 2.5 mm drill bit. It can also be used as an insert sleeve in a 3.5 mm gliding hole to guide the 2.5 mm drill bit into the opposite cortex in the lag screw technique. The serrated end of the double drill sleeve permits a secure hold on the bone surface while drilling. The holes in the handle near the sleeve can be used for Kirschner wires up to 1.6 mm diameter when a parallel screw is to be inserted. The distance of 4.5 mm between Kirschner wire and the screw permits use of a washer if necessary.

Insert Drill Sleeve, 3.5 mm/2.5 mm

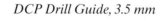

This sleeve is used in lag screw technique if the 30 mm long double drill sleeve is too short. The insert sleeve is pushed into the pre-drilled gliding hole and the 2.5 mm drill bit used to drill the thread hole in the far cortex.

DCP Drill Guide, 3.5 mm

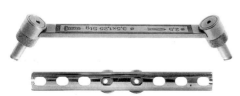

This has a neutral (green) and a load (yellow) guide. The end of each guide fits precisely in the 3.5 mm DCP plate hole and permits pre-drilling for a neutral or a load screw with the 2.5 mm drill bit. The drill hole for the load screw is prepared by placing the guide with the arrow pointing towards the fracture; 1 mm displacement is then achieved. The handle can be rotated into the desired position and is removed for cleaning.

The measurement 3.5 mm refers to the screw size of the screws used with this plate.

Note: The DCP drill guide should only be used with DCP plates.

LC-DCP Drill Guide, 3.5 mm

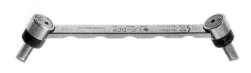

This is the drill guide used with LC-DCP, 3.5 mm. It is similar to the DCP drill guide, in that it has a neutral (green) and a load (yellow) guide, combined on one handle. The inserts will only fit this special handle. It has been designed with the same undercuts as the plate. This allows it to be easily distinguished from the DCP drill guide handle.

The handle is marked with the different positions of the guides. The neutral guide places the screw in a neutral position, if the arrow points towards the fracture. Turned 180°, with the arrow away from the fracture, a buttress position is obtained. The load guide places the screw in an eccentric position for compression when the arrow points towards the fracture.

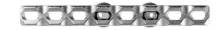

The displacement is 0.75 mm. Because of the hemispherical end of the guides, they have a congruent fit in the plate hole , also when tilted 40° in the longitudinal, and ±7° in the transverse plane.

Note: The LC-DCP drill guide should only be used with LC-DCP plates.

LC-DCP Universal Drill Guide, 3.5 mm

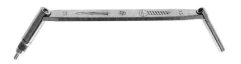

This is as the name indicates a guide for universal use. It is similar in design and function to the LC/DCP drill guide, 4.5 mm. It has two sleeves combined on one handle. One sleeve has an inner diameter of 3.5 mm and is used with the 3.5 mm drill bit and the tap for 3.5 mm cortex screws. The other end consists of two components: an outer sleeve, which has an end that corresponds exactly to the hemispherical undersurface of the screw head, and an inner sleeve with serrated end. This sleeve accepts the 2.5 mm drill bit. The two sleeves are pre-loaded by a spring in such a way, that the inner sleeve protrudes at the tip. By applying pressure the inner sleeve is pushed back into the outer sleeve. When the guide is placed in the plate hole and pressure is applied, the outer end of the sleeve follows the inclined "cylinder" to a neutral position. Here no compression is exerted, and a hole for a neutral screw can be drilled. The load position for a screw is obtained by placing the inner protruding sleeve at the end of the plate hole (far from the fracture). Similarly, the buttress position is obtained when the sleeve is placed at the end of the plate hole nearest the fracture. (See also pp. 88 and 89).

Because of the round end of the guide, which corresponds to the hemispherical undersurface of the screw head, an exact fit between the plate hole and the screw head can be established. This is important because no undesirable torque between bone segments will then occur. It is also possible to place a screw at an angle and still maintain the congruent fit.

The degree of inclination is limited to values that provide an exact fit.

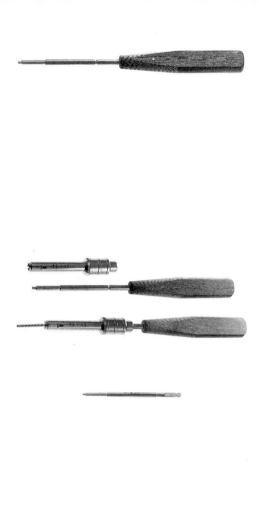

Small Hexagonal Screwdriver

This screwdriver has a hexagonal tip (width across flats 2.5 mm) which fits snugly in the hexagonal head socket of the small fragment screws, allowing easy insertion and removal. The shaft has a groove which is necessary to connect the screw-holding sleeve. The handle is designed so that excessive force cannot be applied when inserting the screws. The old-style screwdriver with simple holding sleeve may still be used.

Note: Never use a screwdriver with a damaged tip. This will then damage the screw head socket and make removal difficult.

Small Screw-Holding Sleeve

This sleeve holds the screw by a self-retaining mechanism. It is slid onto the screwdriver shaft which has a groove to locate it. It is especially useful when removing shaft screws since traction can be applied. The screw-holding sleeve has to be disassembled carefully for cleaning.

Small Hexagonal Screwdriver Shaft

This shaft can be connected to the small air machine for insertion of long screws. This has to be done with great care to avoid stripping of the bone. The shaft may also be connected with the T handle, and used as a reserve screwdriver. It cannot be used with the small screw-holding sleeve, only with the simple sleeve (see p. 186).

Sharp Hook

This hook is used to inspect fracture lines, and to reduce fragments. It can also be used to clean screw head sockets before removal, and to clear threads of bone and tissue debris.

Holding Clip, 3.5 mm

This clip is made of implant material and can be used to hold plates and washers. Regular safety pins cannot be used because of the risk of corrosion being transmitted.

Screw Forceps

This forceps with a simple self-holding mechanism is used to remove screws from the rack.

Bending Templates, 87 mm and 114 mm

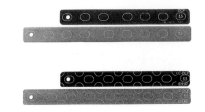

These templates are made of anodised aluminium. They are placed on the bone to determine the shape and position necessary for a plate. They then serve as models when carefully contouring the plates. One side is marked with the hole configuration of a DCP, the other side with that of a LC-DCP. For cleaning, see Sect. 6.22.4.2.

Bending Irons for Small Plates, 2.7 mm and 3.5 mm, 150 mm

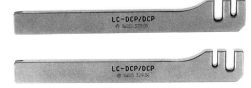

These irons have two slots with different widths to accommodate small fragment plates of various thicknesses. Bending and twisting is performed by placing the two irons opposite each other. The differently orientated slots allow easy overbending of the plate middle. The longitudinal slot at the ends can also be used for twisting and bending.

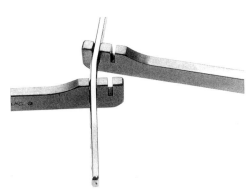

Wire Bending Pliers

These pliers can be used to hold and bend wires (see Sect. 6.17.3). They can also be used to cut wires up to 1.6 mm diameters on the side.

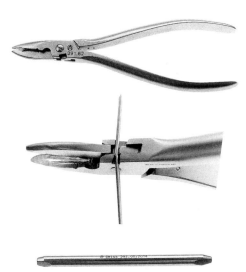

Bending Iron for Kirschner Wires

This iron is used to bend Kirschner wires close to the bone or skin. In tension band wiring technique the iron and a hammer are used to drive the hooked end into the bone. See Sect. 6.17.3

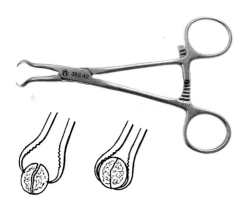

Reduction Forceps with Points, Narrow, 132 mm

This forceps has narrow serrated jaws and points. It can be used to reduce even markedly displaced fragments without causing soft tissue trauma. The main application is in the forearm, clavicle, ankle, metacarpus, and metatarsus. The fine ratchet lock makes handling easy and precise.

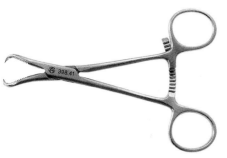

Reduction Forceps with Points, Broad, 132 mm

This forceps has broad, serrated jaws and points. It is used on the same bones and in similar manner as the one mentioned above, but allows space for a plate. It also has a fine ratchet lock.

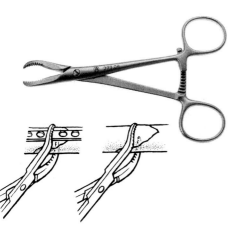

Reduction Forceps with Serrated Jaws, 140 mm

This forceps is excellent for reduction and temporary retention of a plate, e. g. on the forearm or the fibula. The ratchet is easy to handle and to close. The forceps also is available with a speed lock

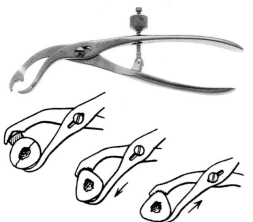

Self-Centering Bone Holding Forceps, 190 mm

This forceps ("Verbrugge") has a sliding joint which permits modification of reduction and plate holding ability. The speed lock allows rapid closure. By squeezing the handles slightly, the locking nut can be unscrewed easily.

Small Retractor, Width 8 mm, 160 mm

This retractor is used to expose the fracture without applying pressure on the wound edges. The small size makes it useful, especially for metacarpal and metatarsal bones.

Retractor for Small Fragments, Width 15 mm, 160 mm

This retractor has a wider blade and is therefore suitable for exposure of fractures of the forearm bones or of the fibula.

Periosteal Elevator, Round Edge, Width 6 mm

This elevator has a slightly curved blade and is used to expose the fracture edges, without widely stripping the periosteum. It is also used to clean the fracture of debris and to reduce fragments.

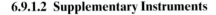

6.9.1.2 Supplementary Instruments

Drill Bit, 2.0 mm

This bit was used formerly to drill the thread hole for small cancellous bone screws. Their core size of 1.9 mm would allow this size of thread hole. However, in dense cortical bone, the 2.3 mm shaft of the screw could crack the bone. (Additionally, oblique drilling with the drill bit 2.0 mm occasionally would result in collision with the endosteal surface of the far cortex at such angle that it skidded. Continued rotation of the drill bit, as it bent, then risked breakage.) Today, therefore, it is recommended that the 2.5 mm drill bit be used instead. The 2.0 mm bit is used to pre-drill for Kirschner and cerclage wires.

Drill Bits, 2.5 mm and 3.5 mm

These bits are available in other lengths, also two- or three-fluted, or with a triangular end to fit the Jacobs chuck. See the SYNTHES catalogue for details.

Tap for 3.5 mm Cortex Screw

This tap is available with a 110 mm long thread for screws longer than 50 mm (as used in pelvic surgery) See Sect. 6.10.1. It is important to use a tap with a thread as long as the screw thread or the pre-cut thread in the bone will be damaged.

Depth Gauge, 3.5 mm – 4.0 mm

This depth gauge is used for measuring small fragment screws up to 110 mm for example in pelvic surgery. The design and function is the same as the shorter depth gauge.

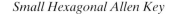

Small Hexagonal Allen Key

This key can be used as a reserve for removing screws with a 2.5 mm hexagonal socket, e. g. 2.7 , 3.5 and 4.0 mm screws.

Reduction Forceps with Points, 130 mm

These "towel clip" style forceps are available with speed lock or ratchet closure.

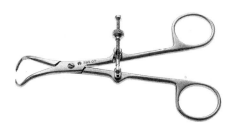

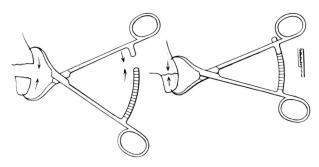

Bending Pliers

These pliers with adjustable anvils for small fragment plates ensures precise bending and requires little force. The large bending pliers for large plates has an anvil suitable also for the small fragment plates.

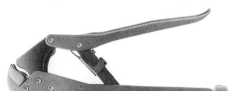

Bending Templates for Reconstruction Plates, 3.5 mm , Straight and Curved

These templates are moulded onto the bone to be used as a model when the plates are contoured. They are made of anodised aluminium and need special care when cleaned. (See Sects. 6.10.1 and 6.22.4.2.)

Bending Irons for Reconstruction Plates, 2.7 mm – 3.5 mm

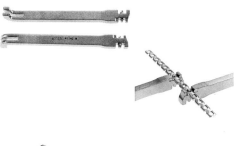

There irons are used in pairs for bending and twisting. By placing the plate onto the special pegs bending "on the flat" can be performed. Twisting can be achieved using the slots in the ends.

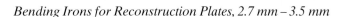

Bending Pliers for Reconstruction Plates 2.7 mm – 3.5 mm

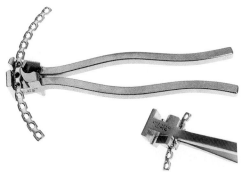

These pliers are designed to allow for three-dimensional bending without exceeding the permitted 15 ° at any one site.

Small Distractor

The small distractor can be used for distraction and reduction of fractures in small bones. The pin holders that are mounted on the carriage have two holes. In one hole, the 2.5 mm threaded Kirschner wire is inserted and fixed with a screw. The second hole may be used for a parallel Kirschner wire or screw to prevent rotation of fragments. The connected wires or screws are at right angles to the spindle, and no corrections can be made with the pin-holders. The Kirschner wires must therefore be parallel, and inserted at right angles to the long axis of the bone. Excursions of 10 mm – 40 mm are possible. See p. 357.

Bone Spreader, 140 mm

The bone spreader for small fragments, is sometimes needed to remove soft tissue trapped between fragments or to inspect the fracture surface.

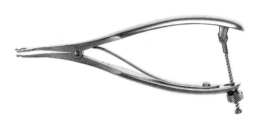

6.9.1.3 Obsolete Instruments

Tap for 4.0 mm Cancellous Bone Screws

This tap with 60 mm thread has been replaced with the new short-threaded tap.

Small Pointed Drill Guide

This drill guide used for reversed lag screw technique has been discontinued, since the technique is rarely indicated.

Tap Sleeve 3.5 mm/2.5 mm Drill Sleeve

This tap sleeve has been replaced by the double drill sleeve, 3.5 mm/2.5 mm.

Tap Sleeve, 3.5 mm

This tap sleeve has been replaced by double drill sleeve, 3.5 mm/2.5 mm.

DCP Drill Guide 3.5 mm

This drill guide for drill bit 2.0 mm is not to be used. The hole for the 3.5 mm cortex screws should be pre-drilled with drill bit 2.5 mm.

Depth Gauge

This depth gauge measuring up to 50 mm has been replaced by the depth gauge with locking screw measuring up to 60 mm.

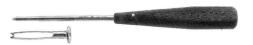

Small Hexagonal Screwdriver with Holding Sleeve

This piece has been replaced by the small hexagonal screw driver with the new screw-holding sleeve.

Bending Templates

These bending templates for small plates without screw hole markings are replaced by the DCP/LC-DCP templates.

6.9.2 Small Fragment Implants

Small fragment implants have been designed for fixation of fractures in the forearm, the distal end of the humerus, the fibula, the ankle, as well as small fragments of large bones. They are also used in acetabular and pelvic fractures. The size and strength of the implants correspond to these specific areas. Therefore, they should not be used where for mechanical and anatomical reasons other sizes are recommended. The evolution of the design and technique of application, as well as new development, of current implants comes from experience and continuous research. Most of the implants are available in both stainless steel and in titanium. See SYNTHES catalogue.
In the following the present standard implants will be discussed, and some earlier versions of implants merely mentioned in Sect. 6.9.2.4.

6.9.2.1 Small Fragment Screws

Small fragment screws are used either as lag screws or as plate fixation screws. The short and fully threaded cancellous bone screws, 4.0 mm diameter are used in the metaphyseal/epiphyseal regions of small bones. The cortex screw and the shaft screw, 3.5 mm diameter are mainly used in the diaphysis. The screw head is the same size for all these screws and has a hexagonal socket to accept the small hexagonal screwdriver. The small cannulated screw is for special applications, and is discussed in Sect. 6.6.3

4.0 mm Cancellous Bone Screw, Partially Threaded

This screw has a smooth shaft and is commonly used as a lag screw in ankle fractures, as well as in fractures of the distal radius. The thread is designed to give good purchase in cancellous bone. The thread length increases from 5 mm to 15 mm in proportion to the screw length. Screw lengths from 10 mm to 50 mm are available.
It is now recommended that the 2.5 mm diameter drill bit be used to pre-drill for the screw, rather than the previously advo-

Small Fragment Instruments and Implants

cated 2.0 mm drill bit. The 2.4 mm shaft of the screw would fit in the hole without risk of cracking, especially in dense, juvenile bone The 4.0 mm cancellous bone screws, partially threaded, are available in lengths from 10 mm to 50 mm, in 2 mm increments up to 30 mm, and then in 5 mm increments to 50 mm.

Important dimensions:
- Head diameter: 6.0 mm
- Hexagonal socket width: 2.5 mm
- Shaft diameter: 2.4 mm
- Core diameter: 1.9 mm (titanium 2.0 mm)
- Thread diameter: 4.0 mm
- Pitch: 1.75 mm
- Drill bit for thread hole: 2.5 mm
- Tap for 4.0 mm cancellous bone screws.

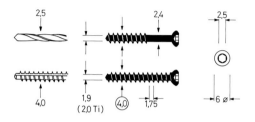

4.0 mm Cancellous Bone Screws, Fully Threaded

These screws are used mainly for the fixation of thin small fragment plates to the metaphysis and are not to be used as a lag screws. The thread profile is the same as that of the partially threaded cancellous bone screw. Its predecessor, the 3.5 mm screw, with 1.75 mm pitch, is discussed in Sect. 6.9.3.

4.0 mm cancellous bone screws, fully threaded, are available in lengths from 10 mm to 60 mm, in 2 mm increments up to 30 mm, and then in 5 mm increments up to 60 mm.

Important dimensions:
- Head diameter: 6.0 mm
- Hexagonal socket width: 2.5 mm
- Core diameter: 1.9 mm (titanium 2.0 mm)
- Thread diameter: 4.0 mm
- Pitch: 1.75 mm
- Drill bit for thread hole: 2.5 mm
- Tap for 4.0 mm cancellous bone screws.

3.5 mm Cortex Screw

Since its introduction in 1983, this is the screw which should be used as a lag screw or for plate fixation in the diaphysis of small bones. Its holding power in dense cortical bone has increased because of the 1.25 mm pitch and the asymmetrical buttress threads. The core diameter of 2.4 mm increases the torsional and bending strength of the screw, preventing shearing when it is used as load screw in self-compression plates. It is not a self-tapping screw and the thread must be cut with the 3.5 mm tap (coloured gold/brown) before insertion.

The 3.5 mm cortex screw is available in lengths from 10 mm to 110 mm, in 2 mm increments up to 40 mm, and then in 5 mm increments up to 110 mm..

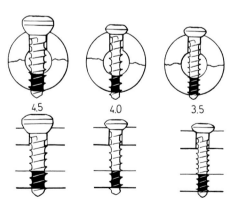

Instrumentation and Techniques

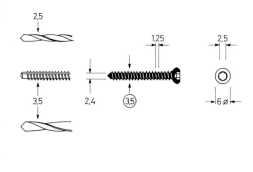

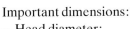

Important dimensions:
- Head diameter: 6.0 mm
- Hexagonal socket width: 2.5 mm
- Core diameter: 2.4 mm
- Thread diameter: 3.5 mm
- Pitch: 1.25 mm
- Drill bit for gliding hole: 3.5 mm
- Drill bit for thread hole: 2.5 mm
- Tap: 3.5 mm

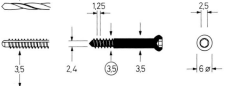

3.5 mm Shaft Screw in Titanium

This screw has been introduced with the LC-DCP system for use as load screw and lag screw. The shaft has the same diameter as the thread, 3.5 mm. It is much stronger than the threaded portion in bending forces. Used as an inclined lag screw, it is 60% more efficient than a fully threaded screw, since the smooth shaft can not produce any undesirable grip in the gliding hole of near fragment. The screw is not self-tapping; the thread must be pre-cut with the 3.5 mm tap (gold/brown colour).
Lengths from 10 mm to 50 mm are available in 2 mm increments up to 40 mm, then in 5 mm increments.

Important dimensions:
- Head diameter: 6.0 mm
- Hexagonal socket width: 2.5 mm
- Shaft diameter: 3.5 mm
- Core diameter: 2.4 mm
- Thread diameter: 3.5 mm
- Pitch: 1.25 mm
- Drill bit for gliding hole: 3.5 mm
- Drill bit for thread hole: 2.5 mm
- Tap: 3.5 mm

Washer, 7 mm

This washer is available to be used with the 4.0 mm cancellous bone screw to prevent the screw head from breaking the cortex in the metaphysis. The flat side is placed on the bone; the countersunk side accepts the hemispherical undersurface of the screw head.

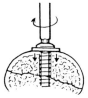
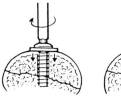

Small Fragment Instruments and Implants

Spiked Washer, 8.0 mm/3.2 mm Diameter

This washer made of polyacetate, and reinforced with stainless steel for X-ray contrast, can be used for reattachment of avulsed ligaments. A 4.0 mm cancellous bone screw is used for the fixation.

The polyacetate washer may be sterilised in temperatures up to 140° C, (or 270° F), allowing a minimum of 8 h for cooling and rehardening. EtO (Ethylene oxide) sterilisation is also possible, followed by a full cycle aeration.

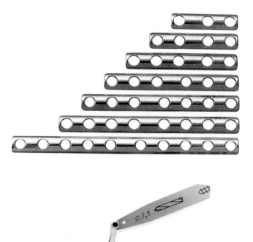

6.9.2.2 Small Fragment Plates

One-Third Tubular Plates

These plates have the form of one-third of the circumference of a cylinder. They have low rigidity since they are only 1 mm thick. The plate is used mainly for the fixation of fractures in the lateral malleolus, the distal ulna, the olecranon, and the metatarsals. The oval holes permit eccentric positioning of the screws, which can be used for axial compression of a fracture. To achieve this, the wide middle section of the plate is placed over the fracture. The screws nearest the fracture in each fragment are inserted eccentrically away from the fracture. The plate is fixed with 3.5 mm cortex screws in diaphyseal bone, and 4.0 mm cancellous bone screws in the metaphyses.

The plate offers good longitudinal stability if in complete contact with the bone, either by the edges along the plate or by the "collar" on the undersurface of each plate hole. The following must be considered: Because of the "one-third of a tube" cross-section, the screw head is almost flush with the plate surface when inserted through the plate hole. As a consequence the undersurface of the screw head protrudes through the undersurface of the plate. If used on a bone with a small circumference the screw head may be in contact with the bone, blocking the plate from being securely fixed. To overcome this problem some plates (titanium plates at present) have a collar around the holes on the underside. These collars prevent the screw head from protruding and secure the plate/bone contact. The plates are available in lengths from 25 mm to 145 mm, with 2 to 12 holes.

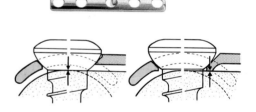

Important dimensions:
- Thickness: 1 mm
- Width: 9 mm
- Hole spacing: 12 mm and 16 mm

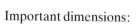

Instrumentation and Techniques

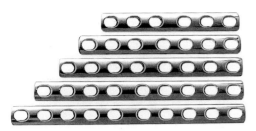

Dynamic Compression Plates, DCP, 3.5 mm

These plates are used with cortex screws 3.5 mm, hence the name. It is the implant of choice for the fixation of fractures in the forearm. It may also be used for distal humerus fractures and the clavicle. The DCP hole design and working principle are analogous to those of the DCP, 4.5 mm. See Sect. 6.5.1.1

The holes allow for 1 mm displacement, if a load screw is used. The 3.5 mm DCP drill guide must be used with this plate to ensure the load effect of the screw. The plate can also be used with the articulated tension device. If necessary, 4.0 mm cancellous bone screws can be inserted in the end holes.

The plates are available in lengths from 25 mm to 145 mm, with 2 to 12 holes.

Important dimensions:
– Profile: See figure
– Thickness: 3.0 mm
– Width: 10   mm
– Hole spacing: 12   mm and 16 mm
– Hole length: 6.5 mm

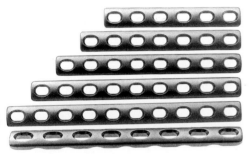

Limited Contact-Dynamic Compression Plate,
3.5 mm in Titanium

The design features of the LC-DCP, 3.5 mm are analogous to those of the LC-DCP, 4.5 mm. See Sect. 6.5.1.1. The plate is smaller in size, and is applied with 3.5 mm titanium cortex screws and 3.5 mm titanium shaft screws in the diaphysis, and with 4.0 mm titanium cancellous bone screws in the metaphysis. The 3.5 mm screws can be inserted in three different positions: neutral, load, or buttress. For this purpose, special drill guides have to be used, either the LC-DCP drill guide, 3.5 mm, or the LC-DCP universal drill guide, 3.5 mm. See Sect. 6.9.1.1. Before applying a LC-DCP, the plate must be contoured. The bending templates are used as models.

The LC-DCP is used for the same indications as the DCP: forearm fractures, fractures of the distal humerus, the clavicle and the pelvis. It can be applied for any desired function as neutralisation, tension band or buttress plate.

The improved design offers certain advantages:
– Structured undersurface: The evenly distributed undercuts reduces to a minimum the contact area between bone and plate. This significantly improves the blood supply of the plated bone segment, and has been shown to prevent local osteoporosis. The undercuts also allow for the formation of a small callus bridge, which increases the strength of the bone at a very critical location. The callus bridge may reduce the risk of refracturing after implant removal.
– The enlarged cross-section at the plate holes and the reduced cross-section between holes offer a constant degree of stiff-

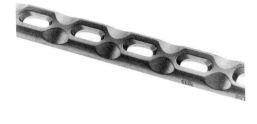

Small Fragment Instruments and Implants

191 ∎

ness along the whole long axis of the plate. No particular stress concentration occurs at the holes when the plate is exposed to a bending load or during contouring of the plate

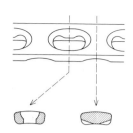

- Trapezoidal cross-section of the plate: The trapezoidal cross-section of the plate results in a smaller contact area between plate and bone. A broad and low bony lamella is formed along the side of the plate, which is less likely to be damaged at plate removal.
- Uniform spacing of plate holes: The plate holes are uniformly spaced, which permits easy repositioning of the plate. The screw holes are 7 mm long.
- Symmetrical spherical gliding holes: The basic principle of spherical gliding of the screw head in the plate hole is preserved, but augmented. Both ends of the plate hole offer the gliding possibility, which means more versatility in use. The holes allow 0.75 mm displacement of the fragment, if a load screw is inserted. Neutral screw placement gives minimal displacement.

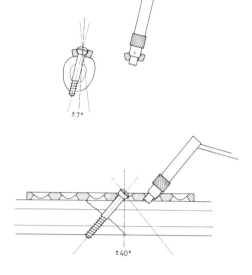

- Undercut plate holes: Undercuts at both ends of the plate hole, allow 40° tilting of screws either way along the long axis of the plate. Lag screw fixation of short oblique fractures is thereby possible. Screws can be tilted ±7° in the transverse plane. Furthermore, the undercuts reduce the contact area between plate and bone even further.
- The articulated tension device may be hooked in the end plate holes if further compression is necessary, i.e. in fractures with a wider gap.
- The LC-DCP, 3.5 mm is available in lengths from 51 mm to 155 mm, with 4 to 12 holes.

Important dimensions:
- Profile: See figure
- Thickness: 4.0 mm
- Width: 11   mm
- Hole spacing: 13   mm
- Hole length: 7   mm

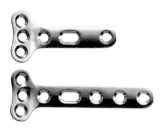

Small T Plate, Right-Angled

This plate is designed for use on the volar aspect of the distal radius. The plate is slightly concave and the head portion bent to accommodate the volar surface of the distal radius. The plate may exceptionally be used in certain fractures of the olecranon, the ankle, and the metatarsals. The head portion has either three or four holes, and the plate shaft three, four, five, or six holes. One hole is elongated to be used for an oblique lag screw, or for preliminary adjustment of the plate. The shaft is fixed with 3.5 mm cortex screws and the head with 4.0 mm cancellous bone screws.

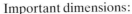

Important dimensions:
- Profile: See figure
- Thickness: 1.2 mm
- Width: 10   mm

Small T Plate, Oblique

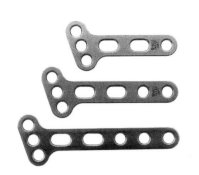

This plate is designed for the dorsal aspect of the distal radius. Its 120°-angled head conforms to the anatomical angle of the bone and fits both the left and the right radius equally well. The holes are made to accept the screw head on both sides. The plate may be contoured by using small pliers and small bending irons. The plate is available with 3 holes in the head and 3, 4, or 5 holes in the shaft. Two shaft holes are elongated for lag screw fixation, and for temporary fixation and adjustment of the plate. The 3.5 mm cortex screws are used in the shaft and 4.0 mm cancellous bone screws in the head.

Important dimensions:
- Shaft profile: See figure
- Thickness: 1.5 mm
- Width: 10   mm

Cloverleaf Plate

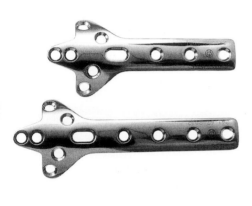

This plate has been developed for comminuted fractures of the distal tibia to buttress its medial side, but may be used also in the proximal humerus. The head portion can be contoured easily to conform to the bone, and can be cut to the desired shape. The holes in the head accept small fragment screws. The shaft is fixed with 4.5 mm screws. In newly developed titanium plates it will accept 3.5 mm cortex screws. In the future these will be available in stainless steel as well. The elongated hole is used for preliminary fixation to permit adjustment of the plate along the axis of the bone.
The plate is presently available with 3 or 4 holes in the shaft, and in lengths of 88 and 104 mm.

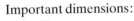

Important dimensions:
- Profile: See figure
- Thickness: 1.2 mm (titanium 2.0 mm)

Kirschner Wires, 150 mm Long

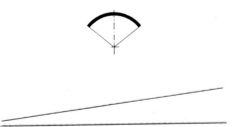

These wires of 1.25 mm diameter and 1.6 mm diameter are available for temporary fixation of small fragments. The trocar tip allows insertion with the small air drill using the Jacobs chuck. Pre-drilling with a drill bit of the nearest dimension is recommended in dense bone. The wires can be cut with a wire cutting forceps if desired. Further sizes of Kirschner wires exist. See SYNTHES catalogue.

6.9.2.3 Supplementary Implants

Reconstruction Plates, 3.5 mm, Straight

These plates are used with 3.5 mm cortex screws. Their main application is in pelvic and acetabular fractures. They may sometimes be used in fractures of the distal humerus (dorsolateral aspect), the clavicle, and the calcaneus. The reconstruction plates have notches alongside the plate, which enables bending in three dimensions. Special bending irons and pliers are available. Bending angles greater than 15° at any one site should be avoided. Note that the already low stiffness of the plate is further diminished by bending. If a strong curvature is needed, e. g. for the pelvis, it is better to choose the pre-bent, curved reconstruction plate. See Sect. 6.10.3.

The oval holes permit some self-compression if the screw is inserted eccentrically. The holes also accept 4.0 mm cancellous bone screws if the plate is placed over cancellous bone area. Screws can be inserted at an angle of approximately 25° longitudinally and 7° sideways. The plates are available in lengths from 58 mm to 262 mm, with 5 to 22 holes.

Important dimensions:
- Profile: See figure
- Thickness: 2.8 mm
- Width: 10 mm
- Hole spacing: 12 mm

Cerclage Wires

These wires in dimensions 1.0 mm and 1.25 mm diameter are sometimes used for the fixation of small fragments in the ankle, the elbow and the wrist. Further sizes cerclage wires exist. See SYNTHES catalogue.

6.9.2.4 Obsolete Implants

3.5 mm Cancellous Bone Screws, Fully Threaded

These screws are no longer manufactured. They have been replaced with the fully threaded 4.0 mm cancellous bone screws.

Y Plate

This plate with side notches was designed for condylar fractures of the humerus. The plate could be bent in three dimensions to conform to the bone. It was also possible to cut the plate to desired size. The oval holes permitted some axial compression. Due to its low stiffness and difficulties in its removal, because of its Y shape, it is no longer manufactured. Fractures of the distal humerus are better fixed with the existing straight small fragment plates.

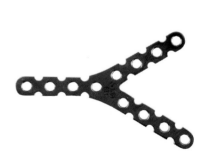

Instrumentation and Techniques

6.9.3 Fixation Techniques with Small Fragment Implants

6.9.3.1 Fixation Techniques with Small Fragment Screws

Small fragment screws are used as lag screws, plate fixation screws, or as transfixing or positioning screws (3.5 mm cortex screw). The principles of the fixation techniques are the same as for the large screws, as are the principles of screw orientation. See Sect. 6.4.1.4. The smaller the size of the instruments and implants, the greater becomes the importance of precise technique.

4.0 mm Cancellous Bone Screw, Partially Threaded, Used as Lag Screw

In fractures of the ankle, the elbow, and the wrist, 4.0 mm cancellous bone screws are often inserted as lag screws, either separately or through a plate hole. Because of its deep thread, smooth shaft and fairly large screw head, substantial interfragmentary compression can be achieved. The thread must have purchase in the far fragment only, the shaft allow gliding in the near fragment, and the screw head must have a secure seat on the bone surface. The position of the screw, if placed separately, is more or less at right angles to the fracture plane.

Lag screw principle: The screw thread must have purchase in the far fragment only.

Step by step procedure for the example of a shear fragment of the lateral malleolus:
– The fracture is reduced with a pointed reduction forceps and temporarily fixed with a Kirschner wire (Fig. 1).
– The thread hole is drilled using the 2.5 mm drill bit in the double drill sleeve, 2.5 mm. If a Kirschner wire has been inserted for reduction, parallel drilling is possible by placing the wire through the hole near the sleeve (Fig. 2).
– A recess is cut in a thick cortex with the countersink (Fig. 3).

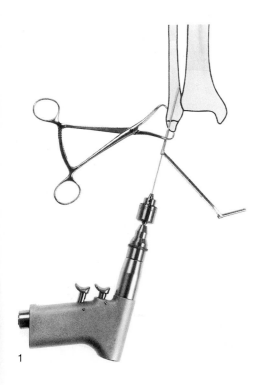

1

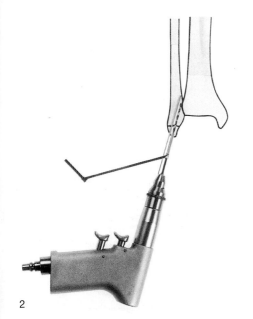

2

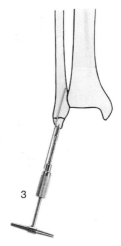

3

- The screw length is measured (Fig. 4).
- In hard, juvenile bone the thread may have to be cut using the tap for 4.0 mm cancellous bone screws in the double drill sleeve end 3.5 mm (Fig. 5).
- The selected screw is inserted with the small hexagonal screwdriver (Fig. 6).
- If the screw is inserted as a separate lag screw and the cortex is thin, a washer is used to prevent the screw head from sinking into the bone. The flat side of the washer is placed on the bone, the recessed side in contact with the head.
- The Kirschner wire is cut, bent , and the end impacted in the bone to secure the fixation (Fig. 7, 8).

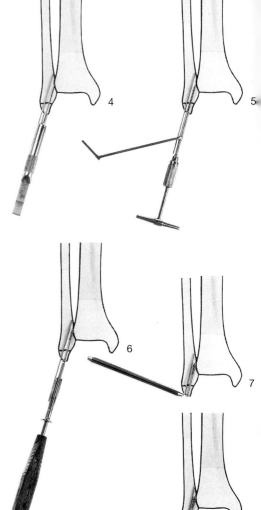

4.0 mm Cancellous Bone Screw, Fully Threaded, Used as Plate Fixation Screw

This screw is mainly used as a plate fixation screw for small fragment plates located over cancellous bone area. Here, the wide thread gives the screw good purchase. This screw is not used as a lag screw, this function being served by the partially threaded screw.

Step by step procedure:
- The thread hole is drilled through the plate hole using the 2.5 mm drill bit in the double drill sleeve end, 2.5 mm.
- The length is measured.
- The cortex is tapped with the tap for 4.0 mm cancellous bone screws in the double drill sleeve end, 3.5 mm.
- The selected screw is inserted with the small hexagonal screwdriver.

3.5 mm Cortex Screw Applied as a Lag Screw

This screw is ideal for fixation of fragments in the diaphyses of small bones such as the forearm, the fibula, and the clavicle. It is also used in larger bones for the fixation of small fragments. A lag screw technique must be used whenever the screw crosses a fracture, even through a plate.

Lag screw principle: The screw thread must have purchase in the far fragment only.

Step by step procedure:
- The fracture is reduced and temporarily fixed.
- The gliding or clearance hole is drilled in the near cortex using the 3.5 mm drill bit and the double drill sleeve end, 3.5 mm (Fig. 1).
- The 2.5 mm end of the double drill sleeve is pushed into the gliding hole until it abuts the far cortex. The thread hole drilled

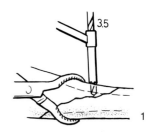

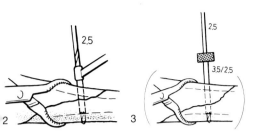

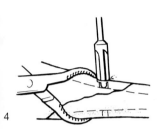
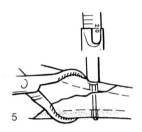

in the far cortex with the 2.5 mm drill bit through the sleeve (Fig. 2). The insert sleeve 3.5 mm/2.5 mm may be used as an alternative (Fig. 3).

– The countersink is used in areas where the screw head is seated upon thick cortex as a separate lag screw (Fig. 4).
– The screw length is measured (Fig. 5).
– The thread hole is tapped with the tap for 3.5 mm cortex screws in the double drill sleeve end, 3.5 mm (Fig. 6).
– The screw is inserted and tightened with the small hexagonal screwdriver. Interfragmentary compression is achieved (Fig. 7).

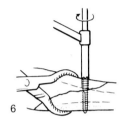
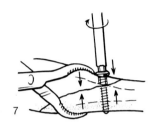

3.5 mm Cortex Screw Applied as a Plate Fixation Screw

Any small fragment plate used for diaphyseal fractures is fixed with 3.5 mm cortex screws. It should ideally have purchase in both cortices, unless the screw crosses a fracture,.

Step by step procedure:
– Using the 2.5 mm drill bit in the double drill sleeve end, 2.5 mm, the thread hole is drilled through both cortices.
– The length is measured.
– The drilled hole is tapped with the tap for 3.5 mm cortex screws in the 3.5 mm double drill sleeve end.
– The screw is inserted with the small hexagonal screwdriver.

3.5 mm Cortex Screw Applied as a Transfixing or Positioning Screw

Transfixing the fibula to the tibia is indicated if, after internal fixation of a fibular fracture in a type C malleolar injury, the syndesmosis remain unstable. It may also be used in the type C subcapital fibular fracture (Maisonneuve fracture), when direct fibular internal fixation is precluded. The screw engages at least three cortices; two in the fibula and one in the tibia (three-point contact). The position of the screw is approximately 4–6 cm proximal to the ankle joint. It is inserted obliquely from back to front at an angle of 25° – 30°. It is directed from the lateral to the medial cortex of the fibula, and into the lateral cortex of the tibia at right angles to the long axis.

A transfixing screw can also be inserted through a plate hole or beside a plate.

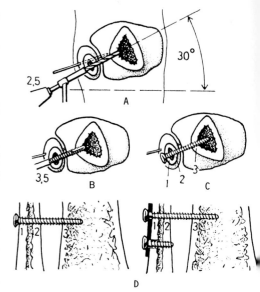

Step by step procedure:
- The fibular fracture is reduced, and provisionally transfixed to the tibia with a horizontal 1.6 mm Kirschner wire.
- Using the 2.5 mm drill bit in the double drill sleeve end, 2.5 mm both cortices of the fibula (1 and 2) and at least one of the tibia (3) are drilled. A recess for the screw head must *not* be cut, since this may weaken the bone (A).
- The length is measured.
- With the fibula carefully held in its fully reduced position, the fibular and tibial cortices are tapped using the tap for 3.5 mm cortex screws in the double drill sleeve end, 3.5 mm (B).
- Insertion of the appropriate cortex screw with the small hexagonal screwdriver (also through a plate if necessary). The screw will not exert any compression as there is no gliding hole, and all cortices have been tapped (D).
- Careful tightening of the screw.

3.5 mm Titanium Shaft Screw Used as a Lag Screw in a LC-DCP, 3.5 mm

The shaft screw is designed as a partially threaded screw with a shaft diameter of 3.5 mm. It therefore can be used as a lag screw gaining purchase only in the far fragment. The smooth shaft ensures gliding in the near fragment. The shaft screw is mainly used in the LC-DCP, 3.5 mm.

Lag screw principle: The screw thread must have purchase in the far fragment only.

Thread Hole First Technique

Preparing the thread hole before the gliding hole ensures exact position of the lag screw in the plate hole.

Step by step procedure:
- The fracture is reduced and the plate fixed to the main fragments.
- The thread hole is drilled through both cortices using the 2.5 mm drill bit in the LC-DCP universal drill guide, 3.5 mm. The drill guide is pressed into the plate hole in the desired direction. The neutral (green) LC-DCP drill guide, 3.5 mm, with the arrow pointing towards the fracture, may also be used.
- The screw length is measured with the depth gauge, 3.5–4.0 mm.

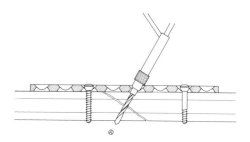

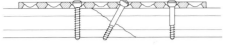

– The thread hole is tapped with the tap for 3.5 mm cortex screws in the 3.5 mm end of the double drill sleeve, or of the universal drill guide.
– Maintaining the direction, the thread hole is carefully over-drilled in the first cortex with the 3.5 mm drill bit in one of the 3.5 mm guides mentioned above.
– The shaft screw is inserted with the small hexagonal screw-driver.

Gliding Hole First Technique

Step by step procedure:
– The fracture is reduced and the plate fixed to the main frag-ments.
– The gliding hole is drilled in the near fragment adjacent to the fracture using the 3.5 mm drill bit in the double drill sleeve, 3.5 mm.
– The double drill sleeve is turned around and the 2.5 mm sleeve pushed into the gliding hole until it abuts the endosteal cortex of the far fragment.
– The thread hole is drilled in the far cortex with the 2.5 mm drill bit through the 2.5 mm sleeve.
– The screw length is measured with the depth gauge, 3.5–4.0 mm.
– The thread hole is tapped with the tap for 3.5 mm cortex screws in the double drill sleeve end, 3.5 mm.
– The selected shaft screw is inserted with the small hexagonal screwdriver. Interfragmentary compression is achieved.

The 3.5 mm Titanium Shaft Screw Applied as a Load Screw in a LC-DCP

Since the smooth shaft has the same diameter as the thread it provides improved stiffness and strength when the screw is used, as load screw, for axial compression. For this application It is possible to use either the LC-DCP drill guide, 3.5 mm, or the LC-DCP universal drill guide, 3.5 mm.

Step by step procedure:
– The plate is fixed to the bone with a neutral screw in the frag-ment whose fracture surface forms an obtuse angle with the underside of the plate.
– On the opposite side of the reduced fracture the LC-DCP drill guide, 3.5 mm for compression is positioned in the plate hole with the arrow pointing toward the fracture. The thread hole is drilled through both cortices with the 2.5 mm drill bit. This hole is now in eccentric position.

Variation:

– The LC-DCP universal drill guide, 4.5 mm is placed with its protruding sleeve in eccentric position in the plate hole, away from the fracture. The thread hole is drilled with the 2.5 mm drill bit.
– The screw length is measured.
– Tapping of the thread hole with the tap for 3.5 mm cortex screw in the double drill sleeve end, 3.5 mm.
– The near cortex is carefully overdrilled with the 3.5 mm drill bit in the double drill sleeve end, 3.5 mm.
– Insertion of the selected 3.5 mm titanium shaft screw with the small hexagonal screwdriver. Interfragmentary compression is achieved.

6.9.3.2 Fixation Technique with Small Fragment Plates

The fixation technique of an implant will depend upon the local anatomy and the fracture type. The following examples serve as guidelines only.

One-Third Tubular Plate Applied as Tension Band Plate

The plate is applied as tension band plate in certain short oblique or transverse fractures, e.g. the fibula, the metatarsus, the distal ulna and the olecranon.

Prerequisites:
– The plate is applied to the tension side of the bone.
– The plate is contoured to the shape of the bone using a template as a model. In transverse fractures the plate is also slightly overbent. See p. 182.
– Axial compression is achieved by eccentric placement of screws in the plate holes adjacent to the fracture.

Plate length:
– Five to six cortices in each main fragment should be engaged.

Step by step procedure:
– After reduction the contoured and slightly overbent plate is applied to the bone with reduction forceps.
– The first screw hole is drilled in one of the plate holes near the fracture using the 2.5 mm drill bit in the double drill sleeve end, 2.5 mm (Fig. 1).
– The screw length is measured (Fig. 2).
– The thread hole is tapped with the tap for 3.5 mm cortex screws in the double drill sleeve end, 3.5 mm (Fig. 3).
– The selected 3.5 mm cortex screw is inserted with the small hexagonal screwdriver, but not fully tightened (Fig. 4).
– The plate is then pulled towards the fracture to place this screw in the eccentric position.

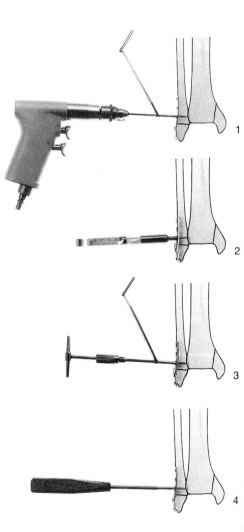

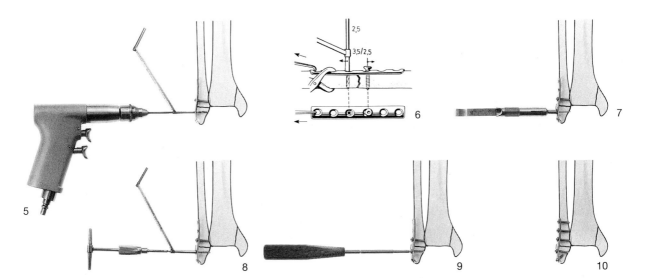

- In the plate hole near the fracture in the opposite fragment, the second screw hole is drilled with the 2.5 mm drill bit and the double drill sleeve end, 2.5 mm. This drill hole is placed in the eccentric (load) position, away from the fracture (Fig. 5, 6).
- The length is measured (Fig. 7).
- If this screw comes to lie in cancellous bone a 4.0 mm fully threaded cancellous bone screw is chosen. Tapping of the thread hole with the tap for 4.0 mm cancellous bone screws in the double drill sleeve end, 3.5 mm (Fig. 8).
- Insertion of the proper length fully threaded cancellous bone screw. The first screw inserted and tightened (Fig. 9).
- The remaining plate screws are inserted alternating from one side of the fracture to the other using the technique described above.
- Final tightening of all screws (Fig. 10).

One-Third Tubular Plate Applied as a Neutralisation Plate

The one-third tubular plate is applied as a neutralisation plate in spiral fractures or fractures with a butterfly fragment, e. g. in the fibula and the distal ulna. It is applied after primary interfragmentary fixation with lag screws. The function of the plate is to neutralise any shearing or bending forces which could disrupt an unprotected lag screw fixation.

Prerequisites:
- Lag screw fixation first separately.
- Contouring of the plate. See p. 182.

Plate length:
- Four to five cortices in each main fragment should be engaged.

Small Fragment Instruments and Implants

Step by step procedure:
- The fracture is reduced and temporary fixation applied.
- A separate 3.5 mm cortex screw is inserted as lag screw in the butterfly fragment using the technique described on p. 196.
- The plate site and shape is determined by means of a template. The plate is then exactly contoured, and fixed to the bone with forceps.
- The drill bit 2.5 mm in the double drill sleeve end, 2.5 mm is used to drill the screw hole.
- The screw length is measured.
- The tap, 3.5 mm in the double drill sleeve, 3.5 mm is used to cut the thread.
- The selected 3.5 mm cortex screw is inserted using the small hexagonal screwdriver.
- The second plate screw is inserted in a similar manner on the opposite side of the fracture.
- Alternating from one side to the other the remaining 3.5 mm cortex screws are inserted.
- Should the plate end lie over cancellous bone, a 4.0 mm fully threaded cancellous bone screw is used in the last plate hole.

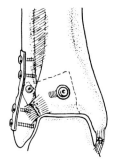

The one-third tubular plate can also be applied as buttress plate in certain fracture situations. All screws are then placed in the buttress position, that is as near the fracture as possible in the plate hole.

The DCP, 3.5 mm Applied as a Self-Compression Plate

The effect of self compression is used for axial compression of short oblique, or transverse fractures of for example, the forearm, clavicle, and pelvis (tension band plating).

Prerequisites:
- The plate is contoured to the bone, and in transverse fractures slightly overbent. See p. 182.
- Axial compression by one or more load screws.

Plate length:
- At least six cortices in each main fragment should be engaged.

Step by step procedure:
- The fracture is reduced. The contoured plate is applied to the bone with the middle portion placed over the fracture, and held with reduction forceps.
- In the plate hole adjacent to the fracture, the first screw hole is drilled using the 2.5 mm drill bit in the DCP drill guide, 3.5 mm (Fig. 1).
- The screw length is measured.
- The tap for 3.5 mm cortex screw in the double drill sleeve end, 3.5 mm is used to cut the thread.

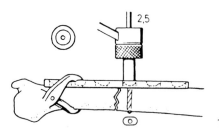

2,5

1

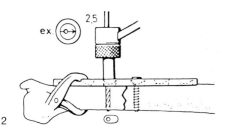

2

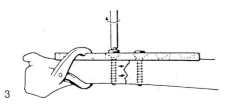

3

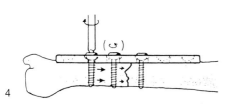

4

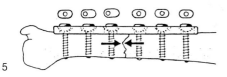

5

– The chosen 3.5 mm cortex screw is inserted with the small hexagonal screwdriver, but not fully tightened.
– The plate is pulled towards the fracture to place the first screw in the eccentric position.
– The second screw hole is prepared in the plate hole adjacent to the fracture in the opposite fragment. The load (yellow) DCP drill guide is placed in the plate hole with the arrow pointing towards the fracture, The thread hole is then drilled with the 2.5 mm drill bit (Fig. 2).
– The screw length is measured.
– The thread is cut with the tap for 3.5 mm cortex screw in the double drill sleeve end, 3.5 mm.
– The 3.5 mm cortex screw is inserted with the small hexagonal screwdriver. Tightening of the two screws produces axial compression (Fig. 3).
– An addition load screw can be inserted if necessary.
– In the next plate hole the load (yellow) DCP drill guide, 3.5 mm is positioned with the arrow towards the fracture. The hole is drilled with the 2.5 mm drill bit.
– The screw length is measured.
– The tap for 3.5 mm cortex screw in the double drill sleeve end, 3.5 mm is used to cut the thread.
– The 3.5 mm cortex screw is inserted until the screw head reaches the plate hole.
– Before the screw is tightened completely, the screw next to it must be loosened to allow for further compression. After tightening of this last load screw, the loosened screw can be retightened (Fig. 4).
– If the compression is sufficient, the remaining screws are inserted alternating from one side to the other: Drill bit 2.5 mm in the neutral DCP drill guide, depth gauge, tap and screw.
– Final tightening of all screws (Fig. 5).
– If any greater displacement is required than can be achieved by three load screws (i. e. >3 mm), the articulated tension device should be used instead.

DCP 3.5 mm Applied as a Self-Compressing Plate with Lag Screw Through the Plate

This technique is used in oblique fractures, where optimal stability can be achieved by combining the self-compressing effect of the DCP for axial compression, and the interfragmentary compression of a lag screw.

Prerequisites:
– The plate is contoured to the bone and placed such that one plate hole can be used for the lag screw.

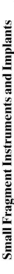

Plate length:
– Six cortices in each main fragment should be engaged by screws.

Step by step procedure:
– The fracture is reduced. The contoured plate is placed on the bone with the wider middle portion over the fracture. A plate hole is left vacant for an angled lag screw through the plate. The plate is held in position by two reduction forceps.
– In the fragment which fracture surface forms an obtuse angle with the undersurface of the plate, the drill bit 2.5 mm in the neutral (green) DCP drill guide, 3.5 mm is used to drill the first hole, near the fracture (Fig. 1).
– The length is measured (Fig. 2).
– The tap for 3.5 mm cortex screws in the double drill sleeve end, 3.5 mm is used to cut the thread (Fig. 3).
– The 3.5 mm cortex screw is inserted but not fully tightened (Fig. 4). The plate is pulled towards the opposite fragment to place the screw in an eccentric position in the plate hole.
– On the opposite side of the fracture the first plate hole is left vacant for the lag screw. In the next hole the load (yellow) DCP drill guide, 3.5 mm is placed with the arrow pointing towards the fracture. The thread hole then drilled with the 2.5 mm drill bit (Fig. 5).
– The screw length is measured (Fig. 6).
– The thread is cut with the tap for 3.5 mm cortex screws in the double drill sleeve, 3.5 mm (Fig. 7).
– The chosen 3.5 mm cortex screw is inserted (Fig. 8). Before the screw is fully tightened, the first screw is driven home. Axial compression is achieved.
– The position for the oblique lag screw through the plate is determined. The angulation of the screw must not exceed ±25° longitudinally and ±7° transversely.
– The gliding hole is drilled in the near cortex using the 3.5 mm drill bit in the double drill sleeve end, 3.5 mm (Fig. 9).
– The 2.5 mm end of this sleeve is then pushed into the hole until it abuts the endosteal cortex of the far fragment. The thread hole is drilled with the 2.5 mm drill bit (Fig. 10).
– After measuring and tapping, the chosen 3.5 mm cortex screw is inserted and carefully tightened. Interfragmentary compression is enhanced (Fig. 11).
– The remaining screws are inserted one by one, alternating from one side to the other: Drilling, measuring, tapping and inserting the screw.
– Final tightening of all screws (Fig. 12).

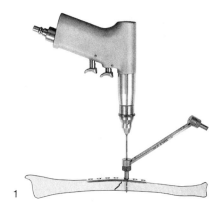

1

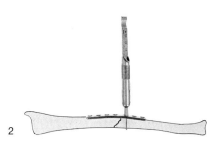

2

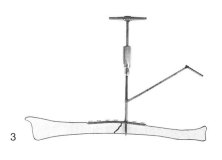

3

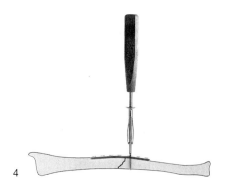

4

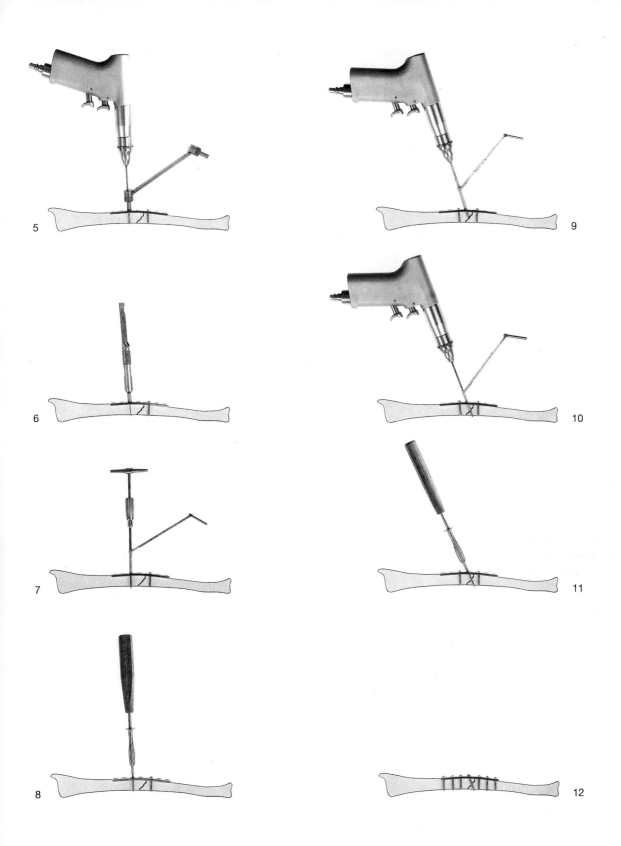

5

6

7

8

9

10

11

12

The DCP 3.5 mm Applied as a Compression Plate Using the Articulated Tension Device. Lag Screw Through the Plate

Axial compression can be achieved by using the articulated tension device instead of the self compressing DCP holes. This is recommended especially if the bone ends are markedly separated. Reduction of interdigitating fragments as well as fine rotational adjustments is easier. If a plate screw crosses the fracture, it should be inserted as a lag screw.

Prerequisites:
- Enough space for the articulated tension device on one side of the fracture.
- Prebending of the plate (see p. 182).

Plate length:
- At least six cortices in each main fragment should be engaged.

Step by step procedure:
- After preliminary reduction, the contoured plate is fixed to the bone with reduction forceps.
- In the fragment which forms an obtuse angle with the undersurface of the plate the first plate hole is drilled with the 2.5 mm drill bit in the neutral DCP drill guide, 3.5 mm. The hole is measured, and then tapped with the tap for 3.5 mm cortex screws in the double drill sleeve end, 3.5 mm. Then the chosen 3.5 mm cortex screw is inserted. A second screw is inserted in this fragment using the same technique

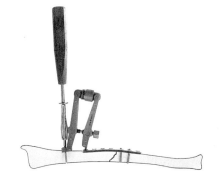

- On the opposite side of the fracture, the opened articulated tension device is hooked into the end plate hole. After drilling, measuring and tapping through the foot-plate, the device is fixed to the bone with a 3.5 mm cortex screw.
- The articulated tension device is carefully tightened using the open end wrench. During tightening the fragments are manoeuvred into correct alignment and rotation until they are compressed.
- If a lag screw is to be inserted, the plate hole nearest the fracture in the opposite fragment is used for this. The gliding hole is prepared in the near cortex with the 3.5 mm drill bit in the 3.5 mm double drill sleeve end. The angulation of the screw must not exceed ±25° longitudinally, and ±7° transversely.
- The 2.5 mm end of the double drill sleeve is pushed into the gliding hole until it abuts the endosteal cortex of the far fragment. The thread hole in the far fragment is prepared with the 2.5 mm drill bit.
- The length is measured.
- The tap for 3.5 mm cortex screws in the double drill sleeve end, 3.5 mm is used to tap the thread hole.
- The chosen 3.5 mm cortex screw is inserted and interfragmentary compression is achieved.

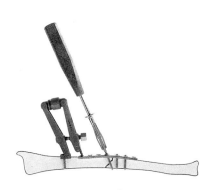

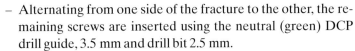

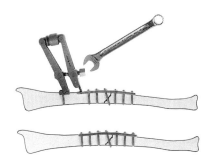

- Alternating from one side of the fracture to the other, the remaining screws are inserted using the neutral (green) DCP drill guide, 3.5 mm and drill bit 2.5 mm.
- The articulated tension device is removed, and the screw in the end plate hole inserted.
- Final tightening of all screws.

DCP, 3.5 mm Applied as a Neutralisation Plate

In spiral fractures of the diaphysis or in a fracture with a wedge fragment, primary stability may be obtained by lag screws. A neutralisation plate is applied to protect the lag screw fixation from bending and shearing forces.

Prerequisites:
- Lag screw fixation of the main fragment.
- Exact contouring of the plate see p. 182.

Plate length:
- Five to six cortices in each main fragment.

Step by step procedure:
- The reduced fracture is fixed with separate 3.5 mm cortex screws as lag screws, using the technique described in Sect. 6.9.3.1.
- The contoured plate is held to the bone with reduction forceps.
- All screws are inserted in the neutral position using the 2.5 mm drill bit in the 3.5 mm DCP neutral (green) drill guide, the depth gauge 3.5 mm – 4.0 mm, the tap for 3.5 mm cortex screws in the double drill sleeve end, 3.5 mm, and the small hexagonal screwdriver.

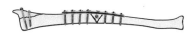

Note: The use of the load (yellow) DCP drill guide is not necessary and may be dangerous. The force exerted could disrupt the interfragmentary compression achieved by the lag screws inserted before applying the plate.

DCP, 3.5 mm Applied as a Buttress Plate

A buttress plate protects a metaphyseal fragment from secondary collapse, or prevents shortening of a comminuted diaphyseal fragment e. g. distal humerus fractures.

Prerequisites:
- Careful contouring of the plate see p. 182.
- All screws are inserted in the buttress position, avoiding compression.

Plate length:
- Depends on the fracture localisation.

Step by step procedure:
- The contoured plate is applied to the reduced fracture using reduction forceps.
- In the main fragment, near the fracture, the double drill sleeve end, 3.5 mm is placed in the plate hole so that it occupies a "buttress" position. This is in the end of the plate hole nearest the fracture. The thread hole is then drilled with the 2.5 mm drill bit in the double drill sleeve end, 2.5 mm.
- The screw length is measured.
- The thread is tapped using the tap for 3.5 mm cortex screw in the double drill sleeve end, 3.5 mm.
- The chosen 3.5 mm cortex screw is inserted with the small hexagonal screwdriver.
- The next screw is inserted in the opposite fragment, in the plate hole nearest the fracture. This screw hole is also prepared in buttress position using the same technique as for the first screw.
- All remaining plate screws are inserted in the buttress position alternating from one side of the fracture to the other.
- If the plate end is positioned over a cancellous bone area, the fully threaded 4.0 mm cancellous bone screw is used.

The LC-DCP, 3.5 mm Applied as Compression Plate with Lag Screw Through the Plate

In an oblique fracture, the plate can be applied to achieve both axial and interfragmentary compression by inserting a load screw and a lag screw through the plate. The uniform hole spacing and the evenly distributed stiffness along the plate makes positioning and contouring of the plate easier. Titanium screws are used in titanium plates.

Prerequisite:
- Prebending of the plate see p. 182.

Plate length:
- Each main fragment must have screws anchored within at least six cortices, and the screws must be spaced as evenly as possible.
- Plate holes can be left free if necessary, or occupied with a short, single-cortex screw.

Step by step procedure:
- The fracture is reduced, and the pre-bent plate temporarily fixed to the bone with reduction forceps. The plate is positioned carefully, and one screw hole in the middle left vacant for the lag screw.
- The first screw is inserted near the fracture in the fragment which fracture surface forms an obtuse angle with the under-

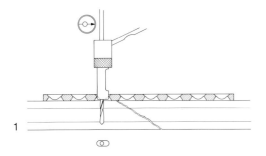

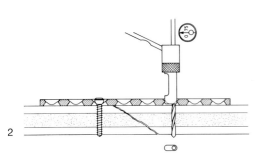

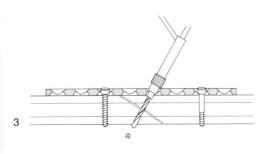

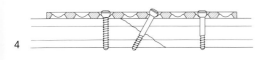

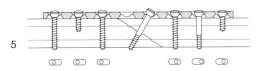

surface of the plate. The neutral (green) LC-DCP drill guide, 3.5 mm is placed in the plate hole with its arrow pointing towards the fracture. The thread hole is drilled with the 2.5 mm drill bit (Fig. 1).

– The screw length is measured.
– The thread hole is tapped with the tap for 3.5 mm cortex screws in the 3.5 mm end of the double drill sleeve.
– The chosen 3.5 mm titanium cortex screw is inserted with the small hexagonal screwdriver, but not fully tightened.
– The plate is pulled towards the fracture, which places this screw in an eccentric (load) position.
– The plate hole nearest the fracture in the opposite fragment is left vacant for the lag screw. In the adjacent, suitable plate hole the LC-DCP load (yellow) guide, 3.5 mm is placed with the arrow pointing towards the fracture. The thread hole is drilled with the 2.5 mm drill bit (Fig. 2).
– After measuring the length, the far fragment is tapped with the tap for 3.5 mm cortex screws in the double drill sleeve end, 3.5 mm.
– The near cortex is then overdrilled with the 3.5 mm drill bit in the double drill sleeve end, 3.5 mm. A shaft screw is used for maximum screw strength for the axial compression.
– The chosen 3.5 mm titanium shaft screw is inserted and fully tightened, but only after the screw in the opposite fragment has been driven home. Axial compression is achieved.

Note: A second and even a third load screw can be inserted if further compression is necessary using the same technique just described. Before tightening the screw, the adjacent load screw has to be loosened.

– The thread hole for the lag screw is now prepared in the plate hole which was left vacant. The LC-DCP universal drill guide, 3.5 mm is pressed into the plate hole in the desired direction. This ensures a congruent fit between screw head and plate hole. Both cortices are drilled with the 2.5 mm drill bit (Fig. 3).
– After measuring, the hole is tapped with the tap for 3.5 mm cortex screws, in the 3.5 mm end of the universal drill guide.
– The near cortex is then overdrilled with the 3.5 mm drill bit in the 3.5 mm end of the universal drill guide.
– The chosen 3.5 mm titanium shaft screw is inserted. Interfragmentary compression is achieved (Fig. 4).
– The remaining screws are inserted using the neutral LC-DCP drill guide, 3.5 mm.
– Final tightening of all screws (Fig. 5).

Variation 1

The LC-DCP universal drill guide, 3.5 mm can be used instead of the LC-DCP drill guide for all screw holes. The neutral position for screws is obtained by pressing the guide into the plate hole. The load position is obtained by positioning the protruding tip of the inner sleeve in the plate hole eccentrically, away from the fracture.

Variation 2

The articulated tension device may be used with the LC-DCP, whenever larger compression is required, i. e. in widely separated fractures, in porotic bone in some pseudarthroses, or in metaphyseal applications. The LC-DCP is fixed first to the fragment whose fracture surface forms an obtuse angle with the undersurface of the plate. The plate is fixed with at least two screws. Then the open articulated tension device is mounted in the opposite end of the plate, and the foot-plate fixed to the bone with a 3.5 mm cortex screw. Axial compression is achieved by carefully tightening the bolt of the device. The remaining screws in this fragment are inserted before the tension device is loosened and removed. The screw used to fix the device should be discarded and not used, as it has been stressed. See also p. 206.

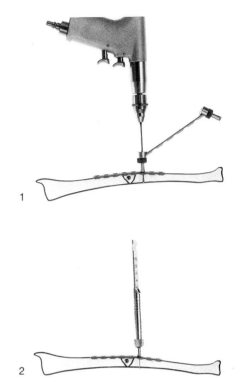

1

LC-DCP, 3.5 mm Applied as a Neutralisation Plate

2

In spiral fractures, or fractures with a wedge fragment, a LC-DCP, 3.5 mm may be used instead of a DCP, 3.5 mm. Because of its uniform hole spacing positioning of the LC-DCP may be easier. Titanium screws are used with titanium plates.

Prerequisites:
– Lag screw fixation of the fracture prior to plate application.
– Exact contouring of the plate see p. 182.

Plate length:
– At least six cortices in each main fragment should be fixed by screws. The quality of the bone finally determines the number of screws.

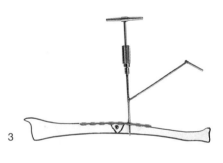

Step by step procedure:
– The fracture is reduced, and fixed with either 3.5 mm or 2.7 mm cortex screws as separate lag screws. See pp. 178 and 249.
– The carefully contoured plate is applied to the bone with two reduction forceps.
– The first screw is inserted in one of the main fragments without crossing the fracture. The 2.5 mm drill bit in the 3.5 mm LC-DCP drill guide is used to drill the thread hole (Fig. 1).
– The screw length is measured with the depth gauge (Fig. 2).
– The hole is tapped with the tap for 3.5 mm cortex screws in the double drill sleeve end, 3.5 mm (Fig. 3).
– Insertion of the 3.5 mm titanium cortex screw with the small hexagonal screwdriver (Fig. 4).

3

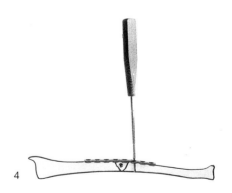

4

Instrumentation and Techniques

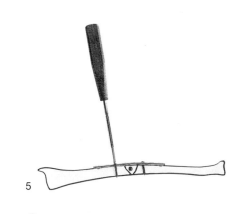

5

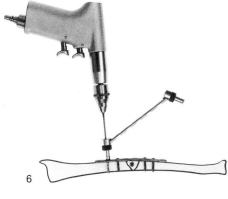

6

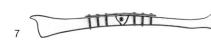

7

– The second 3.5 mm titanium cortex screw is inserted in the opposite main fragment using the same technique (Fig. 5).
– The remaining screws are inserted alternating from one side of the fracture to the other The neutral (green) LC-DCP drill guide, 3.5 mm in the 2.5 mm drill bit is used to drill the thread hole. Measuring and tapping of the thread hole. Insertion of the screw (Fig. 6).
– Final tightening of all screws (Fig. 7).

Note: Not all plate holes need to be occupied with screws. A short screw can be inserted, if the fracture location requires.

LC-DCP, 3.5 mm Applied as a Buttress Plate

Similar to the DCP, 3.5 mm, the LC-DCP, 3.5 mm can be used as a buttress or as a bridging plate to prevent fracture zone collapse in, for example the forearm.

Prerequisites:
– Careful contouring of the plate see p. 182.
– All screws should be inserted in buttress position to avoid compression.

Plate length:
– Depends on the fracture localisation.

Step by step procedure:
– The fracture is reduced and the contoured plate applied to the bone with reduction forceps, holding the bone out to length.
– The first screw is inserted near the fracture using the neutral LC-DCP drill guide, 3.5 mm with the arrow pointing **away** from the fracture. The thread hole is drilled with the 2.5 mm drill bit.
– The screw length is measured and the hole tapped with the tap for 3.5 mm cortex screws in the double drill sleeve end, 3.5 mm.
– The chosen 3.5 mm titanium cortex screw is inserted with the small hexagonal screwdriver and tightened firmly.
– In the opposite fragment the procedure is repeated: Using the neutral (green) LC-DCP drill guide with the arrow pointing *away* from the fracture the thread hole is drilled, measured, tapped, and the 3.5 mm titanium cortex screw inserted.
– If required, a lag screw can be inserted through the plate. Depending on the location it may be a cortex or a cancellous bone screw.
– The remaining screws are inserted in the buttress position using the technique described for the first screw.
– Final tightening of all screws.

Application of Small T Plates

The small T-plates are mainly used for buttressing fractures in the distal radius. If a screw crosses the fracture it should be inserted as a lag screw.

Prerequisites:
– Exact contouring of the plate to the bone surface using pliers.

Plate length:
– Three, four, or five screws in the shaft fragment will depend on the extent of the fracture complex.

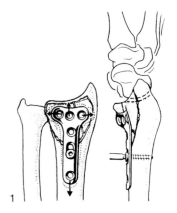

Step by step procedure:
– Preliminary reduction of the fracture, usually with Kirschner wires.
– The contoured plate is temporarily applied to the main fragment with a screw in the oval hole. The drill bit 2.5 mm in the double drill sleeve end, 2.5 mm is used to drill the thread hole.
– The screw length is measured.
– The thread hole is tapped in both cortices with the tap for 3.5 mm cortex screws in the double drill sleeve end, 3.5 mm.
– The 3.5 mm cortex screw is inserted with the small hexagonal screwdriver, but not fully tightened.
– Final reduction is carried out, and the plate position adjusted. The screw in the oval hole is tightened (Fig. 1).
– The plate head is fixed with 4.0 mm cancellous bone screws. The drill bit 2.5 mm in the double drill sleeve end, 3.5 mm is used to prepare the thread hole.
– Measuring and tapping.
– If the screw crosses a fracture, a partially threaded 4.0 mm cancellous bone screw is inserted as a lag screw (screw thread only in the far fragment). If the screw does not cross the fracture a fully threaded 4.0 mm cancellous bone screw is used.
– The shaft is fixed with 3.5 mm cortex screws using the same technique described for the first screw.
– Final tightening of all screws (Fig. 2).

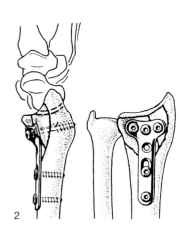

Application of the Cloverleaf Plate

The cloverleaf plate is mainly used as a buttress plate in the distal tibia. Bone graft is inserted in any metaphyseal defect. The plate is fixed with small fragment screws in the head portion and 4.5 mm cortex screws in the shaft. If the recent introduced titanium cloverleaf plate is used, the shaft accommodates 3.5 mm cortex screws in the diaphysis.

Prerequisites:
– Careful contouring and trimming of the plate, to the desired shape. This can be achieved by removing selected lugs with a plate-cutting forceps if necessary.
– Lag screws through the plate whenever possible.

Plate length:
– Three or four holes in the shaft, depending on the fracture pattern.

Step by step procedure:
– The fracture is reduced and temporarily fixed with Kirschner wires.
– The contoured plate is applied and fixed to the shaft with reduction forceps.
– Separate lag screws (mainly 4.0 mm cancellous bone screws) are inserted in the metaphyseal zone, replacing some of the Kirschner wires. (See technique, p. 195.)
– In the distal portion of the plate in one of the holes, the 2.5 mm drill bit in the 2.5 mm double drill sleeve end is used to drill the thread hole.
– The screw length is measured and the near cortex tapped with the tap for 4.0 mm cancellous bone screws in the 3.5 mm double drill sleeve end.
– The chosen 4.0 mm cancellous bone screw is inserted with the small hexagonal screwdriver. A partially threaded 4.0 mm cancellous bone screw is inserted as a lag screw (the thread only in the far fragment), if a fracture line is crossed, otherwise a fully threaded screw is used.
– The plate is fixed to the shaft with either 4.5 mm cortex screws (stainless steel plates) or 3.5 mm cortex screws (titanium plates) (Fig. 1).
– If necessary, bone graft is applied.
– Further plate holes in the head portion are fixed with 4.0 mm cancellous bone screws. It is not always necessary to fill all the holes.
– Constant attention is given to the correct position of each individual fragment while applying the plate.
– If suitable, the oval hole can be used to insert an angled lag screw (Fig. 2).

Note: If stainless steel cloverleaf plates are used, the basic instrumentation is also needed.

Application of 3.5 mm Reconstruction Plate

Although the name implies that the plate is used for reconstruction as a buttress or bridging plate, it can also be used for compression in the diaphysis and especially in pelvic fractures. The oval holes allow eccentric positioning of screws, which can be used to achieve some axial compression as the following example shows.

Prerequisites:

Three-dimensional bending must not exceed 15° at any one site in any plane. The relatively low strength of the plate is otherwise further diminished and the plate holes may be distorted.

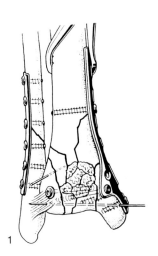

1

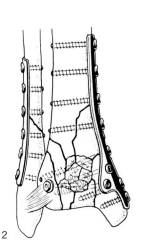

2

Plate length:

In general six cortices in each main fragment.

Step by step procedure:

– The fracture is reduced, and the carefully contoured plate applied to the bone with reduction forceps.
– The 2.5 mm drill bit in the 2.5 mm double drill sleeve end is used to drill the first thread hole near the fracture.
– The screw length is measured.
– The tap for 3.5 mm cortex screws in the 3.5 mm double drill sleeve end is used to cut the thread.
– The chosen 3.5 mm cortex screw is inserted with the small hexagonal screwdriver but not fully tightened. The plate is pulled toward the fracture to place this screw in an eccentric position.
– On the other side of the fracture in the plate hole closest to the fracture the 2.5 mm double drill sleeve end is placed eccentrically away from the fracture. The thread hole is drilled with the 2.5 mm drill bit.
– The length is measured, and the thread hole tapped using the tap for 3.5 mm cortex screws in the 3.5 mm double drill sleeve end.
– The chosen 3.5 mm cortex screw is inserted and fully tightened, once the first screw has been driven home. This produces axial compression.
– The remaining screws are inserted in the neutral position using the 2.5 mm drill bit in the 2.5 mm double drill sleeve end. After measuring and tapping, the screws are inserted.
– Final tightening of all screws.

Note: Any screw crossing the fracture should be inserted as a lag screw (the thread only gripping the far fragment).

Note: If the plate end overlies cancellous bone, a fully threaded 4.0 mm cancellous bone screw is used to fix the plate.

6.9.4 Instruments for Application and Removal of Small Fragment Implants

Instruments for the insertion of 4.0 mm cancellous bone screws

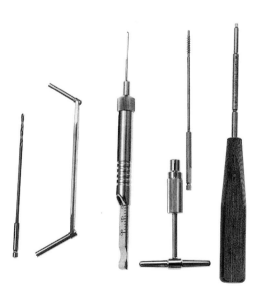

Instrumentation and Techniques

Instruments for the insertion of 3.5 mm cortex screws (fully threaded and shaft screws)

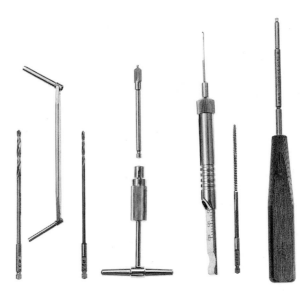

Instruments for the application of DCP, 3.5 mm

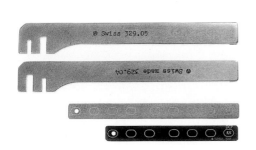
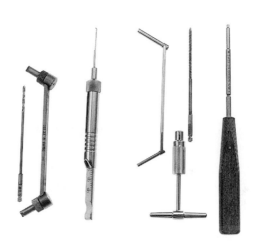

Instruments for the application of LC-DCP, 3.5 mm

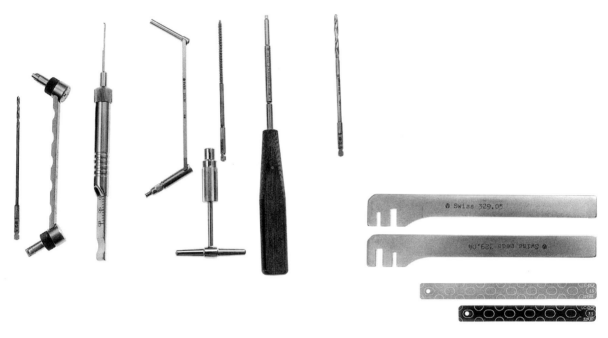

Instruments for the application of one-third tubular plates, small T plates, reconstruction plates, and cloverleaf plates

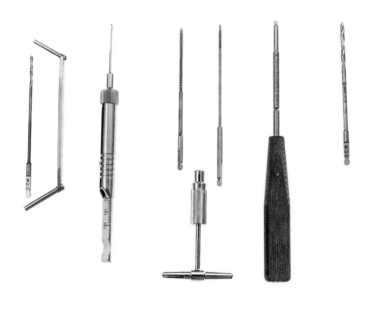

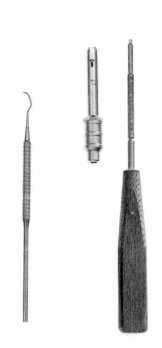

Instruments for the removal of small fragment implants.
- The screw head recess is carefully cleaned of debris, and the small hexagonal screwdriver used to remove the screws. If traction has to be applied to remove, for example, partially threaded screws, the screw-holding sleeve is employed.
- Small fragment plates are in general easy to loosen with a periosteal elevator, and can thereafter be removed.

6.10 Pelvic Instruments and Implants

Since internal fixation of pelvic and acetabular fractures has become more common, special instruments and implants have been developed.

6.10.1 Instruments for Screws and Plates

The instruments listed below will be available in either a graphic case or in a sterilising tray in the future. These sets have to be used in combination with the basic instrument set and the small fragment instrument and implant set.

Drill Bits, 3.5 mm and 4.5 mm Diameter

These bits, 195 mm/170 mm, with quick coupling end, are used to pre-drill for long 3.5 mm and 4.5 mm cortex screws. They are used with the drill guide from the standard sets corresponding in size.

Drill Bits, 2.5 mm and 3.2 mm Diameter, Three-Fluted, and Calibrated

These bits, 230 mm/205 mm, have quick coupling ends. They are used when drilling at oblique angles, since the likelihood of skidding off the bone is reduced by the three cutting edges. The drill bits are used with the drill guides or sleeves from the standard sets corresponding in size. The calibration permits control of the drilling depth from 30 to 200 mm in 10 mm steps. Two ring markings indicate 100, 150 and 200 mm drilling depths. Three rings indicate 250 mm.

Drill Bit, 4.5 mm Diameter, Three-Fluted

This bit, 195 mm/170 mm, with quick coupling end, is used to drill the gliding hole for 4.5 mm cortex screws in a deep wound. The double drill sleeve, 4.5 mm/3.2 mm, from the basic instrument set is used as tap sleeve.

Depth Gauge, 3.5–4.0 mm

This gauge is used for measuring small fragment screws up to 110 mm. The design and function is similar to that of the depth gauges in the basic set or in the small fragment instrument and implant set.

Tap for 3.5 mm Cortex Screws, Calibrated

This tap is 175 mm long and has a 50 mm thread length. It is used to cut the thread before inserting 3.5 mm cortex screws longer than 50 mm. The double drill sleeve, 3.5 mm/2.5 mm, from the small fragment instrument and implant set is used as tap sleeve. The tap has a quick coupling end and is used with the T handle in the standard sets. The calibration permits control of the tapping depth from 60 to 140 mm in 10 mm steps.

Tap for 4.5 mm Cortex Screws, Calibrated

This tap is 175 mm long and has a 50 mm thread length. It is used to cut the thread in bone when inserting long 4.5 mm cortex screws. The double drill sleeve, 4.5 mm/3.2 mm, from the standard basic set is used as tap sleeve. The tap has a quick coupling end and is used with the T handle from the basic set. The calibration permits control of the tapping depth from 60 to 140 mm in 10 mm steps.

Large Hexagonal Pelvic Screwdriver, 300 mm

This screwdriver, 3.5 mm in width across flats, is used to insert 4.5 mm cortex screws and 6.5 mm cancellous bone screws in deep wounds. The screwdriver shaft has a groove to lock the large holding sleeve.

Large Holding Sleeve

This is a self-retaining screw-holding sleeve which connects to the large hexagonal pelvic screwdriver and large shaft. The holding sleeve holds the large screws securely during insertion in a deep wound.

Large Hexagonal Pelvic Screwdriver Shaft

This shaft, 3.5 mm in width across flats and 165 mm long, may be connected to the small air drill and used to insert 4.5 mm cortex screws and 6.5 mm cancellous bone screws in deep wounds.

Small Hexagonal Pelvic Screwdriver, 270 mm

This screwdriver, 2.5 mm in width across flats, is used when inserting small fragment screws in a deep wound. The screwdriver shaft has a groove to lock the small holding sleeve in position.

Small Holding Sleeve

This is a self-retaining screw-holding sleeve which connects to the small hexagonal pelvic screwdriver and the small shaft. The small fragment screws are securely held by the sleeve during insertion in a deep wound.

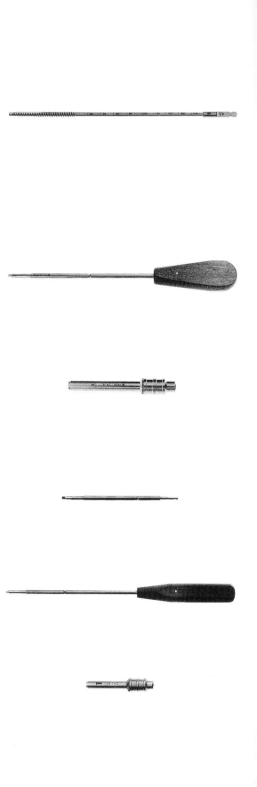

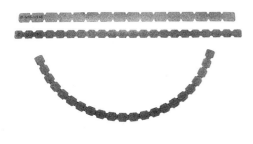

Small Hexagonal Pelvic Screwdriver Shaft

This shaft, 2.5 mm in width across flats and 165 mm long, may be connected to the small air drill and used to insert small fragment screws in deep wounds.

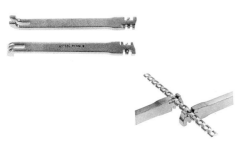

Bending Template for Straight Reconstruction Plates, 4.5 and 3.5 mm, and for Curved Pelvic Reconstruction Plates, 3.5 mm

These templates are made of anodised aluminium and easily moulded to conform to the shape of the bone. They are used as models when contouring reconstruction plates. They have indentations at the edges similar to those of the reconstruction plates corresponding in size.

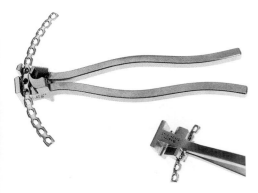

Bending Irons for Reconstruction Plates, 3.5 mm and 4.5 mm

These irons are used in pairs for two-dimensional contouring and twisting of 3.5 mm and 4.5 mm reconstruction plates. Bending "on the flat" can be performed by placing the plate onto the special pegs. Twisting can be achieved using the other end.

Bending Pliers for Reconstruction Plates 2.7 mm and 3.5 mm

These pliers are designed to allow three-dimensional bending without exceeding the permitted 15° at any one side.

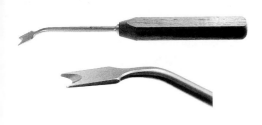

Pelvic Osteotomy Chisels

These chisels, 304 mm with 15 mm and 20 mm blade widths, are designed for periacetabular osteotomies in the treatment of hip dysplasia. The chisel is angulated 4 cm beyond the cutting end. It has a half-moon shaped groove with blunt ends on the tip of the blade, which helps to protect the soft tissue when cutting osteotomies blind. For cutting, the chisel has to be pushed towards the bone in a direction parallel to the blade.

Pelvic Instruments and Implants

6.10.2 Supplementary Instruments

Combined Depth Gauge for 3.5–6.5 mm Screws

This depth gauge measures up to 150 mm. It is used to measure the length for the long 3.5 mm and 4.5 mm cortex screws and the long 6.5 mm cancellous bone screws included in the pelvic implant set.

6.10.3 Pelvic Reduction Instruments

Pelvic reduction instruments are available in either a graphic case or in a sterilising tray.

Straight Ball Spike, 300 mm

This spike is used to push bone fragments carefully into place.

Blunt Pelvic Retractor

This retractor has a round tip to prevent any damage to viable structures when used in pelvic surgery.

Oblique Pelvic Reduction Forceps, Small, 190 mm,
and Large, 230 mm, Pointed Ball Tips

The oblique jaws of these forceps permit reduction while positioning the handles away from the centre of the wound, and the line of vision. The *pointed ball tips* of all these forceps provide a secure hold in bone, while the 8 mm balls prevent over-penetration of thin bone. In addition, the balls fit in the holes of a 4.5 mm DCP or LC-DCP. This allows the use of the plate as a reduction aid to distribute forces over a larger area. The point projects beyond the undersurface of the plate into the bone to prevent slipping.

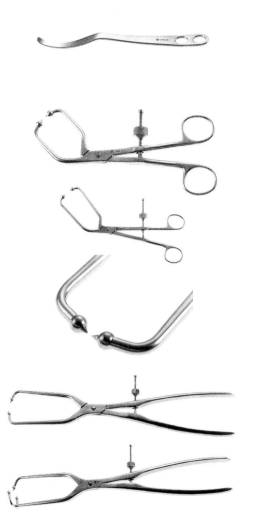

Pelvic Reduction Forceps, 400 mm, Pointed
and Three Pointed Ball Tips

The long jaws of these two forceps permit reduction deep into the pelvis around large fragments of the ilium. The long handles increase the leverage.

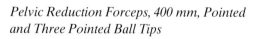

Instrumentation and Techniques

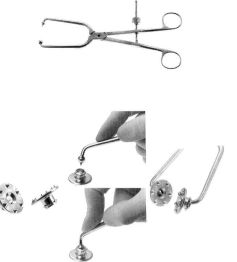

*Pelvic Reduction Forceps, 250 mm,
with Angled Pointed Ball Tips*

This forceps is applied when reducing fractures of relatively flat bones where soft tissue limits access to the fracture. The angled tips afford better grip and prevent slippage.

Spiked Disc

This disc attaches to the ball tip of any of the above reduction forceps. It disperses the forces of the forceps by providing a greater contact area, reducing the risk of penetrating thin bone. The disc swivels on the ball-tip; the seven points prevent slippage. It is attached by placing the disc on a hard surface and pushing the tip of the forceps through the centre hole.

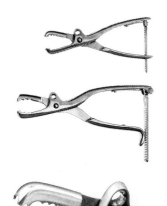

Small Pelvic Forceps, 190 mm, and Medium Pelvic Forceps, 250 mm

These forceps are reduction forceps of Faraboeuf type used for reduction by applying the forceps to screws inserted in the different fragments. The jaws have a cut-out to grip around the screw head.

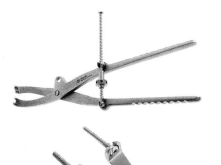

Pelvic Reduction Forceps, 330 mm

This forceps is used in conjunction with two screws for reduction, for example, of pelvic and acetabular fractures and for symphysis ruptures. Two screws are fully inserted in the two fragments at a distance of no more than 80 mm apart. After releasing the screws slightly the tips of the forceps may be attached.
Both compression and distraction can be exerted by changing the speed-lock from the outer side of the handle to the inner side.

Pelvic Instruments and Implants

Reduction Forceps with Points, 200 mm

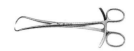

This forceps with ratchet may be used for the reduction of pelvic and acetabular fractures, applied directly to the bone surface, to shallow drill holes through the cortex or to the anchoring rings or hooks.

Anchoring Hooks, Small and Large

These hooks may be hooked around the iliac crest or in the bone and hold one arm of the pointed reduction forceps when reducing a pelvic fracture.

Anchoring Ring

This ring, 20 mm in diameter, made of polyoxymethacrylate (POM) is used with the pointed reduction forceps to reduce pelvic fractures. It is fixed with either a 4.5 mm cortex screw or 6.5 mm cancellous bone screw to the iliac wing fragment, where placing a pointed reduction forceps is difficult. If necessary, a second ring may be placed in the other fragment. The pointed reduction forceps is then attached to the two rings and used to squeeze the fragments together.

Bone Hook

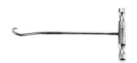

The hook, medium and large, may be used for reduction of pelvic fractures. See also p. 361.

Universal Chuck with T Handle

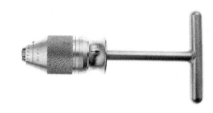

This chuck is used with the Schanz screw, 6.0 mm, to reduce fragments.

Schanz Screw, 6.0 mm Diameter, 190 mm

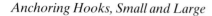

This flat-tipped screw, with a core size of 4.1 mm and a 50 mm thread length, is used with the universal chuck with T handle to reduce fragments. Inserted into the ischium, it can be used to control rotation of the posterior acetabular column.

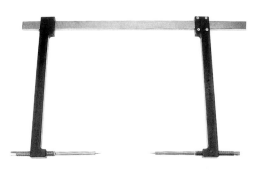

6.10.4 Pelvic C Clamp

This clamp may be applied in unstable injuries to the pelvic girdle associated with massive blood loss to prevent fatal shock before adequate therapeutic measures can be initiated. It permits rapid reduction and stabilisation of the posterior part of the pelvic girdle. It is not intended for use as a permanent or definitive fixation device. In case of fracture of the sacrum or rupture of the sacroiliac joint with concomitant blood loss from the fracture surface, the use of the emergency pelvic C clamp can save life. Direct transverse compression of the sacroiliac joint reduces the bleeding. The rare case of arterial bleeding, however, is hardly affected. In such a case interventional radiology or even internal iliac ligation may be needed.

The pelvic C clamp can be applied as an emergency measure in the emergency room, too, on any table. Its application, however, requires experience, and great care is recommended when handling the instrument.

The components of the pelvic C clamp can be obtained in a sterilising tray. The components are:

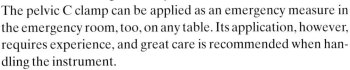

– Two pointed nails, 223 mm long, 10 mm in diameter, with collar and two nail elongations

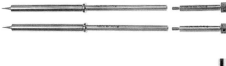

– Two 40 cm long side struts with threaded tubes

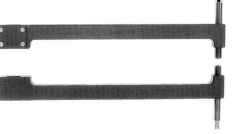

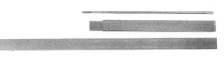

– A 50 cm rail, a 25 cm extension rail, and a connecting screw

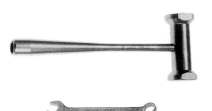

Instruments necessary for application:
– Socket wrench with hammer

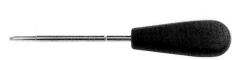

– Combination wrench, 11 mm

– Large hexagonal screwdriver

Step by step application:

- The patient is in supine position, with pelvis and hips prepared and draped, if possible.
- The posterior superior iliac spine (PSIS) is palpated, and an imaginary line drawn between the PSIS and anterior superior iliac spine (ASIS). The nail insertion point is on this line, approximately 3 to 4 fingerwidths anterolateral to the PSIS in the average patient. This point is also on an extension of the line of the proximal femur and of the greater trochanter in neutral hip rotation (Fig. 1).
- The nails are inserted into the threaded tubes in the side struts of the assembled C clamp (Fig. 2) and pushed through the stab incisions until the nails engage the bone. This will prevent dorsal slippage on the sharp iliac edge.

Note: The nails must not be placed too ventrally, as this may cause perforation of the thin part of the ilium.

- The side struts are pressed together by applying force on the struts near the rail (Fig. 3).
- At this stage a cranial displacement can be simultaneously reduced by pulling on the leg.
- Dorsal displacement may be reduced by inserting a Steinmann pin into the ASIS and rotating one side of the pelvis (one of the pelvic fragments).
- The nails, with the nail elongations, are further inserted using the socket wrench hammer and the struts adjusted until stopped by the shoulders (Fig. 4).
- The threaded tubes are tightened using the combination wrench or, after removal of the nail elongation, with the socket wrench. This locks the side struts on the rail and compresses the dorsal segment of the pelvic ring (Fig. 5).
- The extension rail may be removed if the struts are placed on the main rail (necessary in, for example, CT scanning). The large hexagonal screwdriver is used to tighten and retighten the connecting screws.
- The pelvic C clamp can be positioned either caudally, e. g., for a laparotomy, or cranially for angiography (Fig. 6).

Note: The pelvic C clamp is not designed for comminuted fractures of the ilium in the proximity of the sacroiliac joint because the nails cannot be adequately secured in the comminuted area. There is also a danger of pressing the fractured ilium medially across the sacrum.

- Insertion of the nail too distally endangers the sciatic nerve and the gluteal vessels.
- In the case of osteoporotic bone and incorrect positioning of the nails excessive compression can force the nail too far into the bone.

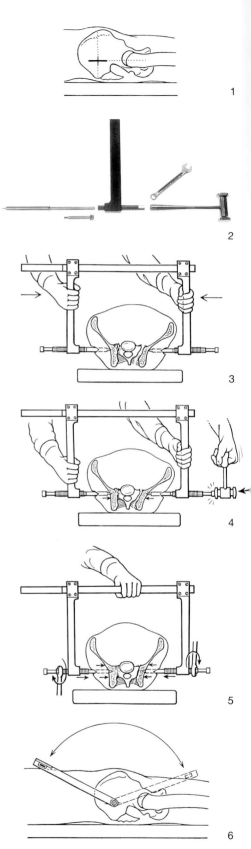

1

2

3

4

5

6

- The nail insertion sites must be meticulously disinfected and dressed. The pelvic C clamp should be replaced as soon as possible by a definitive fixation.
- Should the patient have to be moved he/she should on no account be placed on the side as this could cause one of the nails to penetrate the bone excessively.

6.10.5 Pelvic Implants

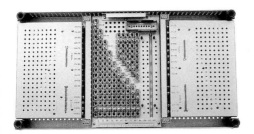

For the fixation of pelvic and acetabular fractures the standard implants contained in the basic implant sets and the small fragment instrument and implant set (see Sect. 6.9) are used. In addition to these implants, longer screws and a variety of plates are available in a special pelvic implant set. The application of these implants is similar to that of their counterparts. See Sects. 6.4., 6.5 and 6.9. They do, however, sometimes require the longer instruments described in Sect. 6.10.1.

These additional pelvic implants are available in either a graphic case or in a sterilising tray.

Cortex Screws, 3.5 mm

These 3.5 mm cortex screws in lengths from 55 to 110 mm, in 5 mm increments, are used separately or for the fixation of 3.5 mm implants in pelvic fractures where deep anchoring of the implant is necessary. The long drill bits and taps are used. For details see Sect. 6.9.2.1

Cortex Screws, 4.5 mm

The 4.5 mm cortex screws are available in lengths from 72 to 80 mm, in 4 mm increments, and from 85 to 110 mm, in 5 mm increments. The long instruments are required for the insertion. For details see Sect. 6.4.1.

Cancellous Bone Screws, 6.5 mm, with 16 mm and 32 mm Thread Length

These screws are available in lengths of 115 mm and 120 mm. For details see Sect. 6.4.1.

Cancellous Bone Screws, 6.5 mm, Fully Threaded

These screws are available in lengths of 45, 50, 55, and 60 mm. For details see Sect. 6.4.1.

Reconstruction Plates, 3.5 mm, Straight

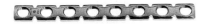

These plates are used with 3.5 mm cortex screws. Their main application is in pelvic and acetabular fractures. They may also be used in fractures of the distal humerus (dorsolateral aspect), the clavicle and of the calcaneus.

The reconstruction plates have lateral notches between the holes, which enables twisting and bending in two dimensions. Special bending irons and pliers are available. Bending angles greater than 15° at any one site should be avoided. Note that the already low stiffness of the plate is further diminished by bending. If a strong curvature is needed, for example, for the pelvis, it is better to choose a prebent, curved reconstruction plate. See below.

The oval holes permit some self-compression if the screw is inserted eccentrically. The holes also accept 4.0 mm cancellous bone screws if the plate is placed over cancellous bone area. Screws can be inserted at an angle of approximately 25° longitudinally and 7° sideways.

The plate is available in lengths from 58 to 262 mm, with 5 to 22 holes.

Important dimensions:
- Profile: See figure
- Thickness: 2.8 mm
- Width: 10   mm
- Hole spacing: 12   mm

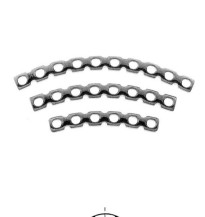

Reconstruction Plates, 3.5 mm, Curved

These plates are especially designed for fractures of the anterior column of the pelvis. They are slightly thicker than the straight plate and are precurved. The design and application is otherwise similar to that of the straight reconstruction plate.

The curved reconstruction plate, 3.5 mm, is available with 6 to 18 holes, in lengths from 70 to 214 mm.

Important dimensions:
- Profile: See figure
- Thickness: 3.6 mm
- Width: 10   mm
- Hole spacing: 12   mm
- Bending radius: 100 mm

Reconstruction Plates, 4.5 mm, Straight

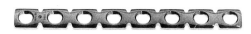

These plates are similar in design to the 3.5 mm reconstruction plates, only larger and used with 4.5 mm cortex screws. This plate is chosen in very tall or heavy patients instead of the smaller one.

The reconstruction plate, 4.5 mm, is available with 3 to 16 holes, in lengths from 45 to 253 mm.

Important dimensions:
- Profile: See figure
- Thickness: 2.8 mm
- Width: 12   mm
- Hole spacing: 16   mm

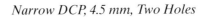

Narrow DCP, 4.5 mm, Two Holes

This is a regular DCP, 39 mm long, used for the treatment of, for example, symphyseal ruptures. It is fixed with fully threaded 6.5 mm cancellous bone screws on the superior aspect of the symphysis pubis.

Important dimensions:
– Profile: See figure
– Thickness: 3.6 mm
– Width: 12   mm
– Hole spacing: 25   mm

6.11 Mini Fragment Instruments and Implants

6.11.1 Mini Fragment Instruments

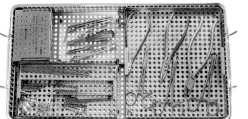

The instruments used for the reduction and temporary fixation of fragments of diminutive size, and for the application of mini implants, are similar in design to instruments used for large and small fragments. Their size is reduced to accommodate tiny fragments. Handles, however, are not always proportionally smaller since surgeons' hands remain the same size.

Great care is required in the use and handling of these delicate instruments. The small diameters of drill bits and taps, as well as the fine points and delicate jaws of reduction forceps, make them susceptible to breakage if misused.

The mini fragment instruments and implants can be obtained in either a graphic case or in a sterilising case.

6.11.1.1 Standard Instruments

Standard Instruments for 2.7 mm Implants

Drill Bit Design (see Sect. 6.2)

Drill Bit, 2.0 mm Diameter

This drill bit, 100 mm/75 mm (total and effective lengths), is used to prepare the thread hole for 2.7 mm cortex screws, and also the gliding hole for 2.0 mm cortex screws. It has a quick coupling end to fit the small air drill. Drill bits should always be used with a drill sleeve or guide of the same size to protect both the drill bit and surrounding soft tissue. Drill bits must be sharp when used.

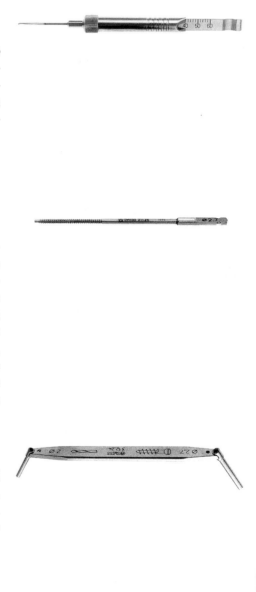

Drill Bit, 2.7 mm Diameter

This drill bit, 100 mm/75 mm (total and effective lengths), is used to prepare the gliding hole for 2.7 mm cortex screws, when they are used as lag screws. It has a quick coupling end to fit the small air drill. The 2.7 mm drill bit should be used with the double drill sleeve end, 2.7 mm to protect both the drill bit and surrounding soft tissue.

Small Countersink, 2.7 mm

This countersink is used to cut a recess in a thick cortex. This allows accommodation of the screw head and distributes the pressure over a greater area, when the screw is inserted as a single lag screw. The 2.0 mm diameter tip centres the countersink in the pre-drilled thread hole. It is used with the handle with quick coupling. Countersinks of current manufacture have five cutting edges instead of four. This increases the cutting capability.

Note: Always countersink before measuring

Depth Gauge, 2.7–4.0 mm

This gauge measures the drilling depth for 2.7 mm screws up to 60 mm. The hook must engage the opposite cortex securely before the sleeve is pushed onto the bone or the plate and the measurement taken. If the drill hole is at an angle, the longest depth must be measured. Depth gauges of recent design have a locking screw.

Note: Always measure before tapping.

Tap Design (see Sect. 6.2).

Tap for 2.7 mm Cortex Screws

This tap is used to pre-cut the thread in the bone before the cortex screw can be inserted. The 33 mm long thread has the same configuration as the screw thread, but only the first two conically increasing threads are cutting. The flutes extend from the tip as far as the first ten threads only. The long threaded portion protects the newly cut path as the tap is advanced. The tap is used with quick coupling handle and the double drill sleeve end, 2.7 mm. The handle is turned clockwise and anti-clockwise once until the tip has passed through the far cortex. This action allows bone debris to be deposited in the flutes. Tapping must be done by hand and not with a power machine.

Double Drill Sleeve, 2.7 mm/2.0 mm

This drill sleeve has a sleeve on each end of the handle, and should be used for the protection of tissues and instruments. The 2.7 mm sleeve is used with the corresponding tap and drill bit. The 2.0 mm sleeve is used with the 2.0 mm drill bit. It may be used through plate holes or separately, and it is steadied by pressing the serrated end onto the bone. The 2.0 mm sleeve can be used as an insert sleeve in lag screw technique with 2.0 mm cortex screws. The hole in the handle adjacent to the sleeve can be used over a previously inserted Kirschner wire (up to 1.6 mm diameter) to permit parallel drilling. The distance of 4.5 mm between the wire and the screw allows the use of a washer.

Handle with Quick Coupling

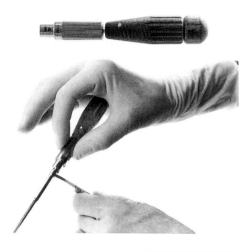

This handle is used with the countersink, the tap, 2.7 mm, and with the small hexagonal screwdriver shaft. The rotating end of the handle permits support in the palm and precise turning of the instrument with two fingers.

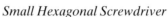

Small Hexagonal Screwdriver

This screwdriver has a hexagonal tip (width across flats 2.5 mm) which fits snugly in the hexagonal socket of the small fragment screws allowing easy insertion and removal. The shaft has a groove which is necessary to connect the screw-holding sleeve. The handle is designed so that excessive force cannot be applied when inserting the screws.

Note: Never use a screwdriver with a damaged tip. This will then damage the socket of the screw head and make removal very difficult.

Small Screw-Holding Sleeve, 2.7 mm

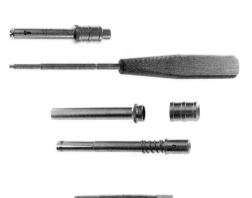

This sleeve holds the screw by a self-retaining mechanism. It is slid onto the shaft of the small hexagonal screwdriver which has a groove to receive it. It is especially useful when removing shaft screws, as traction can be applied. The screw-holding sleeve has to be disassembled carefully for cleaning.

Small Hexagonal Screwdriver Shaft

This shaft can be connected to the handle with quick coupling, and used to insert screws, if the regular screwdriver is unavailable. The screwdriver shaft can also be coupled with the small air drill and used for removal of screws, but only after they have first been loosened by hand.

Standard Instruments for 2.0 mm and 1.5 mm Implants

Drill Bit, 2.0 mm

See under "Standard Instruments for 2.7 mm Implants" (p. 227).

Drill Bit, 1.5 mm Diameter

This drill bit, 85 mm/60 mm (total and effective lengths), is used to prepare the gliding hole for the 1.5 mm cortex screw, and the thread hole for the 2.0 mm cortex screw. It has a quick coupling end to fit the small air drill. This fine diameter drill bit is also susceptible to breakage and must be used with great care to avoid damage. The use of the corresponding size drill sleeve is recommended.

Drill Bit, 1.1 mm Diameter

This drill bit, 60 mm/35 mm (total and effective lengths), is used to prepare the thread hole for the 1.5 mm cortex screw. It has a quick coupling end for use with the small air drill. Due to its very small diameter it must be used with great care lest it break, especially when coupled with the drill. The use of the correct size drill sleeve helps to protect the drill bit as well as the soft tissue.

Mini Countersink, 1.5 mm/2.0 mm

The mini countersink, for the handle with mini quick coupling, is used to cut a recess in dense cortical bone to intensifier the screw head and to distribute the pressure over a greater area. The 1.1 mm tip centres the countersink in the pre-drilled hole, and the five cutting edges enable easy cutting when turned clockwise.

Note: Countersink before measuring.

Depth Gauge, 1.5–2.0 mm

The depth gauge measures up to 38 mm. The fine and delicate probe is protected by a screw-on sleeve, which should be removed only when measuring and cleaning. The hook should engage the far cortex before the sleeve is pushed onto the bone and the measurement taken.
The depth gauge must be carefully disassembled before cleaning.

Tap for 2.0 mm Cortex Screws

This tap has a 24 mm thread length, and is used to cut the thread in the bone before inserting 2.0 mm cortex screws. It couples

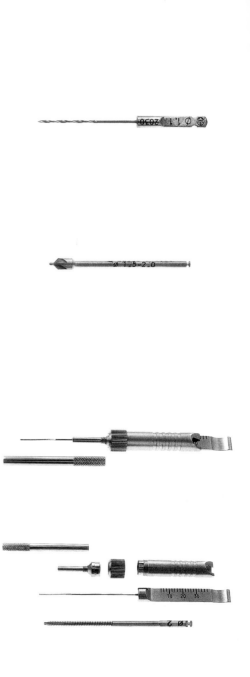

with the handle with mini quick coupling. The 2.0 mm double drill sleeve end is used for protection of the tap.

Note: The tap is always used after measuring.

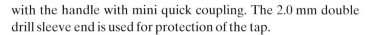

Tap for 1.5 mm Cortex Screws

This tap has a 20 mm thread length, and is used to cut the thread in bone before inserting 1.5 mm cortex screws. It is used with the handle with mini quick coupling and the 1.5 mm double drill sleeve end for protection. As a general rule the tap is turned twice clockwise and once anti-clockwise to allow bone debris to collect in the flutes. The tip should pass through the far cortex before the tap is removed.

Note: The tap is always used after measuring.

Double Drill Sleeve, 2.0 mm/1.5 mm

This sleeve is similar in design and function to the double drill sleeve described above (2.7 mm/2.0 mm). It is the sleeve necessary when drilling 1.5 mm or 2.0 mm, and tapping for a 2.0 mm screw. The handle has a hole for a previously inserted Kirschner wire (up to 1.25 mm diameter) if parallel drilling is necessary. The distance between wire and the screw is 4.0 mm to allow the use of a washer.

Double Drill Sleeve, 1.5 mm/1.1 mm

This sleeve has a 1.5 mm sleeve on one end of the handle and a 1.1 mm sleeve on the other end. The 1.5 mm sleeve is used with the 1.5 mm tap and drill bit, and the 1.1 mm sleeve with the 1.1 mm drill bit, for the insertion of 1.5 mm cortex screws. The serrated end allows secure purchase on the surface of the bone, and the thin-walled sleeve permits exact placement of screws in a plate hole. The hole in the handle near the sleeve allows use over a previously inserted Kirschner wire (up to 1.25 mm diameter) for parallel drilling. The distance of 2.8 mm between the wire and the screw permits the use of a washer.

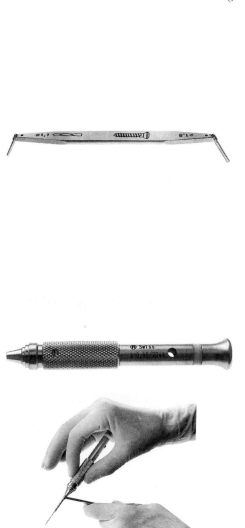

Handle with Mini Quick Coupling

This handle is used with the mini countersink, the taps for 1.5 mm and 2.0 mm screws, and the mini hexagonal screwdriver shaft. The rotating end of the handle allows support in the palm while turning the instrument using two fingers.

Handle with Mini Quick Coupling and a Plastic Handle

This is an alternative to the handle with mini coupling described above. The handle may be supported in the palm, while turning the front part of the handle with two fingers.

Mini Hexagonal Screwdriver

This screwdriver, with holding sleeve, has a hexagonal tip (1.5 mm width across the flats) to fit the stainless steel mini screws. The removable holding sleeve grips the screw during insertion, but is pushed back for the final tightening.

Mini Hexagonal Screwdriver Shaft

This screwdriver shaft, with holding sleeve, has a hexagonal tip (1.5 mm width across the flats) to fit the stainless steel mini screws. It can be used with the handle with mini quick coupling instead of the regular screwdriver. The removable holding sleeve grips the screw during insertion, but is pushed back for the final tightening.

Cruciform Screwdriver Shaft

This screwdriver shaft is used with the handle with mini quick coupling, for the insertion of titanium 1.5 mm and 2.0 mm cortex screws that have a cruciform head slot. (In the USA it is also used for stainless steel mini screws.) The removable holding sleeve grips the screw during insertion, but is pushed back for the final tightening.

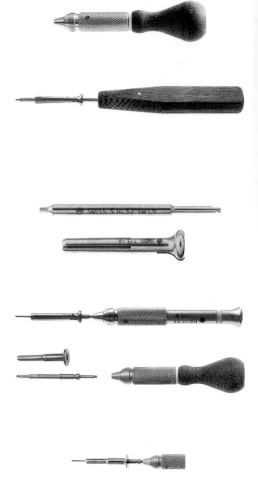

General Instruments

Small Retractors, Widths 6 and 8 mm

Small retractors, 160 mm long, are used to expose fractures of the metacarpals and the metatarsals. Excessive pressure on the soft tissue must not be applied.

Periosteal Elevator, Straight Edge, Width 3 mm

This elevator, with a slightly curved blade, is used to aid reduction, cleaning of fracture fragments, and for preparation of screw and plate sites. It is *not* used to *strip* the bone widely of the periosteum.

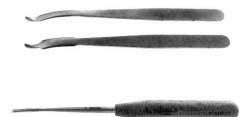

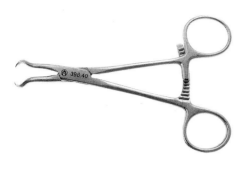

Reduction Forceps with Points, Narrow

This forceps, 132 mm, has narrow serrated jaws and fine points to allow for exact reduction of fractures of small bones, as in the hand and the foot, for example. The narrow jaws do not compromise the soft tissue. A fine ratchet lock permits easy and even closure.

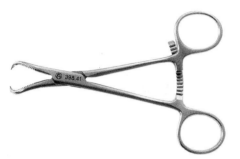

Reduction Forceps with Points, Broad

This forceps, 132 mm, has broad serrated jaws and points and is used in similar manner on the same bones as mentioned above, but allows room for a plate. The forceps has a fine ratchet lock for easy and even closure.

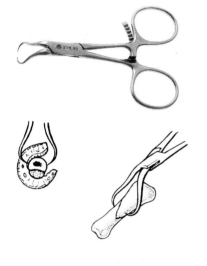

"Stag beetle" Forceps

This forceps, 120 mm, has jaws that resemble the antler-like mandible of the male stag beetle. The fine points of this forceps makes it possible to fix bone on one side either through the soft tissues, without having to strip them aside, or even percutaneously. This has practical value in the phalanges. The fine ratchet lock permits controlled closure.

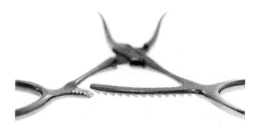

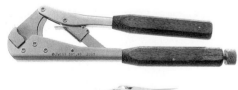

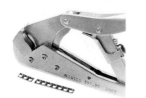

Plate Cutting Forceps

This forceps, 256 mm, for 1.5 mm – 2.7 mm plates (except DCP, 2.7 mm), is used to cut the plates to the desired length and shape. The mechanism enables clear cutting, without leaving sharp edges, and extra trimming is not necessary.

Sharp Hook

This hook is used to inspect fracture lines, and to reduce fragments. It can also be used to clean screw head sockets before removal, and to free instruments with threaded parts of bone and tissue debris.

Screw Forceps

These forceps, with a simple self-holding mechanism, are used to remove screws from the rack.

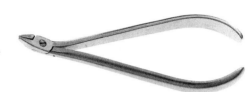

Plate-Bending Forceps

These forceps, 140 mm, are used in pairs for precise bending or twisting of 1.5 mm 2–7 mm plates.

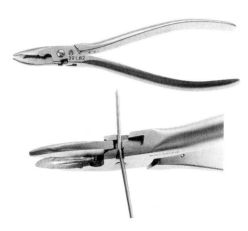

Wire-Bending Pliers

These 155 mm pliers can be used to hold and bend wires. They can also be used to cut wires up to 1.6 mm in diameter.

Small Wire Cutter

This 175 mm wire cutter for cutting cerclage and Kirschner wires up to 1.25 mm in diameter. The oblique jaws permit cutting at their very tip.

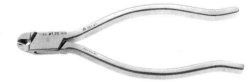

Bending Iron, for Kirschner Wires 0.8, 1.0 and 1.25 mm Diameter

This bending iron has been designed to permit bending of Kirschner wires close to the bone or skin surface.

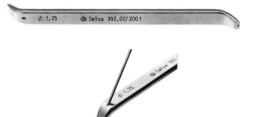

6.11.1.2 Supplementary Instruments

Drill Bits, 1.1, 1.5, 2.0 and 2.7 mm Diameter

These bits are also available with three flutes, in different lengths, and also with triangular end to fit Jacobs chuck. See SYNTHES catalogue for further details.

Taps for 1.5, 2.0 and 2.7 mm Screws

Taps longer than those described in Sect. 6.11.1.1 are available. The thread length of the tap should be at least as long as that of the screw, or else the pre-cut thread in the near cortex will be damaged by the unthreaded shaft of the tap. See SYNTHES catalogue for details.

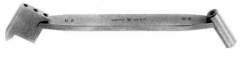

Triple Wire Guide, 2.0 mm

This guide wire can be used as a guide for the insertion of Kirschner wires. The three holes on one side allow parallel placement of wires, which is necessary in tension band wiring technique.

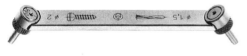

DCP Drill Guide, 2.0 mm

This drill guide, neutral and load, is used when applying a DCP, 2.0 mm, for the placement of neutral screws (green end), and load screws (yellow end) The 1.5 mm drill bit is used. The self-compression distance achieved with the load screw is 0.6 mm (arrow towards the fracture).

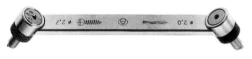

DCP Drill Guide, 2.7 mm

This drill guide, neutral and load, is used when applying a DCP, 2.7 mm. The drill bit 2.0 mm is used to pre-drill for 2.7 mm cortex screws either in neutral position (green end), or in load position (yellow end). The self-compression achieved with the load screw is 0.8 mm (arrow towards the fracture).

Holding Sleeves

These sleeves for the mini and small screwdrivers can be obtained separately, if they are lost or damaged. See p. 232.

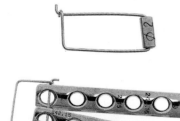

Holding Clips

These clips, marked 2.0 or 2.7 mm, are made of implant material and can be used to hold plates and washers. Regular safety pins cannot be used because of the risk of corrosion being transmitted.

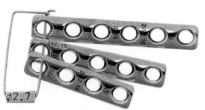

Bending Irons for Small Plates, 2.7 and 3.5 mm, 150 mm

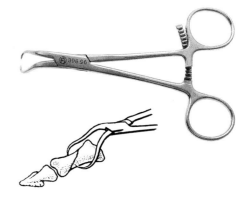

These bending irons have two slots with different widths to bend plates of various thicknesses. Bending and twisting is performed by placing the two irons opposite each other. The differently orientated slots allow easy overbending at the middle section of the plate. The longitudinal slots at the end can also be used for twisting and bending.

"Termite" Forceps

This forceps, 90 mm, is a lightweight (15 g) reduction forceps used especially for fractures of the phalanges and small metacarpal fragments. It has flared jaws, very fine points and a fine ratchet lock. The fine points allow percutaneous fixation. Because of its light weight, the forceps remains in position once it has been locked.

Forceps with Sliding Jaws

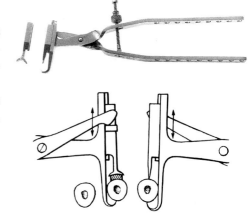

This forceps has an angulated handle with speed lock, and jaws that move parallel to each other. The upper jaw is interchangeable; one has a point and one a foot plate. They oppose a stationary pointed hook.

The forceps is used for reduction and provisional fixation of the third and fourth metacarpal, where access is often a problem. The foot plate can be used to hold a mini plate against the bone.

Self-Centring Bone Holding Forceps, 150 mm

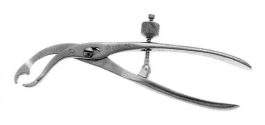

This forceps, with speed lock, has its application mainly in metacarpal or metatarsal fractures; sometimes also in fine forearm bones. The self-centring jaws make application easy even in small wounds.

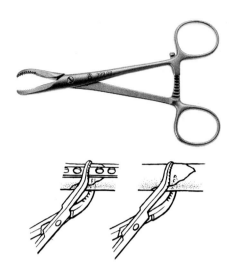

Reduction Forceps with Serrated Jaws, 140 mm

This forceps is excellent for reduction and temporary retention of a plate, such as on the forearm, the fibula, or the metacarpal and metatarsal bones. The ratchet is easy to handle and to close. The forceps are also available with a speed lock.

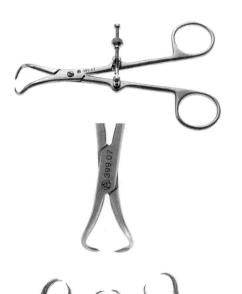

Reduction Forceps with Points, 130 mm

This forceps may be used for reduction of the metatarsal and metacarpal bones. However, its wide jaws makes it more difficult to apply, than the narrow reduction forceps described in Sect. 6.11.1.1. The forceps are available with both ratchet and speed-lock closure.

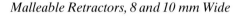

Malleable Retractors, 8 and 10 mm Wide

These retractors, 230 mm long, can be moulded to the desired shape.

Periosteal Elevators

Different sizes of these elevators are available. See SYNTHES catalogue.

Holding Forceps for Small Plates

This forceps is used to provisionally hold small plates when planning the correct site, or while drilling.

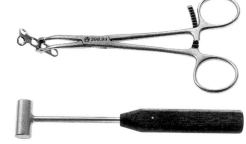

Hammer, 100 g

This hammer is to be used with fine osteotomes for osteotomies in, for example, the hand.

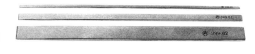

Osteotomes, 2, 5, 10 mm Wide

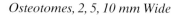

These osteotomes, 150 mm, are used for osteotomies in the hand.

Small Distractor

See Sect. 6.14.2

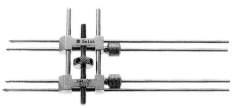

Mini Air Drill

See Sect. 6.21.3.4. See also the SYNTHES catalogue.

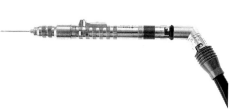

6.11.1.3 Obsolete Instruments

Mini Drill Sleeve, 1.1 and 1.5 mm

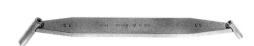

This sleeve has been replaced by double drill sleeve, 1.5 mm/1.1 mm.

Tap Sleeve, 3.5 mm

This sleeve, used as tap sleeve for the 2.7 mm tap, has been replaced by double drill sleeve, 2.7 mm/2.0 mm

Insert Sleeve, 2.7 mm/2.0 mm

This sleeve is no longer necessary since its function is taken over by the double drill sleeve, 2.7 mm/2.0 mm.

Small Hexagonal Screwdriver with Holding Sleeve

This screwdriver has been replaced by the small hexagonal screwdriver with groove in the shaft for the screw-holding sleeve.

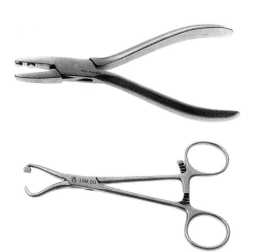

Bending Pliers for Small Plates

These pliers, with one or two "warts", have been replaced with the two small plate-bending forceps described in Sect. 6.11.2.

Holding Forceps for Finger Plates

It has been found that too extensive an incision is required for the holding forceps for finger plates to be of practical use in the hand.

Retractor for Small Fragments, 120 mm

This retractor, with a ring handle, has been replaced with the 160 mm long retractor, that has a 15 mm wide blade.

6.11.2 Mini Fragment Implants

Internal fixation of fractures in the hand and the foot has gained favour in recent years. The goal of providing the stability needed for early postoperative mobilisation in large bones also applies to smaller bones. The same basic principles of open reduction and stable internal fixation apply, only the size of implants varies. The trend towards using small implants has led to the development of a large number of different types and sizes. All the implants are now available in titanium as well as in stainless steel.

The implants are delicate as are the instruments needed for their application. They are designed to be handled with skill rather than force.

6.11.2.1 The Mini Fragment Screws

The mini fragment screws, 2.7, 2.0, and 1.5 mm cortex screws, are used as lag screws or as plate fixation screws. In small-sized bones the cancellous bone is rather dense, allowing the use of cortex screws also in the metaphyseal and epiphyseal areas. The screws are available in both stainless steel and titanium.

2.7 mm Cortex Screw

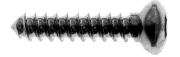

This screw is used for lag screw fixation of metacarpal and metatarsal fractures, as well as of small fragments in the forearm and the ankle. The 2.7 mm cortex screw is also used for the application of 2.7 mm plates in these bones. It can also be used with a spiked plastic washer to reattach avulsed ligaments.

The asymmetrical, buttress thread of the screw permits excellent hold in the bone. The bone has to be tapped before screw insertion. The screw head has the same sized hexagonal socket as the small fragment screws (2.5 mm), and the same core diameter as that of the 4.0 mm cancellous bone screws (1.9 mm). Therefore the same depth gauge and screwdriver is used for 2.7 mm screws as for the small fragment screws. The screw head has a spherical undersurface.

The 2.7 mm cortex screws are available in lengths from 6 mm to 40 mm, in 2 mm increments.

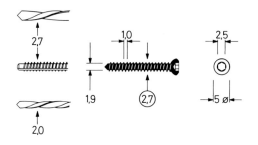

Important dimensions:
- Head diameter: 5.0 mm
- Hexagonal socket: 2.5 mm
- Core diameter: 1.9 mm
- Thread diameter: 2.7 mm
- Pitch: 1.0 mm
- Drill bit for gliding hole: 2.7 mm
- Drill bit for thread hole: 2.0 mm
- Tap: 2.7 mm

2.0 mm Cortex Screw

This screw is used for lag screw fixation of fragments in the proximal and middle phalanx, in small metacarpals and in fractures of small radial heads. It is also used for the application of 2.0 mm mini plates in these bones.

The screw has an asymmetrical buttress thread for sound purchase in the bone after tapping. The screw head has a spherical undersurface. The head of the 2.0 mm screw is available with either a hexagonal socket (stainless steel screws), or a cruciform recess (titanium screws, and in the USA the stainless steel screws.). Care must be taken to have the correct screwdriver available.

The 2.0 mm cortex screws are available in lengths from 6 mm to 38 mm, in 2 mm increments.

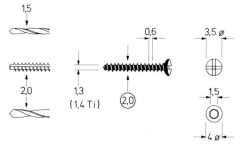

Important dimensions:
- Head diameter: 4.0 mm (titanium 3.5 mm)
- Hexagonal socket: 1.5 mm
- Core diameter: 1.3 mm (titanium 1.4 mm)
- Thread diameter: 2.0 mm
- Pitch: 0.6 mm
- Drill bit for gliding hole: 2.0 mm
- Drill bit for thread hole: 1.5 mm
- Tap: 2.0 mm

1.5 mm Cortex Screw

This screw is suitable for lag screw fixation of tiny fragments of the phalanges, the metacarpals and the radial head. It is also used for the application of 1.5 mm mini plates.

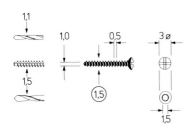

Considering the size of this very small screw it has excellent purchase in the bone thanks to its asymmetrical buttress thread. The bone has to be pre-tapped. The screw head has a spherical undersurface.

The 1.5 mm cortex screw is also available with either a hexagonal socket head (stainless steel screws), or a cruciform recess (titanium screws, and in the USA also the stainless steel screws). The correct screwdriver must be selected.

The 1.5 mm cortex screw exists in lengths from 6 to 20 mm; 6–12 mm in 1 mm increments, and 14–20 mm in 2 mm increments.

Important dimensions.
- Head diameter: 3.0 mm
- Hexagonal socket: 1.5 mm
- Core diameter: 1.0 mm
- Thread diameter: 1.5 mm
- Pitch: 0.5 mm
- Drill bit for gliding hole: 1.5 mm
- Drill bit for thread hole: 1.1 mm
- Tap: 1.5 mm

Washer, 7.0 mm Outer Diameter

This washer, available in both stainless steel and titanium, may be used to prevent the head of the 2.7 mm screw from splitting the cortex and sinking into the bone.

Washer, 4.5 mm Outer Diameter

This washer may be used with 1.5 or 2.0 mm cortex screws to prevent their heads from splitting the cortex and sinking into the bone.

Spiked Washer, 8.0/3.2 mm Diameter

This washer is made of polyacetate and stainless-steel reinforced for X-ray contrast. It can be used with a 2.7 mm cortex screw for the reattachment of an avulsed ligament.

The washer is autoclavable (maximum 140 °C, or 280 °F) up to 30 times. It must be left to recrystallize at least 8 h before use.

6.11.2.2 Mini Fragment Standard Plates

The Standard Plates for 2.7 mm Screws

Quarter-Tubular Plates

These plates are mainly used as tension band plates in fractures of metacarpal and metatarsal bones. The plate offers good longitudinal stability if in complete contact with the bone. This is achieved either by the edges along the plate or by the "collars" around the plate holes. Due to the "one-quarter of a tube" cross-section, the screw head is almost flush with the plate surface when inserted through the plate hole. As a consequence the undersurface of the screw head protrudes through the undersurface of the plate. If used on a bone with small circumference, the screw head may be in contact with the bone, preventing the plate from being securely fixed. To overcome this problem newer stainless steel plates have a collar around the holes on the underside. These collars prevent the screw head from protruding and secure the contact with the bone.

The plates are available in lengths from 23 mm to 63 mm, with 3 to 8 holes.

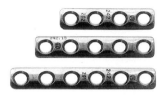
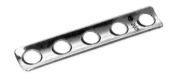
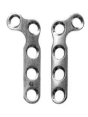

Important dimensions:
- Profile: See figure
- Thickness: 1 mm
- Width: 7 mm
- Hole spacing: 8 mm

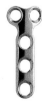

Small L Plates, 2.7 mm Oblique

These plates are mainly used in fractures of the distal or proximal ends of the metacarpal bones. The thin plates are easily contoured with two bending pliers. The head is placed over the wider metaphysis. The slightly oval holes permit eccentric placement of screws to produce some compression.

The plates are available in left and right oblique versions, with 3 holes in the shaft and 2 in the head.

Important dimensions:
- Profile: See figure
- Thickness: 2 mm
- Width: 7 mm
- Hole spacing: 8 mm
- Length: 35 mm

Small T Plates, 2.7 mm

These plates are similar to the L plate in use and design, but the head is T-shaped rather than L-shaped.

There are 3 holes in the shaft and 2 in the head.

Instrumentation and Techniques

Important dimensions:
- Profile: See figure
- Thickness: 2 mm
- Width: 7 mm
- Hole spacing: 8 mm
- Length: 32 mm

Small Condylar Plates, 2.7 mm

These plates are designed to be used in periarticular fractures in metacarpal and metatarsal bones. The plates have a 2.7 mm wide and 20 mm long pin at 90° in one end, positioned either to the left or to the right of a coaxial plate hole. The pin is cut to the desired length with a plate cutting forceps. The implant provides firm fixation in the fragment adjacent to the joint with minimal space requirement. The plate is notched to allow easy contouring.

The small condylar plates, 2.7 mm are available with 6 holes in the shaft and 1 beside the pin. At present the plate is only manufactured in titanium.

Important dimensions:
- Profile: See figure
- Thickness: 1.6 mm
- Width: 7 mm
- Hole spacing: 8 mm
- Plate length: 55 mm

The Standard Plates for 2.0 mm Screws

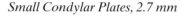

Straight Mini Plates, 2.0 mm

Straight mini plates, with 20 holes, can be cut to the desired length with the plate-cutting forceps. The unused portion may be used for other applications. The plate is mainly used in phalangeal fractures. It is easily contoured with two plate-bending forceps. Some compression is possible by eccentric placement of the screws in the oval holes.

Important dimensions:
- Profile: See figure
- Thickness: 1.2 mm
- Width: 5 mm
- Hole spacing: 5 mm
- Length: 10 mm

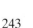

Mini T Plates, 2.0 mm

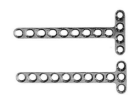

These plates are T-shaped, and can be cut to the desired length and shape with the plate-cutting forceps. The plate is used in the distal or proximal ends of phalanges. The head portion is placed over the metaphysis.

Contouring is easy using two plate-bending forceps. Some compression can be achieved by placing the screws eccentrically in the oval plate holes.

The 2.0 mm mini T plate is available with 9 holes in the shaft, and with either 3 or 4 holes in the head.

Important dimensions:
- Profile: See figure
- Thickness: 1.2 mm
- Width: 5   mm
- Hole spacing: 5   mm
- Length: 50 mm

Mini Condylar Plates, 2.0 mm

These plates are designed to be used in fractures or osteotomies near the metacarpophalangeal (MP) or proximal interphalangeal (PIP) joints. At one end, the plates have a 2.0 mm wide pin, 14 mm in length, set at 90° either to the left or right of a coaxial plate hole. The pin is cut to the desired length with a plate-cutting forceps before insertion into the metaphyseal bone. The implant provides firm fixation in the fragment adjacent to the joint with minimal space requirement. The plate is notched to allow easy contouring.

The 2.0 mm small condylar plates are available with 6 holes in the shaft, and 1 beside the pin. The plates with the pin to the left are available in both stainless steel and titanium, plates with the pin to the right are available only in titanium.

Important dimensions:
- Profile: See figure
- Thickness: 1.2 mm
- Width: 5   mm
- Hole spacing: 5   mm
- Plate length: 29 mm

Standard Plates for 1.5 mm Screws

Straight Mini Plates, 1.5 mm

These plates, with 20 holes, can be cut to the desired length with the plate-cutting forceps. The remaining portion may be left for other applications. The plate is mainly used in phalangeal fractures. It is easily contoured with the two plate-bending forceps. Some compression is possible by placing the screws eccentrically in the oval holes.

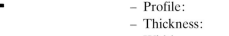

Important dimensions:
- Profile: See figure
- Thickness: 0.9 mm
- Width: 3.8 mm
- Hole spacing: 5   mm
- Length: 100   mm

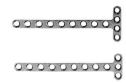

Mini T Plates, 1.5 mm

These plates are T-shaped and can be cut to the desired length and shape with the plate-cutting forceps. The plate is used in the distal or proximal ends of phalanges. The head portion is placed over the metaphysis.

Contouring is easily achieved with the two plate-bending forceps. Some compression can be achieved by placing the screws eccentrically in the oval plate holes.

The mini T plates, 1.5 mm are available with 9 holes in the shaft, and with either 3 or 4 holes in the head.

Important dimensions:
- Profile: See figure
- Thickness: 0.9 mm
- Width: 3.8 mm
- Hole spacing: 5   mm
- Length: 50   mm

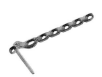

Mini Condylar Plates, 1.5 mm

These plates are designed to be used in fractures or osteotomies near the metacarpophalangeal (MP) or proximal interphalangeal (PIP) joints. At one end, the plates have a 1.5 mm wide pin, 14 mm in length, set at 90° either to the left or to the right of the coaxial plate hole. The pin is cut to the desired length with a plate-cutting forceps before insertion into the metaphyseal bone. The implant provides firm fixation in the fragment adjacent to the joint with minimal space requirement. The plate is notched to allow easy contouring.

The 1.5 mm mini condylar plates exist with 6 holes in the shaft, and 1 beside the pin. The plates with the pin to the left are available in both stainless steel and titanium, plates with the pin to the right only in titanium.

Important dimensions:
- Profile: See figure
- Thickness: 0.9 mm
- Width: 3.5 mm
- Hole spacing: 5   mm
- Plate length: 26   mm

Mini Fragment Instruments and Implants

Kirschner Wires

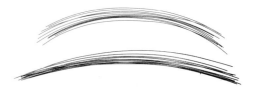

Kirschner wires in stainless steel and titanium alloy are available with a diameter of 0.8 mm and a length of 70 mm, with a diameter of 1.0 mm and a length of 150 mm, or with a diameter of 1.25 mm and a length of 150 mm, and with a trocar tip. They are used for reduction and temporary, or definitive fixation of fractures in the hand and foot, or in other small bones.

They are inserted with either the mini air drill or the small air drill with Jacobs chuck. The different lengths should help in identifying the diameter of the wire. Further sizes are available.

Cerclage Wires

Cerclage wires, 0.6 mm in diameter and 175 mm long, and 0.8 mm in diameter and 200 mm long, are sometimes used for tension band wiring of mini fragments. The wire has excellent tensile strength and is easy to handle. The pre-cut lengths help to identify the different diameters of wires.

6.11.2.3 Supplementary Implants

DCP, 2.7 mm

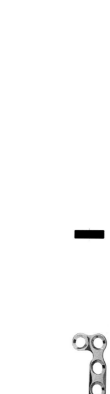

This plate is similar in design to its larger counterparts, DCP, 4.5 mm and 3.5 mm, and is used in mandibular and veterinary surgery, but has also found application in metacarpal and metatarsal fractures. The DCP drill guide, 2.7 mm, neutral (green) and load (yellow), is used to drill for the 2.7 mm cortex screw. Self-compression can be obtained by using the load drill guide (arrow towards the fracture) for eccentric placement of the screw in a plate hole. The axial displacement is 0.8 mm. To obtain further compression, the articulated tension device can be used. The plate is contoured with the small bending irons.

The DCP, 2.7 mm is available in lengths from 20 mm to 100 mm, with 2 to 12 holes. The two-hole plate with longer hole spacing is used in mandibular surgery.

Important dimensions:
– Profile: See figure
– Thickness up to 6 holes: 2.0 mm (titanium 2.2 mm)
– Thickness 7–12 holes: 2.5 mm (titanium 2.7 mm)
– Width: 8   mm
– Hole spacing: 8 and 12 mm

Small L Plate, 2.7 mm, Left and Right Angled

These plates are similar in design and use to the oblique L plate (see above).

Instrumentation and Techniques

DCP, 2.0 mm

This plate is similar in design and use to the other DCPs. It is used in the hand or the foot, especially in secondary procedures, when an extra strong implant is required. The DCP drill guide, 2.0 mm is used to drill for the 2.0 mm screws. Axial self-compression of 0.8 mm can be obtained if the load (yellow) drill guide is used (arrow towards the fracture).

The DCP, 2.0 mm is available in lengths from 22 to 42 mm, with 4 to 8 holes.

Important dimensions:
– Profile: See figure
– Thickness 4–6 holes: 1   mm
– Thickness 7, 8 holes: 1.5 mm
– Width: 5   mm
– Hole spacing: 7   mm

Straight Plate, 2.0 mm

This plate is used for diaphyseal fractures of the phalanges. Some axial compression may be obtained by eccentric placement of screws in the oval plate holes.

The plate is available in lengths from 17 mm to 35 mm, with 3 to 6 holes.

Important dimensions:
– Profile: See figure
– Thickness: 1.2 mm
– Width: 5   mm
– Hole spacing: 6   mm

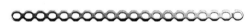

Adaptation Plate, 2.0 mm

The adaptation plate, with 20 holes, is a very thin and malleable plate which has edge indentations between holes that allow bending in two planes. It can be cut to the desired length with the plate-cutting forceps. The plate may be used in the reconstruction of fingers.

Important dimensions:
– Profile: See figure
– Thickness: 0.9 mm
– Width: 5   mm
– Hole spacing: 5   mm
– Length: 100 mm

Mini T Plate, 2.0 mm , and Mini L Plates, 2.0 mm,
Oblique and Right Angled

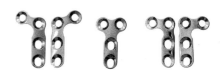

These plates are similar in design to their 2.7 mm counterparts, but smaller. Their main application is in fractures near joints, where the head is fixed first in the metaphysis and its shaft in the diaphysis. Some axial compression can be achieved with eccentric placement of the screw in the first shaft hole.
The plates are available with 2 holes in the shaft and 2 in the head.

Important dimensions:
– Thickness: 1 mm
– Width: 5 mm
– Hole spacing: 6 mm

H Plate, 2.0 mm

This plate is used mainly for reimplantation of transversely amputated fingers, where extensive exposure is not desirable. It is fixed with 2.0 mm screws.

Important dimensions:
– Profile: See figure
– Thickness: 1 mm
– Width: 11 mm
– Length: 12 mm
– Hole spacing: 7 and 6 mm

H Plate, 1.5 mm

This plate is similar in use to the 2.0 mm H plate, but fixed with 1.5 mm screws.

Important dimensions:
– Profile: See figure
– Thickness: 0.9 mm
– Width: 9   mm
– Length: 8.2 mm
– Hole spacing: 5   and 4.2 mm

Kirschner Wires with Double Tip

These wires, available with diameters of 0.6 and 0.8 mm and 70 mm in length, and with diameters of 1.0 mm and 1.25 mm and 150 mm in length, may be useful in the fixation of phalangeal and metacarpal fractures. Further sizes are available (see SYNTHES catalogue).

6.11.3 Fixation Techniques with Mini Fragment Implants

6.11.3.1 Fixation Techniques with Mini Fragment Screws

As with the larger screws sizes, the mini fragment screws can be used as lag screws, separately or through a plate, or as plate fixation screws. The principles of insertion are the same as are the principles of screw orientation (see Sect. 6.4.4). The very small dimension of the implants and instruments demands an absolutely precise insertion technique and is difficult.

2.7 mm Cortex Screw Used as a Lag Screw, Separately or Through a Plate Hole

Lag screw fixation with 2.7 mm cortex screws is used, for example, in spiral or oblique fractures of metacarpal or metatarsal bones. These are cylindrical bones with a small medullary cavity. Thanks to the introduction of the double drill sleeve system, the standard lag screw "gliding hole first" technique may also be employed (see next page).

Lag screw principle: The screw thread must have purchase in the far fragment only.

Step by step procedure:
"Thread hole first" technique:
– After anatomical reduction and temporary fixation, the thread hole is drilled through both cortices with the 2.0 mm drill bit in the double drill sleeve end, 2.0 mm (Fig. 1).
– The countersink is used to cut a recess for the screw head. (Not if a plate is used.)
– The screw length is measured (Fig. 2).
– The 2.7 mm tap in the 2.7 mm double drill sleeve end is used to cut the thread in both fragments (Fig. 3).

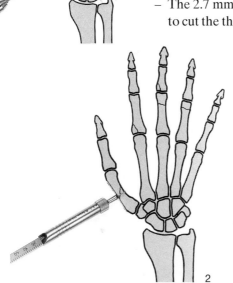

1

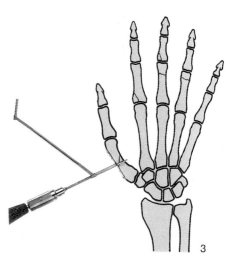

2   3

- The gliding hole is drilled with great care in the near cortex, using the 2.7 mm drill bit in the 2.7 mm double drill sleeve end. *Note*: The drilling axis must be the same as that of the thread hole to avoid any displacement (Fig. 4).
- The selected 2.7 mm cortex screw is inserted with the small hexagonal screwdriver and firmly tightened (Fig. 5).

Variation: "Gliding hole first" technique:
- Anatomical reduction and temporary fixation.
- The gliding hole is drilled in the near cortex using the 2.7 mm drill bit in the 2.7 mm double drill sleeve end.
- The 2.0 mm end of the double drill sleeve is carefully inserted into the gliding hole until it abuts the far cortex. The thread hole is drilled with the 2.0 mm drill bit (Fig. 6).
- The countersink is used to cut a recess for the screw head. If the screw is inserted through a plate this step is omitted.
- The screw length is measured with the 2.7–4.0 mm depth gauge.
- The 2.7 mm tap in the 2.7 mm double drill sleeve end is used to tap the thread hole in the far cortex.
- The selected 2.7 mm cortex screw is inserted using the small hexagonal screwdriver and firmly tightened. Interfragmentary compression is achieved.

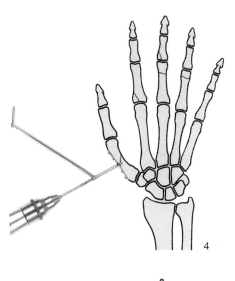

4

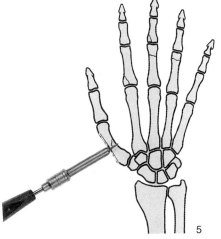

5

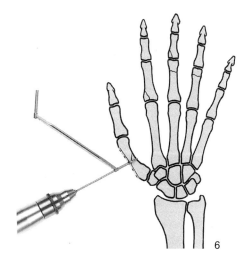

6

2.7 mm Cortex Screw Used as a Plate Fixation Screw

The 2.7 mm plates are fixed with 2.7 mm cortex screws both in the diaphysis and the metaphysis.

Step by step procedure:
- The 2.0 mm drill bit in the 2.0 mm double drill sleeve end is positioned in the plate hole and the thread hole drilled through both cortices.
- The screw length is measured.
- The 2.7 mm tap in the 2.7 mm double drill sleeve end is used to cut the thread hole in both cortices.
- The selected 2.7 mm cortex screw is inserted with the small hexagonal screwdriver.

2.0 mm Cortex Screw Used as a Lag Screw, Separately or Through a Plate Hole

In spiral or oblique fractures of the phalanges, 2.0 mm cortex screws may be used as lag screws. The insertion techniques are similar to those described above for 2.7 mm screws; both the "gliding hole first" and "thread hole first" techniques are used.

Lag screw principle: The screw thread must have purchase in the far fragment only.

Step by step procedure:
"Gliding hole first" technique:
- The fracture is reduced and temporarily fixed with a fine pointed reduction forceps (Fig. 1).
- The gliding hole is carefully drilled in the near cortex using the 2.0 mm drill bit in the 2.0 mm double drill sleeve end (Fig. 2).
- The 1.5 mm double drill sleeve end is pushed into the gliding hole until it abuts the far cortex. The thread hole is drilled with the 1.5 mm drill bit (Fig. 3).

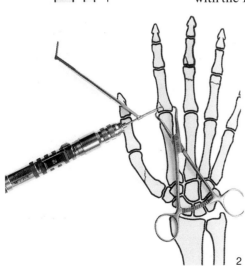

1

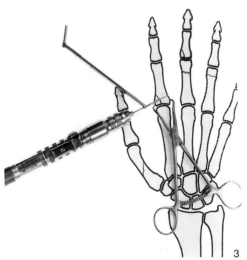

2   3

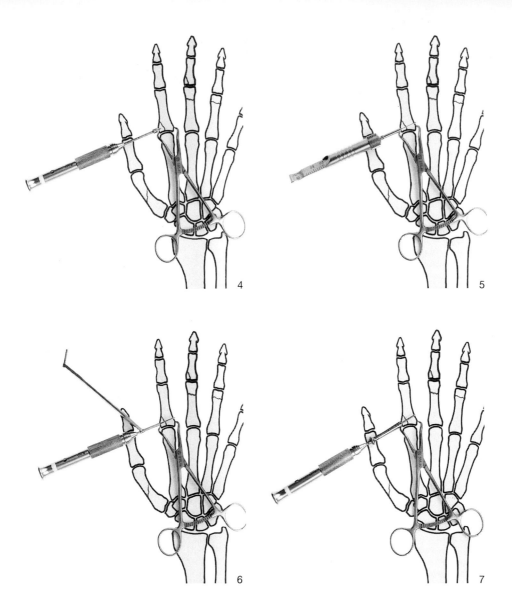

- If necessary, a recess for the screw head is cut with the mini countersink (Fig. 4).
- The 1.5–2.0 mm depth gauge is used to determine the screw length (Fig. 5).
- The 2.0 mm tap in the 2.0 mm double drill sleeve end is used to cut the thread in the far cortex (Fig. 6).
- The selected 2.0 mm cortex screw is inserted with the mini hexagonal screwdriver, and tightened (Fig. 7). (For screws with a cruciform recess the cruciform screwdriver shaft and handle are used.)

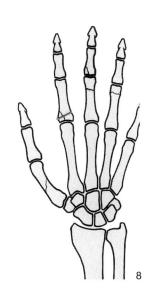

8

Variation: "Thread hole first" technique:
– After reduction and temporary fixation, the thread hole is drilled with the 1.5 mm drill bit in the double drill sleeve end, 1.5 mm through both cortices.
– Countersink, if necessary.
– The screw length is measured.
– The thread hole is tapped in both cortices with the 2.0 mm tap and the 2.0 mm double drill sleeve end.
– The gliding hole is carefully drilled in the near cortex with the 2.0 mm drill bitin the 2.0 mm double drill sleeve end.
– The 2.0 mm cortex screw of appropriate length is inserted with the mini hexagonal or cruciform screwdriver and gently tightened (Fig. 8).

2.0 mm Cortex Screw Used as a Plate Fixation Screw

The 2.0 mm mini plates are fixed with 2.0 mm cortex screws both in the diaphysis and the metaphysis.

Step by step procedure:
– The 1.5 mm drill bitin the 1.5 mm double drill sleeve end is positioned in the plate hole and the thread hole drilled through both cortices.
– The screw length is measured with the 1.5–2.0 mm depth gauge.
– The 2.0 mm tap in the 2.0 mm double drill sleeve end is used to cut the thread hole in both cortices.
– The selected 2.0 mm cortex screw is inserted with the mini hexagonal screwdriver or the cruciform screwdriver shaft and handle.

Cortex Screw 1.5 mm Used as a Lag Screw, Separately or Through a Plate Hole

For the fixation of very small fragments in the hand or the foot, the 1.5 mm cortex screw may be the implant of choice. The same techniques as described above also apply to this very small screw.

Lag screw principle: The screw thread must have purchase in the far fragment only.

Step by step procedure:
"Gliding hole first" technique:
– The fracture is reduced and temporarily fixed with a fine Kirschner wire or a fine pointed reduction forceps (Fig. 1).

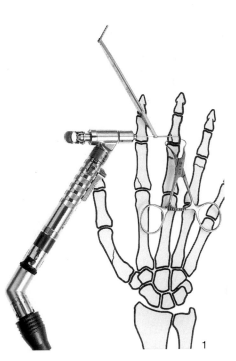

1

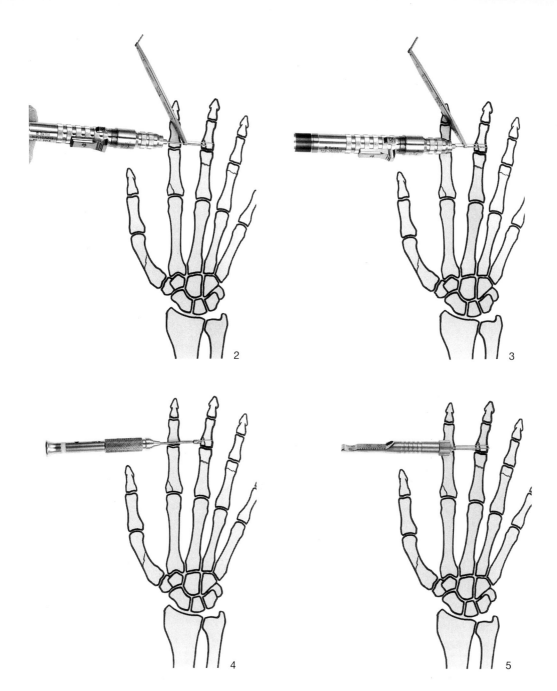

- The gliding hole is drilled in the near fragment using the 1.5 mm drill bit in the 1.5 mm double drill sleeve end (Fig. 2).
- The 1.1 mm double drill sleeve end is carefully inserted into the gliding hole until it abuts the far cortex. The 1.1 mm drill bit is used to drill the thread hole in the far cortex (Fig. 3).
- If necessary, a recess is cut for the screw head with the mini countersink (Fig. 4).
- The screw length is measured with the 1.5–2.0 mm depth gauge (Fig. 5).

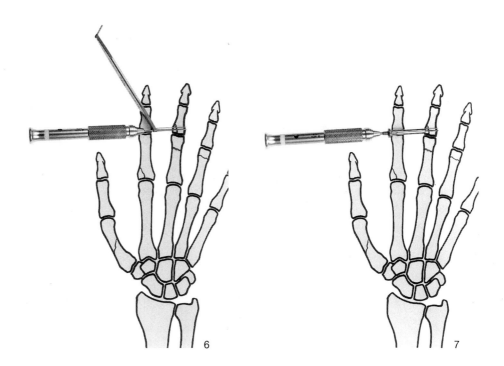

6

7

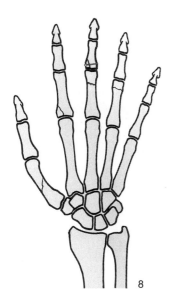

8

- The 1.5 mm tap is used in the 1.5 mm double drill sleeve end to cut the thread in the far fragment (Fig. 6).
- The selected 1.5 mm cortex screw is inserted with the mini hexagonal screwdriver, or cruciform screwdriver shaft and handle, and the screw gently tightened (Fig. 7).

Variation: "Thread hole first" technique:
- The fracture is reduced and temporary fixed with a fine Kirschner wire. The thread hole is drilled through both cortices using the 1.1 mm drill bit in the 1.1 mm double drill sleeve end.
- The mini countersink is used to cut a recess, if necessary.
- The screw length is measured.
- The 1.5 mm tap in the 1.5 mm double drill sleeve end is used to cut the thread in both cortices.
- The gliding hole is carefully drilled in the near cortex with the 1.5 mm drill bit in the 1.5 mm double drill sleeve end.
- The selected 1.5 mm cortex screw is inserted with the mini hexagonal screwdriver or the cruciform screwdriver shaft and handle (Fig. 8).

Cortex Screw, 1.5 mm Used as a Plate Fixation Screw

The 1.5 mm mini plates are fixed with 1.5 mm cortex screws both in the diaphysis and the metaphyses of the small phalangeal bones.

Step by step procedure:
– The 1.1 mm drill bit in the 1.1 mm double drill sleeve end is positioned in the plate hole and the thread hole drilled through both cortices.
  The screw length is measured with the 1.5–2.0 mm depth gauge.
  The 1.5 mm tap in the 1.5 mm double drill sleeve end is used to cut the thread hole in both cortices.
  The selected 1.5 mm cortex screw is inserted with the mini hexagonal screwdriver, or the cruciform screwdriver shaft and handle, and gently tightened.

6.11.3.2 Fixation Techniques with Mini Fragment Plates

The fixation technique of an implant will depend upon the local anatomy and the fracture type. The following examples serve only as guidelines.

Quarter-Tubular Plate Applied as a Neutralisation Plate

The quarter-tubular plate is mainly applied as a neutralisation plate in lag screw fixation of spiral, or oblique, fractures of the metacarpal bones to protect against shearing and bending forces. The technique of application follows the same principles as for the larger one-third tubular plates.

Prerequisites:
– Lag screw fixation at an appropriate angle, beside or through the plate.
– All screws are placed in central (neutral) position in the plate holes.

Plate length:
– In each main fragment four or five cortices should be engaged by screws.

Step by step procedure:
– The fracture is reduced. The plate site is determined, the plate exactly contoured and fixed provisionally to the bone with forceps.
– If the apex of the fracture is directly beneath the plate, a 2.7 mm cortex screw is inserted as a lag screw through the plate (see p. 249). In other instances a separate lag screw, beside the plate, is inserted using the same technique.

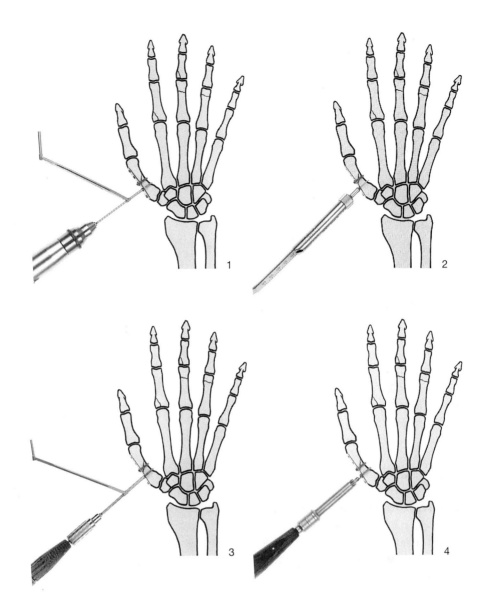

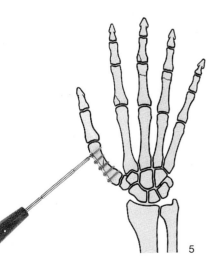

- The drill bit 2.0 mm in the 2.0 mm double drill sleeve end is then used to drill through both cortices for the first plate fixation screw (Fig. 1).
- The screw length is measured (Fig. 2).
- The 2.7 mm tap in the 2.7 mm double drill sleeve end is used to cut the thread hole (Fig. 3).
- The selected 2.7 mm cortex screw is inserted using the small hexagonal screwdriver (Fig. 4).
- The second plate fixation screw is inserted in similar manner on the opposite side of the fracture.
- Alternating from one side to the other, the remaining 2.7 mm cortex screws are inserted (Fig. 5).

Quarter Tubular Plate Applied as a Tension Band Plate

The plate is applied as tension band plate in short oblique, or transverse, fractures of mainly the metacarpal bones.

Prerequisites:
– The plate is applied to the tension side of the bone.
– The plate is contoured to the shape of the bone; in transverse fractures also slightly overbent.
– Axial compression is achieved by eccentric placement of the screws in those plate holes nearest the fracture on each side.

Plate length:
– Five to six cortices in each main fragment should be engaged by screws.

Step by step procedure:
– After reduction and provisional fixation, the contoured plate is applied to the bone with reduction forceps.
  The first screw hole is drilled through one of the plate holes near the fracture using the 2.0 mm drill bit in the 2.0 mm double drill sleeve end.
– The screw length is measured.
– The thread is cut in both cortices with the 2.7 mm tap in the 2.7 mm double drill sleeve end.
– The selected 2.7 mm cortex screw is inserted with the small hexagonal screwdriver, but not fully tightened.
– The plate is pulled towards the fracture to place this first screw in the eccentric position.
– In the plate hole near the fracture in the opposite fragment, the second screw hole is drilled using the 2.0 mm drill bit in the 2.0 mm double drill sleeve end. The drill hole is placed in the eccentric position, away from the fracture.
– After measuring and tapping the second 2.7 mm cortex screw is inserted and tightened. The first screw is then tightened, compressing the fracture (Fig. 1).
– The remaining plate screws are inserted alternating from one side to the other using the technique described for the first screw.
– Final tightening of all screws (Fig. 2).

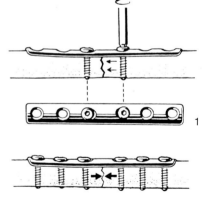

1

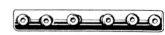

2

Instrumentation and Techniques

Application of the Small T and L Plates, 2.7 mm

Oblique or transverse metaphyseal fractures of metacarpal and metatarsal bones can be fixed with small 2.7 mm T or L plates.

Prerequisites:
– Exact contouring of the plate to the bone is mandatory, especially of the head portion.
– Axial compression by the eccentric placement of one of the shaft screws.
– If possible, a lag screw should be inserted through the plate, after axial compression has been applied. In such a case the plate functions as a neutralisation plate

Plate length:
– Only one length is available.

Step by step procedure:
– Axial and rotational alignment is verified.
– Exact contouring of the plate, especially the head portion.
– The first plate screw is prepared in the head by drilling with the 2.0 mm drill bit in the 2.0 mm double drill sleeve end as a guide (Fig. 1).
– The screw length is measured with the small depth gauge, 2.7 mm – 4.0 mm.
– The thread hole is tapped with the 2.7 mm tap in the 2.7 mm double drill sleeve end.
– The selected 2.7 mm cortex screw is inserted with the small hexagonal screwdriver through the plate hole (Fig. 2).
– The axial and rotational alignment, as well as the precise fit of the plate, is rechecked.
– Insertion of the second 2.7 mm cortex screw in the head as described above. To avoid collision with the previous screw, the screwdriver shaft can be inserted in its head to indicate its direction. Drill for the second screw either parallel to the first screw, or obliquely, but on a different plane.
– The correct alignment of the plate shaft is verified before drilling for the first shaft screw. The 2.0 mm drill bit in the 2.0 mm double drill sleeve end is positioned eccentrically in the plate hole, away from the fracture, and the thread hole drilled.
– The screw length is measured.
– The 2.7 mm tap in the 2.7 mm double drill sleeve end is used to cut the tread hole in both cortices.
– The selected 2.7 mm cortex screw is inserted and carefully tightened. This screw should achieve axial compression (Fig. 3).
– If possible, a lag screw is inserted through the plate.
– The remaining shaft screws are inserted in the neutral position using the same technique as described for the first screw. Final tightening of all screws (Fig. 4).

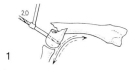

1

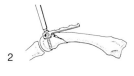

2

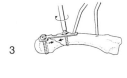

3

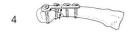

4

Application of the Small Condylar Plate, 2.7 mm

The small 2.7 mm condylar plate can be used for the fixation of periarticular fractures, with or without intra-articular extensions of metacarpals and metatarsals.

Prerequisites:
– Placement of the pin parallel to the joint.
– Exact contouring of the plate.
– Axial compression by eccentric placement of one screw in the plate shaft.

Plate length:
– In the plate shaft, screws should engage four to five cortices in oblique fractures, and five or six in transverse fractures.

Step by step procedure:
– The technique of application is similar to that of the 2.0 mm condylar plate, except that the 2.7 mm instrumentation is used (see below).

DCP, 2.7 mm Applied as a Self-Compression Plate

The DCP 2.7 mm may be inserted as a self-compression plate for axial compression in short oblique, or transverse, fractures of metacarpals and metatarsals. The 2.7 mm cortex screws are used for the fixation of the plate.

Prerequisites:
– The plate is contoured to the bone; in transverse fractures also slightly overbent.
– Axial compression by one or more load screws.
– Stability is augmented if a lag screw can be inserted through the plate.

Plate length:
– In each main fragment four to five cortices should be engaged by screws.

Step by step procedure:
– The fracture is reduced. The contoured plate is applied to the bone with the middle portion placed over the fracture and held with reduction forceps.
– In the plate hole adjacent to the fracture the first screw hole is drilled using the 2.0 mm drill bit and the DCP drill guide, 2.7 mm.
– The screw length is measured.
– Tapping with the tap for 2.7 mm cortex screw in the 2.7 mm double drill sleeve end.
– The selected 2.7 mm cortex screw is inserted with the small hexagonal screwdriver, but not completely tightened.

- The plate is pulled towards the fracture to place the first screw in eccentric position.
- The second screw hole is prepared in the opposite fragment in the plate hole adjacent to the fracture. The load (yellow) DCP drill guide is placed in the plate hole with the arrow pointing towards the fracture and the hole drilled with the 2.0 mm drill bit.
- The screw length is measured.
- The thread is cut with the tap for 2.7 mm cortex screw in the 2.7 mm double drill sleeve end.
- Insertion of the 2.7 mm cortex screw with the small hexagonal screwdriver. Tightening of both screws produces axial compression.
- If the compression is sufficient, the remaining screws are inserted in the neutral position, alternating from one side of the fracture to the other: drill bit 2.0 mm in the neutral DCP drill guide, measure, tap and insert the screw.
- Final tightening of all screws.
- A third load screw can be inserted if necessary:
- In the second plate hole the 2.7 mm load (yellow) DCP drill guide is positioned with the arrow towards the fracture. The hole is drilled with the 2.0 mm drill bit.
- The screw length is measured.
- The tap for 2.7 mm cortex screw in the 2.7 mm double drill sleeve end is used to cut the thread.
- The chosen 2.7 mm cortex screw is inserted until the screw head reaches the plate hole.
- Before this screw is tightened completely, the adjacent screw must be loosened to allow further compression. After tightening of the third load screw the other screw can be retightened.

**Straight Mini Plate, 2.0 mm,
Applied as a Self-Compression Plate**

Straight mini plates are applied for axial compression in short oblique, or transverse, diaphyseal fractures of the phalanges. The plate is cut to the desired length with the plate-cutting forceps and fixed to the bone with 2.0 mm cortex screws.

Prerequisites:
- Contouring of the plate with two plate-bending forceps.
- Axial compression by inserting screws in the eccentric position.

Plate length:
- In each main fragment four cortices should be engaged by screws.

Mini H Plate, 2.0 mm Applied as a Compression Plate

The mini H plate may be used for compression of transverse fractures of the phalanges, or for y-shaped metaphyseal fractures, when extensive exposure is undesirable. The 2.0 mm cortex screws are used for fixation.

Prerequisites:
– Contouring of the plate.
– Compression by eccentric placement of screws.

Plate length:
– The plate is available only with four holes.

Step by step procedure (for example, for a transverse fracture):
– The fracture is reduced, and axial and rotational alignment verified.
– The 1.5 mm drill bit in the 1.5 mm double drill sleeve end is used to drill the first screw hole.
– The length is measured with the 1.5–2.0 mm depth gauge.
– The 2.0 mm tap in the 2.0 mm double drill sleeve end is used to cut the thread.
– The first 2.0 mm cortex screw is inserted with the mini hexagonal (or cruciform) screwdriver.
– The second screw in the same fragment is inserted in similar manner.
– In the opposite fragment the 1.5 mm drill bit and the 1.5 mm double drill sleeve end are positioned eccentrically in the plate hole, away from the fracture, and the thread hole drilled.
– After measuring and tapping, the third 2.0 mm cortex screw is inserted.
– The fourth screw is also inserted in an eccentric position using the same technique. Collision with the third screw, owing to convexity of the bone, should be avoided by placing a screwdriver shaft in its head to indicate its direction.
– Final tightening of all screws.

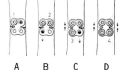

A   B   C   D

Application of Mini Plates, 1.5 mm

The 1.5 mm mini plates are used for the same indications as the 2.0 mm mini plates only in smaller bones. Since the shapes of the plates are identical, the technique of application is similar, except that the 1.5 mm instrumentation is used instead.

6.11.4 Instruments for Application and Removal of Mini Fragment Implants

Instruments for insertion of 2.7 mm screws

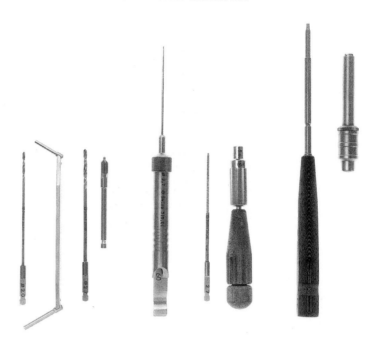

Instruments for application of 2.7 mm plates, for DCP, 2.7 mm below to the right

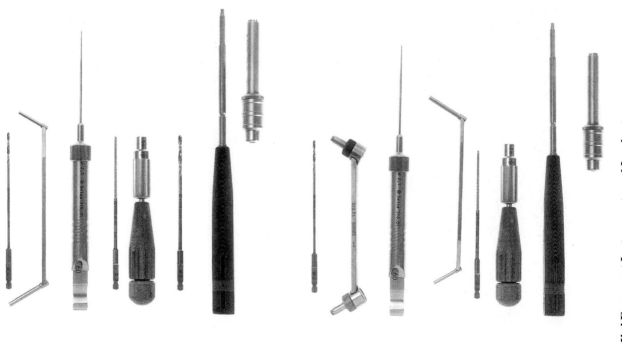

Instruments for insertion of 2.0 mm screws

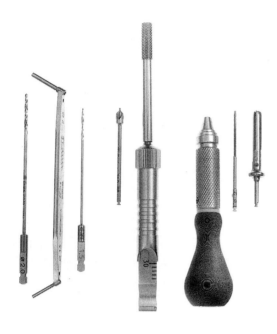

Instruments for application of 2.0 mm plates

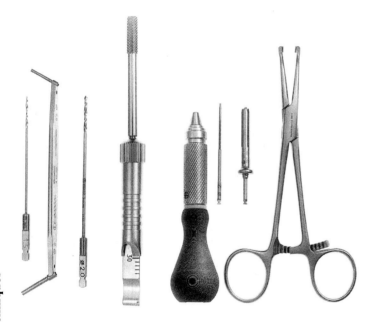

Instruments for insertion of 1.5 mm screws

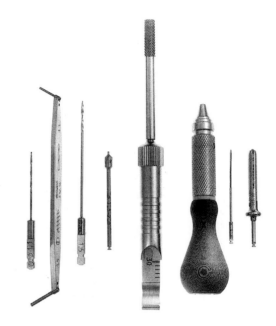

Instruments for application of 1.5 mm plates

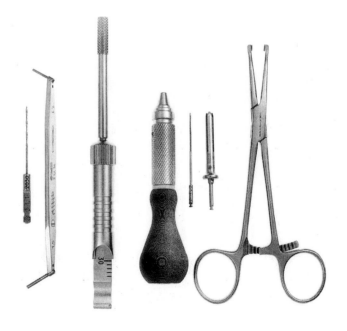

Mini Fragment Instruments and Implants

Instruments for removal of 2.7 mm implants

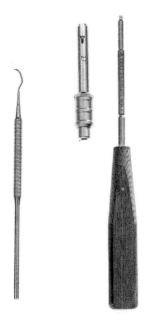

Instruments for removal of 2.0 mm and 1.5 mm implants

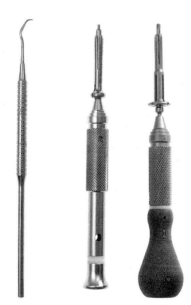

6.12 Intramedullary Nailing Instruments and Implants

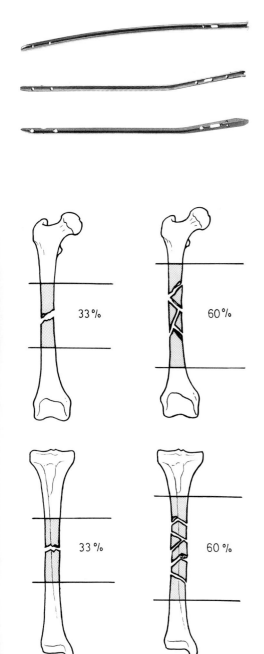

Intramedullary nails of various different designs have been used for the stabilisation of long bone fractures since their introduction by Küntscher in the late 1930s. In the early 1950s, he also introduced reaming of the medullary cavity, and, around the same time, the concept of interlocking.

AO adopted the nailing concept and developed femoral and tibial nailing systems which were used for many years and finally led to the introduction of the present AO/ASIF universal nailing system, which can be used with or without locking. This system has now been supplemented with the unreamed solid tibial nail with locking possibilities. Intramedullary nails of earlier design, thin-walled and partially slotted, are still in use, but will not be discussed in this book (for details, see the previous edition).

The medullary nail is a load-sharing device, much stronger than a plate. It can thus permit an early return to weight-bearing, if axial and rotational stability is ensured. Depending on the fracture pattern, this can be achieved by different means. The AO/ASIF universal nail may be used after reaming of the cavity in transverse or short oblique fractures with cortical stability in the middle third of femur or tibia. Open or "closed" nailing is possible. Interlocking is employed if the fracture is axially and/or rotationally unstable, e. g. long spiral fractures, multifragmentary or segmental fractures, or fractures of the proximal and distal ends of the diaphysis. Reaming is then limited to a minimum.

The AO/ASIF unreamed tibial nail (UTN), which was introduced more recently, finds its (locked) application in fresh fractures of the diaphysis with severe soft tissue injuries. An unreamed femoral nail is currently under development.

Indications for Universal Nailing of Femur and Tibia, With and Without Locking

Conventional nailing without locking for stable fractures with bony support in the middle third of the bone, such as:
– Transverse fractures
– Short oblique fractures
– Delayed union or nonunion

Locked medullary nailing for unstable fractures without bony support in approximately the middle 60 % of the bone, where axial and rotational stability has to be achieved, such as:
– Fractures near the metaphysis
– Long torsional fractures
– Segmental fractures
– Multifragmentary fractures
– Fractures with bone defects

6.12.1 Standard Instruments for Universal Nailing

The instruments necessary for the insertion of the universal femoral and tibial nails can be obtained either in graphic cases or in sterilising trays.

6.12.1.1 Reaming Instruments

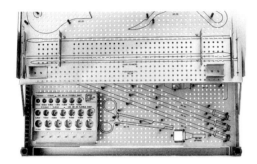 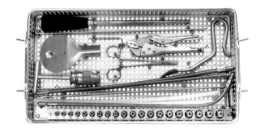

Centring Pin, 4 mm Diameter, 400 mm

This pin is introduced about 50 mm into the medullary canal at the point of insertion and at the correct angle to guide the cannulated cutter. The universal chuck is used for insertion.

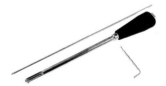

Cannulated Cutter, 11 mm Diameter, 350 mm

This cutter is used with the centring pin to open the medullary canal for both femoral and tibial nailing. The centring pin can be locked to the cutter with the Allen screw. The cannulated cutter has a special sharpened tip to allow cutting/carving while rotating the instrument by hand. It should be rotated 180°, and then turned back. Some older instruments had a metal plate at the end of the handle, inviting use of the hammer, but this is *not recommended*, since damage to the delicate cutting edge may result. The cutting edge may be resharpened.

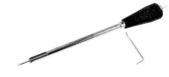

Large Hexagonal Allen Key

This key is used to tighten the Allen screw on the cannulated cutter (see above).

Instrumentation and Techniques

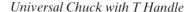

Universal Chuck with T Handle

This handle is used to insert the centring pin, and also the reaming rod, into the medullary canal.

Small Awl

This awl may be used to open the medullary canal of both femur and tibia by twisting movements. Great care must be taken not to slip off the bone and damage soft tissue, or to split the cortex. Since the introduction of the cannulated cutter, the use of the small awl has decreased.

Hand Reamers, 6 mm, 7 mm, and 8 mm Diameter

These hand reamers can be used to broach the medullary canal if it is obstructed by pseudarthrosis or callus. Further sizes are available. See SYNTHES catalogue for details.

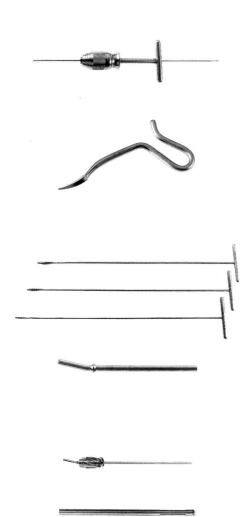

Reaming Rod, 3 mm Diameter, 950 mm

This rod, with an offset ball tip and slightly curved, is introduced into the medullary canal and used as a guide when reaming is performed with the flexible shafts. The ball, offset 2 cm from the tip, prevents the flexible shaft from reaming past the rod. It is also used when removing a jammed reamer. The curved tip facilitates passage of the reaming rod through the fragments, especially in closed nailing. The proximal end of the of the rod has two flats to accommodate the holding forceps (or the holder). The 950 mm long rod is used to ensure that the proximal end protrudes and can be held while reaming with the flexible shafts with reaming depth up to 440 mm.

Note: The reaming rod must be checked for damage. Proper passage of the reamer heads and flexible shafts may otherwise be impossible and force the rod forwards into the joint.

Holding Forceps

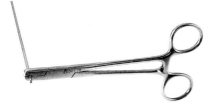

This forceps holds the reaming rod in place during the reaming process. It is attached at the proximal end while reaming, and where the reaming rod enters the medullary canal when reamer heads and flexible shafts are exchanged.

Intramedullary Nailing Instruments and Implants

Flexible Shaft with Front Cutting Reamer, 9 mm Diameter

This shaft has the reamer fixed to it. It is the first to be used when reaming the medullary canal. It cuts at the front, and is stopped only by the offset ball tip of the reaming rod, which, therefore, must always be used with this instrument.

Note: All three flexible shafts are connected to the universal air machine with the right-angle drive for reaming.

Note: The flexible shafts are made of three coaxially arranged coils with soldered end pieces. This ensures great flexibility and easy use, but makes them difficult to clean. See Sect. 6.22.5.2.

Never pull on the shaft since this could damage the coil or the soldered connections.

Never drive the shafts in reverse, or they will uncoil!

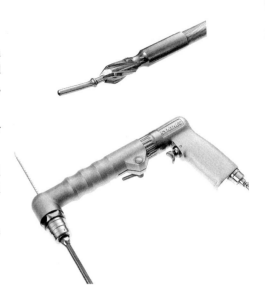

Flexible Shaft, 8 mm Diameter, Reaming Depth up to 440 mm

This shaft is used to continue the reaming process with the separate reamers 9.5–12.5 mm (engraved on the end piece) in 0.5 mm increments. It must be used with the reaming rod.

Flexible Shaft, 10 mm Diameter, Reaming Depth up to 440 mm

This shaft is used with reamers 13.0–19.0 mm (engraved on the end piece), also in 0.5 mm increments, in the same manner as the above.

Medullary Reamers, 9.5–19.5 mm Diameter

These reamers are used with the 8 mm and 10 mm flexible shafts for reaming the medullary canal. The reamers are inserted from the side onto the dovetail end of the flexible shaft, and held in place with two fingers until slid over the reaming rod. The conically shaped corners and the sides of the reamers are cutting. These must be constantly checked for damage, or else use may lead to heat necroses of the inner cortex. Due to the time and cost involved, they cannot be resharpened but must be replaced when damaged (see Sect. 6.22.5.2).

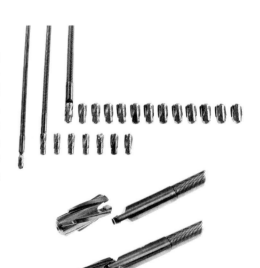

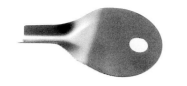

Tissue Protector

The tissue protector protects the soft tissue from being injured during the reaming process. The tissue protector is held between the soft tissue and the flexible shaft at the entry point.

Medullary Tube

This tube is inserted over the reaming rod and holds the reduced fragments in place when exchanging the reaming rod for the guide rod. It has a marker at the tip for X-ray control. The plastic tube is autoclavable, but has to be checked for elasticity, since frequent sterilisation makes the tube brittle.

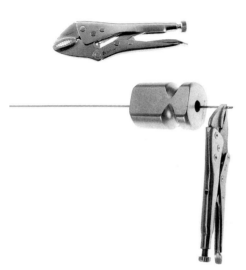

Locking Pliers

These pliers are useful if a jammed reamer has to be removed. After uncoupling the air machine and sliding the ram over the reaming rod, the rod is gripped at the end with the locking pliers. By striking the ram against the pliers, the reamer should disengage. The pliers may also be used to grip the nail end to loosen a jammed conical bolt.

Air Jet, for Cleaning Instruments

This air jet, made of a non-autoclavable plastic, is used together with the air tube to clean the flexible shafts. It can be connected to a compressed air source, or to a water tap via a quick coupling hose.

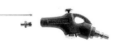

Air Tube, 2.0 mm Diameter, for Air Jet

This tube is connected to the air jet by removing the nozzle head. After inserting the tube into the head it is screwed back into the nozzle.

6.12.1.2 Insertion Instruments

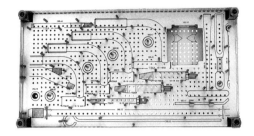
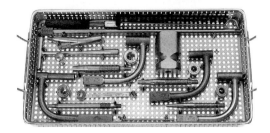

Guide Rod, 3 mm Diameter, 950 mm, with Flattened Ends, for Tibial Nails

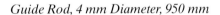

This rod is exchanged with the reaming rod, using the medullary tube, before inserting the universal tibial nail. It is more flexible than the 4 mm guide rod and can therefore "guide" the curved tibial nail. The flattened ends prevent the guide rod from being used as a reaming rod. The flattened distal end also allows removal from the nail without getting the rod stuck in the slot of the nail. The guide rod has two flats at the end for the holding forceps (or for the old style holder).

Guide Rod, 4 mm Diameter, 950 mm

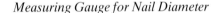

This rod is used to "guide" the femoral nail during insertion. First the medullary tube is slid over the reaming rod, which can then be removed without loss of reduction. The guide rod is inserted and the medullary tube removed. The guide rod has two flats at the proximal end for the holding forceps or the holder.

Measuring Gauge for Nail Diameter

This gauge is used to check diameters of nails and reamers. For correct measurement, the nail must be slid in as far as its middle.

Insertion Handles for Universal Femoral Nails, 9–12 mm, 13–16 mm, 17–19 mm Diameter

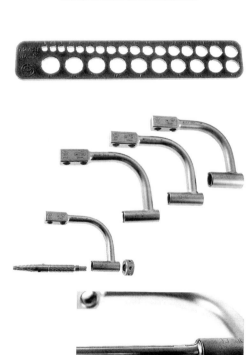

These handles are used for the insertion of nails within the size range marked on the instrument. It is used together with the corresponding size threaded conical bolt and locking nut. The lugs on the handle must engage the positioning notches at the upper end of the nail for insertion in either the left or the right leg (see marking). The handle is also used for proximal locking of the nail. The holes in the handle position the locking instruments. See Sect. 6.12.5.3.

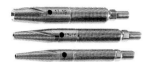

Threaded Conical Bolts for Universal Femoral Nails,
9–12 mm, 13–16 mm, 17–19 mm Diameter

These bolts are screwed by hand into the nail within the size range marked on the bolt, and then assembled with the insertion handle. Once the lugs of the handle have engaged the notches, firm tightening is achieved with the cannulated socket, or combination wrench. The grooves of the bolt collect any ingrown tissue when removal is performed.

Note: The threaded conical bolt can only be removed from the universal nail when the handle is positioned with the lugs in the notches of the nail. See Sect. 6.12.6.6.

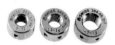

Locking Nuts for Universal Femoral Nails,
9–12 mm, 13–16 mm, 17–19 mm Diameter

These nuts are screwed onto the bolt of corresponding size (see engravings on bolts and nuts). They lock the handles in position in the nail with the lugs engaging the notches. Firm tightening is performed with the pin wrench.

Note: Some earlier handles, bolts and locking nuts for the universal femoral nail were marked 9–12, 12–16, and 16–19. This no longer applies.

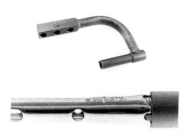

Insertion Handle for Universal Tibial Nails,
10–14 mm Diameter

This handle is used for insertion and for locking of universal tibial nails. Its lugs have to engage in the notches of the nail for insertion either in the left or in the right leg (see engravings). The handle is also used for proximal locking of the nail, for which it has to be placed on the medial side. The three holes in the handle position the locking instruments for static or dynamic locking (see engravings).

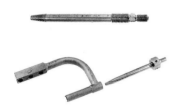

Threaded Conical Bolt for Universal Tibial Nails,
10–14 mm Diameter

This bolt is pushed through the handle and screwed into the nail end for insertion. It is tightened with the cannulated socket wrench, or the combination wrench. The grooves of the conical threaded end collect any ingrown tissue when the nail is removed.

Intramedullary Nailing Instruments and Implants

Locking Nut for Universal Tibial Nails, 10–14 mm Diameter

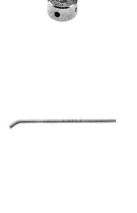

This nut is screwed onto the bolt and locks the insertion handle for universal tibial nails in position in the nail. The lugs of the handle sleeve must engage the notches in the nail end. The holes in the side are used to tighten or loosen the locking nut with the pin wrench.

Pin Wrench

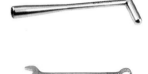

This wrench is used to tighten the locking nuts on the threaded conical bolts. It can also be used to tighten and loosen the driving head from the curved driving piece, and to loosen the ram guide from the threaded conical bolts after insertion.

Cannulated Socket Wrench, 11 mm

This wrench is used to tighten or loosen instruments with a socket 11 mm in width.

Combination Wrench, 11 mm

This wrench is used to tighten or loosen instruments with a nut 11 mm width across flats. The open end can be used if already assembled instruments have to be retightened or loosened.

Curved Driving Piece

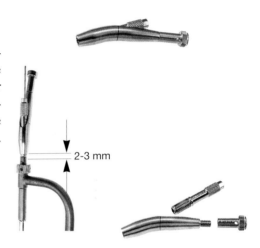

2-3 mm

This piece can be used together with the driving head for insertion of the universal nails with a hammer. It is screwed onto the threaded conical bolt, leaving a 3 mm gap between the rear threads of the bolt and the striker receptacle of the curved driving piece. This distance is necessary to reduce the risk of damage to the initial threads by hammer blows when driving in the nail. The instrument is disassembled for cleaning.

Driving Head

This driving head is screwed onto the proximal end of the curved driving piece for insertion of universal nails with a hammer. The hole in the neck allows insertion of the pin wrench, or similar instrument, to unscrew a tight driving head.

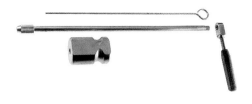

Ram Guide

This piece is used for insertion and extraction of universal nails with the ram. It is hollow to allow passage of the guide rod during insertion. The hole in the distal end is used to unscrew a tight ram guide with the pin wrench, or similar instrument. The threaded proximal end accepts the flexible grip.

Guide Rod Retainer

This retainer is used to prevent the guide rod from backing out during insertion of the nail.

Ram

This ram, 1300 g in weight, is slid over the ram guide and used to insert universal nails. By simply letting it fall a short distance, the nail is inserted 5–10 mm at a time. The ram is also used for the removal of nails.

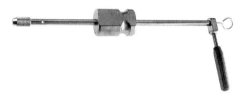

Flexible Grip

This grip is screwed onto the proximal end of the ram guide to protect the ram from disengaging during insertion. When extracting the nail the flexible grip is necessary to receive the blows of the ram.

6.12.1.3 Locking Instruments

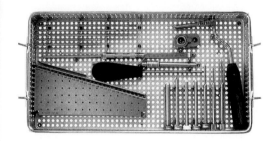 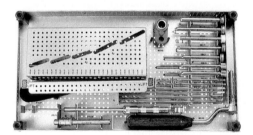

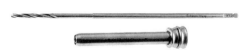

Drill Bit, 4.0 mm Diameter, Shaft 4.5 mm, Two-Fluted

This bit, 225 mm/75 mm (total length/effective length), has a quick coupling end. It is used to drill the pilot hole for the 4.9 mm diameter locking bolts. The 4.5 mm shaft ensures accurate guidance of the drill bit in the 8.0 mm/4.5 mm protection sleeve. A *three-fluted drill bit* with depth markings from 25–100 mm, in 5 mm increments, has recently been introduced. This drill bit allows determination of the screw length, but only if used with the 8.0 mm/4.5 mm protection sleeve.

Drill Bit, 4.5 mm Diameter

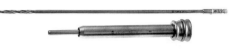

This 145 mm/120 mm bit for quick coupling, may be used to drill the near cortex for the 4.9 mm locking bolt if the distal aiming device assembly is used. Thanks to its short length, it allows drilling if the distance between the bone and the image intensifier head does not, for some reason, permit the use of the longer 4.0 mm/4.5 mm drill bit. It is a regular two-fluted drill bit.

Drill Bit, 3.2 mm Diameter

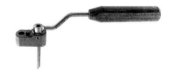

This 225 mm/200 mm bit for quick coupling is used to drill the far cortex if the technique mentioned for the 4.5 mm drill bit is employed. The two-fluted drill bit is then guided by the 4.5 mm/ 3.2 mm insert drill sleeve.

Distal Aiming Device

This aiming device can be used to position accurately the instruments needed for distal locking of the universal nails, if an image intensifier is used. The X-ray source must be placed underneath the leg and the receiver head above. It connects with the direction finder, which is held in place by a ball bearing. The 11 mm sleeve accepts the 11 mm/8 mm protection sleeve, the aiming trocar, and the fixation bolts. The depth gauge and the screwdriver are also used through the sleeve. Its two sharp points can be anchored in the bone with light taps from a hammer. See also technique described in Sect. 6.12.5.3.

Direction Finder

This direction finder is connected to the distal aiming device for the locking procedure. It has a round radiolucent circle with a central radio-opaque dot, and two metal rings. With the dot centred in the two concentric circles, the direction finder's axis is parallel to the image intensifier's beam. It automatically corrects for the 4° divergence of the X-ray beams. The second hole accepts the drill sleeve, 8 mm/4.5 mm, which is the same distance from the axis of the distal aiming device as the distance between the two locking holes in the nail. The direction finder is made of a heat-resistant (thermosetting) plastic.

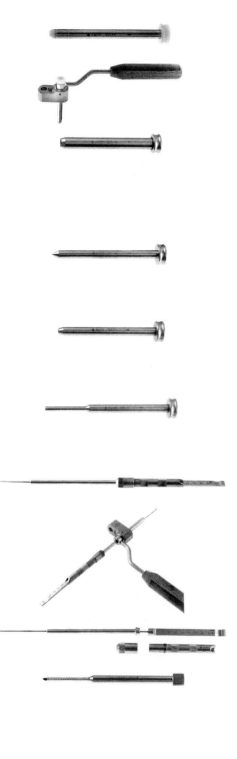

Aiming Trocar

The trocar is used through the distal aiming device sleeve to centre the trocar exactly in the locking hole with the help of the built-in metal dot. When centred, the position of the distal aiming device is correct in the long axis.

Protection Sleeve, 11 mm/8 mm Diameter

The protection sleeve is inserted through either the distal aiming device sleeve, or the direction finder, to guide the different instruments used for distal locking. It is also used for the same purpose for proximal locking through the insertion handle.

Trocar, 8.0 mm Diameter

This trocar is used with the 11 mm/8 mm protection sleeve for insertion through the soft tissue.

Drill Sleeve, 8 mm/4.5 mm Diameter

This drill sleeve accepts the 4.0 mm/4.5 mm and the 4.5 mm drill bits.

Insert Drill Sleeve, 4.5 mm/3.2 mm Diameter

This drill sleeve is used to guide the 3.2 mm drill bit when the far cortex is drilled.

Depth Gauge for Locking Bolts

This depth gauge measures up to 115 mm. It has a long neck allowing measuring for the locking bolt through the distal aiming device and the insertion handle. It must be disassembled for cleaning.

Femoral Fixation Bolt

This bolt is used to hold the distal aiming device in position in the first drill hole while drilling for the second locking bolt for the universal femoral nail. It has a long threaded portion.

Tibial Fixation Bolt

This bolt is inserted through the distal aiming device to hold it in position in the first drill hole while drilling for the second locking bolt for the universal tibial nail. It has a shorter thread than the femoral fixation bolt.

Intramedullary Nailing Instruments and Implants

Large Hexagonal Screwdriver

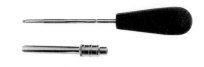

The large hexagonal screwdriver is needed for the insertion of the 4.9 mm locking bolts. It is also used to lock the direction finder in the correct position on the distal aiming device when drilling for the second locking bolt.

Large Holding Sleeve

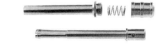

This is a self-retaining screw-holding sleeve necessary to grip and pull locking bolts when they are removed. It consists of three parts and must be disassembled for cleaning.

Radiation Shield

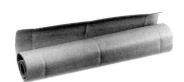

This shield, 400 mm/600 mm, is made of double-layered lead foil covered with natural rubber. The equivalent lead thickness is 0.25 mm. The radiation shield is used to protect the surgeons hands while drilling for the locking bolts under image intensification. The shield is placed on the patient's leg outside the X-ray screen to prevent scattering of rays between the surgeons hands and the X-ray source. The shield may be sterilised in steam autoclaves at 134° C (or approximately 280° F).

6.12.2 Supplementary Instruments

Holder

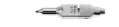

The holder can be clipped onto the reaming rod and used as a handle in stead of the holding forceps when inserting the rod into the medullary canal. It also has a hexagonal projection at one end which can be used instead of a screwdriver, for example when fitting the old-style right-angle drive onto the universal air machine.

Guide Handle for Nails

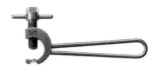

This guide handle is employed only if earlier, thin-walled and partially slotted medullary nails are used. It is fixed to the proximal end of the nail, its two lugs fitting into the nail slots, and used as an anti-rotational guide while the nail is inserted.

Connector for Extraction Hooks

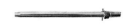

This connector is screwed into the extraction hook and connected with the ram guide, ram, and flexible grip for extraction of universal femoral nails, if the standard technique has failed, or if the thread of the proximal end is damaged.

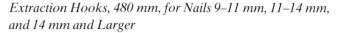

Extraction Hooks, 480 mm, for Nails 9–11 mm, 11–14 mm, and 14 mm and Larger

These hooks may have to be employed if the standard technique for femoral nail extraction has failed. It is assembled with the connector for extraction hooks, the ram guide, ram and flexible grip, and pushed into the nail. Once hooked onto the nail end, extraction is performed by striking the ram onto the flexible grip.

Radiolucent Drive

This drive allows drilling under image intensifier control, without exposing the hands to high doses of radiation. It is made of radiolucent synthetic material, and enables safe, effective aiming and drilling without the need for aiming devices. It attaches to the small air drill and is used with special drill bits (see below) to drill for the locking bolts for both the universal and the unreamed nailing system.

The drill bit is inserted by pushing the quick coupling of the radiolucent drive forward and inserting the plastic coupling end of the drill bit. The drill bit is turned in order to seat the end completely, then the coupling is pulled back into its locked position. To detach the drill bit the reversed procedure is used.

The radiolucent drive can be autoclaved to a maximum of 134° C (290° F). After sterilisation the drive *must* be allowed to cool to room temperature, since using the drive whilst hot or warm will result in jamming. The cooling process should *not* be accelerated as this will cool the casing but not the gears within. See also Sect. 6.22 for care and maintenance.

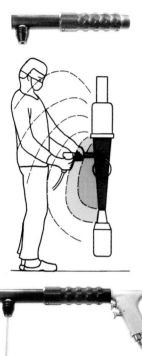

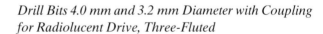

Drill Bits 4.0 mm and 3.2 mm Diameter with Coupling for Radiolucent Drive, Three-Fluted

These bits minimise the tendency to slip off the bone surface. The short spiral portion reduces the likelihood of soft tissue spooling, eliminating the need for a drill sleeve. Two sizes of drill bit are used for the nailing systems:
– Drill bit, 4.0 mm diameter, 150 mm/120 mm (effective and total length) for the 4.9 mm locking bolts (universal femoral and tibial nails),
– Drill bit, 3.2 mm diameter, 150 mm/120 mm (effective and total length) for the 3.9 mm locking bolts (UTN).

Further sizes are available: see SYNTHES catalogue for details.

Other Items

Other necessary items include the universal air drill, the right-angle drive and the small air drill; see Sect. 6.21. Regarding the distractor for reduction see Sect. 6.14.

Intramedullary Nailing Instruments and Implants

6.12.3 Obsolete Instruments

The large awl has been replaced by the cannulated cutter. The reaming rod with olive tip, 950 mm, has been replaced by the reaming rod with offset ball tip.

6.12.4 Universal Femoral and Tibial Nails, and Locking Bolts

Universal Femoral Nail

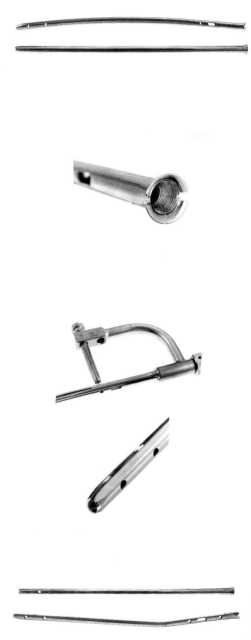

This nail, introduced in 1987, is a tube with a cloverleaf cross-section and 1.2 mm wall thickness. It has a continuous longitudinal slot on its anterior aspect. The nail has thus a certain flexibility under bending and torsion, and provides the necessary strength under functional stress. The complete longitudinal slot prevents stress concentration, particularly under torsion, and promotes an even distribution of stress over the length of the nail.

The proximal end has an internal thread which allows use of the threaded conical bolt for insertion and extraction of the nail. This rigid connection between nail and the instruments used for insertion and extraction ensures an accurate and efficient transmission of forces.

The slightly flared proximal end of the nail has two notches to receive the lugs of the insertion handle positioning it for insertion in either the left or the right leg. The keystone configuration of the slot in the proximal cylindrical section of the nail prevents spreading of the nail end when tightening the threaded conical bolt. For proximal locking, two holes are available: a 5 mm diameter round hole for static locking, and a second slotted hole for dynamic locking. The curvature of the nail corresponds to an average anatomical curvature of the adult femur of 1.5 m radius.

The distal end of the nail is rounded to allow smooth insertion over the guide rod. For distal locking, the femoral nail has two 5 mm diameter locking holes for medial or lateral locking; the most distal hole is 20 mm from the tip of the nail, the second 30 mm from the first, measured from the centres of the holes.

The AO/ASIF universal femoral nails can be used for either the right or the left leg. It is currently available with a diameter of 11 to 18 mm in lengths from 300 to 480 mm in 20 mm increments, and with a 19 mm diameter in lengths from 380 mm to 480 mm.

Universal Tibial Nail

This nail was introduced shortly after the universal femoral nail, also following extensive clinical and biomechanical studies. The characteristic features of this nail are similar to those of the

femoral nail. It is made of a tube with 1.2 mm wall thickness and a cloverleaf cross-section. It has a continuous longitudinal slot on the dorsal aspect, formed as a keystone at the proximal end. The full-length slot prevents stress concentration, particularly under torsion, and ensures an even distribution of stress over the whole length of the nail. The keystone slot prevents widening of the nail end when tightening the threaded conical bolt. The inner conical thread of the proximal end has the same configuration for all nail sizes. This allows the same insertion/extraction instruments to be used for all nail diameters.

The anterior aspect of the proximal end is bevelled to prevent irritation of the overlying soft tissue and patellar tendon. The two notches accept the lugs of the insertion handle, positioning the handle for right or left leg insertions. The nail has a bend at the transition between the middle and the proximal third. This bend takes into account the anatomical angle of about 11° formed by the axis of the access canal, and that of the medullary canal. The bend greatly facilitates insertion. The tapered tip of the nail ensures sliding of the nail along the guide rod without penetration of the posterior cortex.

For locking of the nail, there are three holes both proximally and distally. The proximal three holes are used for mediolateral locking. The middle, slotted one is used for dynamic locking, and the two 5 mm diameter round holes for static locking. Two of the distal holes, the most distal and the most proximal, are orientated mediolaterally, and the middle hole antero-posteriorly. The antero-posterior (AP) hole is used if medial soft tissue coverage is inadequate or if the proximal mediolateral hole is too close to the fracture site. The most distal mediolateral hole is 20 mm from the nail end, and the second mediolateral hole 30 mm from the first hole.

The universal tibial nail is at present available with diameters of 11 mm, 12 mm, and 13 mm lengths from 285 mm to 360 mm in 15 mm increments, and from 380 mm to 400 mm in 20 mm increments. A 10 mm diameter nail with round cross-section is being introduced. This nail is *only* used for interlocking.

Locking Bolts, 4.9 mm Diameter

These bolts have a core diameter of 4.3 mm and are fully threaded. The 8 mm diameter head profile is low, 2.5 mm, to ensure better soft tissue coverage. The 3.5 mm hexagonal socket allows the use of the large hexagonal screwdriver. The self-cutting trocar tip of the bolt permits easy insertion into the 4.0 mm drill hole. The flat thread safely engages in both the nail and the bone, if the 4.0 mm drill bit is used to pre-drill for the slightly larger core size. Backing out of the bolt is thus prevented. Tapping is not necessary. When measuring the length for the locking bolt, a 2 mm longer locking bolt than measured must be chosen. The tip of the bolt will then pass through the bone on the oppo-

L
+2mm

Determining the Nail Length and Diameter

The nail length can be determined prior to surgery by measuring the uninjured leg from the knee joint line to the tibiotarsal joint and subtracting 30–40 mm (*a*). The length may also be determined by measuring the exposed portion of the reaming rod (*b*). Length *A* is subtracted from the rod's total length of 950 mm (*b*). Comparative measurement can be made by holding a guide rod (*c*) of the same length parallel to the exposed rod. The tip of the rod is aligned with the point of insertion (*i*). The length from the free end of the reaming rod to the end of the guide rod is the nail length *L*. Nails of this length, one 15 mm longer and one 15 mm shorter are prepared.

The nail diameter depends on the fracture pattern and localisation. In simple transverse or short oblique fractures where reaming is used, the largest reamer used will indicate the diameter. If necessary, a nail of 0.5 mm smaller diameter is chosen.

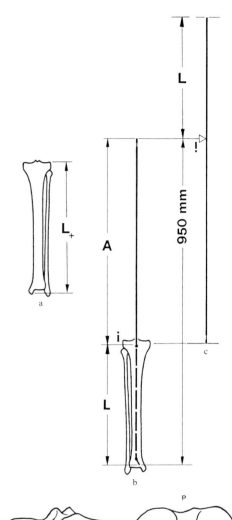

Point of Insertion

The point of insertion lies slightly offset medially, and slightly proximal to the tibial tuberosity in line with the medullary canal. It must be sufficiently below the intercondylar area to avoid damage to the joint. A 60 mm longitudinal incision is made medial to the patellar ligament. The tendon is then retracted laterally.

Insertion Technique

Opening the Medullary Canal:
- The 4 mm centring pin is mounted in the universal chuck with T handle and positioned over the insertion point. The universal tibial nail is placed alongside the tibia to act as an "angle guide".
- The pin is inserted in the medullary canal parallel to the upper end of the nail by turning and pressing simultaneously. The handle is removed.

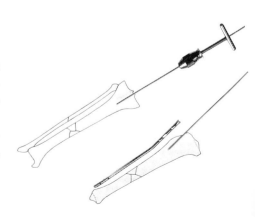

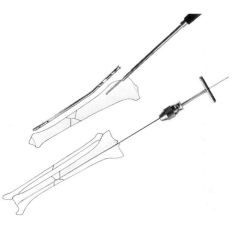

- The cannulated cutter is passed over the pin and the Allen screw tightened with the large hexagonal screwdriver. To open the medullary canal, the cannulated cutter is rotated 180° and then turned back. It must *not* be hammered.
- The reaming rod with offset ball tip is mounted in the universal chuck with T handle, and inserted under image intensification across the fracture site as far as the distal metaphyseal mass. Its correct position is checked with the image intensifier in both planes.

Reaming the Medullary Canal:
- The flexible shaft with fixed front-cutting reamer, 9 mm in diameter, is pushed over the reaming rod, and connected to the right-angle drive assembled on the universal air machine.
- The holding forceps (or old style holder) is used to hold the rod in position and prevent rotation during the reaming procedure. The tissue protector is placed between the soft tissue and the flexible shaft at the insertion point.

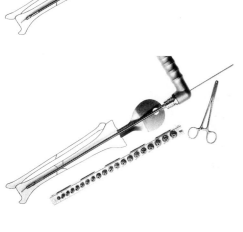

- Reaming starts only when the reamer is in the medullary canal. Reaming speed should be about 300–350 rpm. The reaming progresses slowly and is interrupted by occasional backward movement to clear the canal of debris. The reamer is halted by the offset ball tip of the reaming rod. Reamer depth is checked with image intensification.
- The flexible shaft is removed. The reaming rod is held in place with the holding forceps at the entry of the medullary canal after the reaming head has been withdrawn from the bone. If the reaming rod backs out the reduction may be lost.
- The 9.5 mm diameter reamer is mounted on the 8 mm flexible shaft and held with two fingers until placed over the reaming rod. The power drill is connected, and reaming to the desired size is continued as described above.

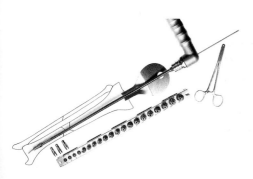

- The reamers should be used in increments of 0.5 mm to minimise heat generation and to reduce the risk of jamming. If the 13 mm diameter reamer is used (rare in tibial nailing), the 8 mm flexible shaft has to be exchanged for the 10 mm shaft or else the reamer will jam. If a reamer jams, reaming must be stopped immediately. For technique of removal of a jammed reamer, see illustration on p. 275.
- If not measured prior to surgery, the correct length and diameter of the universal tibial nail is determined (see p. 298).

– The medullary tube is passed over the reaming rod to hold reduction.

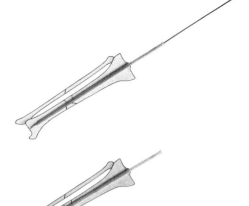

– The reaming rod is then removed.

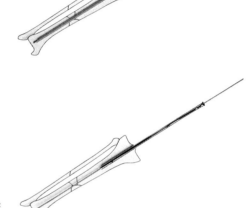

– The 3 mm guide rod with flattened ends is inserted.

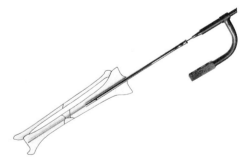

Insertion of the Universal Tibial Nail:
– The nail is passed over the guide rod and pushed into the medullary canal by hand as far as possible.
– The threaded conical bolt for tibial nails is pushed through the insertion handle, the assembly slid over the guide rod and tightened slightly by the combination wrench. The lugs of the insertion handle sleeve must engage the notches of the nail end before the threaded conical bolt can be firmly tightened, followed by the locking nut. For insertion of the nail, the handle can be positioned either medially or laterally.

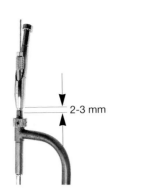

2-3 mm

– For insertion, the curved driving piece is screwed on the threaded conical bolt leaving 3 mm clearance between the curved driving piece and the first thread of the threaded conical bolt. This is necessary to avoid jamming. The guide rod protrudes at the hexagonal socket end. The angled end of the curved driving piece is pointing posteriorly.

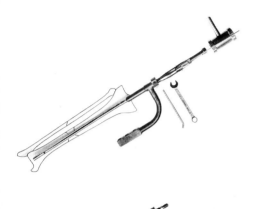

– The driving head is screwed on, and the 800 g hammer used to insert the nail with controlled blows, while the guide rod is held in place with the holding forceps. Each blow should advance the nail further into the medullary canal.
– If insertion is difficult, reaming 0.5–1 mm further may be necessary.
– The nail is inserted until the proximal end of the nail is flush with the surface of the cortex at the point of insertion. If the correct length has been chosen, the tip of the nail should lie in the distal metaphysis.
– The curved driving piece, the driving head, and the guide rod are removed.
– If locking of the nail is planned, the insertion handle, threaded conical bolt, and locking nut are left in place. The handle must then be placed medially for locking.

The insertion handle, threaded conical bolt and locking nut are removed as follows:
– The locking nut is loosened by a half turn.
– The insertion handle is held firmly with the lugs in the notches
– The threaded conical bolt is now detached using the combination or socket wrench.

Note: This technique must always be employed when removing the threaded conical bolt or else the nail end may distort and cause jamming of the bolt.

Note: The nail may be inserted by using the ram guide and the ram. The following technique is then employed:
– The ram guide is screwed on the threaded conical bolt, the ram passed over the ram guide and the flexible grip screwed on the ram guide.
– The nail is inserted with controlled blows by the ram, using the insertion handle to control rotation. Letting the ram fall from a distance should actually move the nail 5–10 mm. The flared end of the nail should not be driven into, but should "sit" on the top of the bone.
– The ram guide, ram, flexible grip, and guide rod are removed.

6.12.5.4 Locking of the Universal Tibial Nails

The locking procedure is carried out using the special instruments for distal and proximal locking. The distal locking is performed when control of a short distal fragment is required. It is also used when static locking is required to control tendency to shorten or rotate at the fracture site. In general, distal locking is performed first, because if the distal fragment has to be manipulated after locking this is best done by using the insertion handle from the proximal end.

**Distal Locking of the Universal Tibial Nail
Using the Radiolucent Drive**

Simple free-hand locking technique may be performed by using the radiolucent drive attached to the small air drill, and the 4.0 mm diameter three-fluted drill bit for radiolucent drive.

Step by step procedure:
- The image intensifier is aligned until the locking hole is absolutely round (Fig. 1).
- After the incision, the radiolucent drive is positioned with the tip of the 4.0 mm drill bit centred on the locking hole. Only the drill bit and the centring ring are visible, whilst all other parts of the gear housing remain invisible (Fig. 2).
- Still under image intensification, the drill bit is tilted until the drill bit appears as a single dot in the centre of the locking hole. The centring ring acts as an additional reference for positioning (Fig. 3).

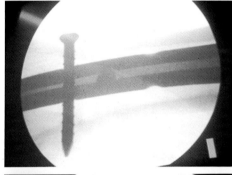

1

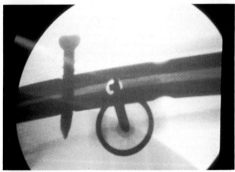

2

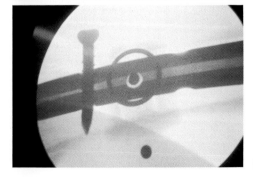

3

Instrumentation and Techniques

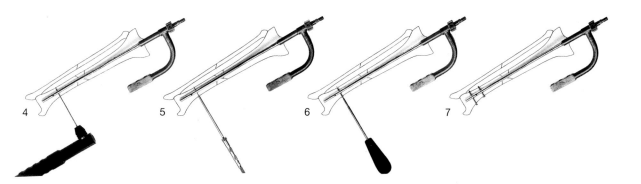

– The drill is held firmly in this position, while drilling both cortices. The drill bit should not be forced through the bone, but cut its way through. Image intensification may be needed to assure that the drill bit stays centred (Fig. 4).
– The depth gauge is used to measure the length. The hook must engage the far cortex and not only the nail (Fig. 5).
– A 4.9 mm locking bolt, 2 mm longer than measured, is inserted using the large hexagonal screwdriver and firmly tightened. The tip of the locking bolt should then protrude out of the far cortex to provide reliable support (Fig. 6).
– A second locking bolt is inserted using the same technique (Fig. 7).

Proximal Locking of the Universal Tibial Nail

The proximal locking bolts are inserted using the insertion handle for aiming. Image intensification is not necessary. For locking of tibial nails the handle must be turned medially.

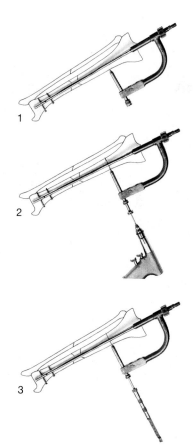

Step by step procedure:
– The 11 mm/8 mm protection sleeve and trocar are inserted through the desired hole of the insertion handle to mark the stab incision. The middle hole is for dynamic locking and is clearly marked. The sleeve and trocar are pushed onto the bone. The trocar is then removed (Fig. 1).
– The 8 mm/4.5 mm drill sleeve is inserted and the 4.0 mm/4.5 mm drill bit used to drill through both cortices (Fig. 2).
– The drill bit and drill sleeve are removed and the depth gauge inserted through the protection sleeve to measure the length. The hook must engage the far cortex, not the nail (Fig. 3).

- A 4.9 mm locking bolt, 2 mm longer than measured, is inserted using the large hexagonal screwdriver, and tightened firmly. The tip of the bolt should protrude out of the far cortex to provide reliable support (Fig. 4).
- The second, and, if necessary for stability, a third bolt are inserted using the same technique (Fig. 5).
- Removal of the insertion handle, threaded conical bolt and locking nut as follows:

  The locking nut is loosened by a half turn.

  The insertion handle is held firmly with the lugs in the notches.

  The threaded conical bolt is now unscrewed using the combination wrench, or the socket wrench and the assembly removed (Fig. 6).

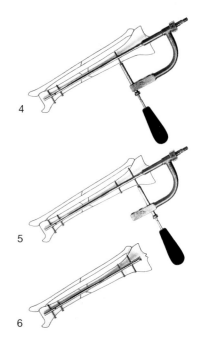

Distal Locking of the Tibial Nail Using the Distal Aiming Device Assembly and 4.0 mm/4.5 mm Drill Bit

By using the distal aiming device assembly accurately, aiming for the locking holes is quite simple. Image intensification is necessary also for this technique. The leg of the patient must be placed between the X-ray source and the aiming device because of the device's built in correction of the converging X-ray beam.

Step by step procedure:
- The image intensifier is positioned so that the picture on the monitor and the orientation of the leg correspond. The nail should be shown in the lower half of the monitor with the more proximal hole in the middle. The image intensifier is moved until this hole appears absolutely round on the monitor, and is then fixed in this position. On no account should the C arm or the leg be moved again until drilling is finished.
- The radiation shield is placed on the patient's leg to protect the surgeon's hands. The shield, however, should not extend into the window of the monitor, to prevent the radiation level from being automatically raised.
- The tip of a scalpel is placed over the locking hole under image intensification to mark the incision.
- The distal aiming device and trocar are pressed onto the cortex (Fig. 1).
- The trocar is removed and replaced with the aiming trocar (Fig. 2).
- The axis of the aiming device is then adjusted to centre the direction finder's central dot in the circle.
- The device is then moved along the long axis of the bone until the second dot of the aiming trocar is located in the centre of the locking hole. This position should be maintained throughout the drilling procedure.

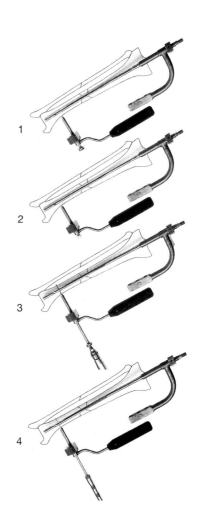

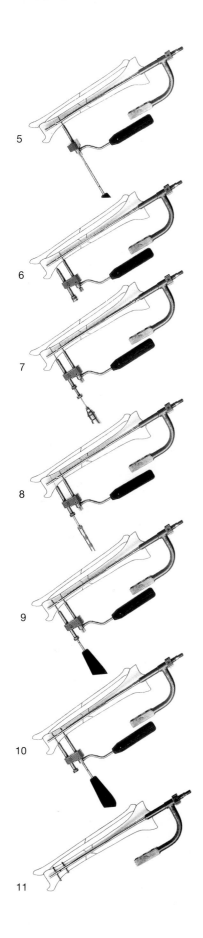

5

6

7

8

9

10

11

– Accidental displacement of the distal aiming device is prevented by tapping the sharp tips slightly in the bone, once it is in the correct position.
– The aiming trocar is removed and the 8 mm/4.5 mm drill sleeve inserted. Image intensification is used to verify that the hole in the nail is circular and concentric with the drill sleeve.
– The 4.0 mm/4.5 mm drill bit is used to drill both cortices, passing through the locking hole. The direction is controlled by checking that the central dot of the direction finder remains centred in the circle (Fig. 3).
– After removal of the drill sleeve and the protection sleeve, the depth gauge is used to measure the length directly through the distal aiming device. The hook must engage the far cortex, not the nail, before the outer sleeve is pushed onto the bone and the measurement read (Fig. 4).
– The tibial fixation bolt is inserted through the aiming device and tightened. It holds the distal aiming device in a fixed position while preparing for the second locking bolt (Fig. 5).
– The large hexagonal screwdriver is used to loosen one of the Allen screws of the direction finder, and to turn it until its two straight metal markers are parallel with the nail on the monitor. The exact distance between the two locking holes is determined by correct placement of the direction finder. The hole of the direction finder will not therefore appear coaxial with the second locking hole.
– The 11 mm/8 mm protection sleeve and trocar are inserted into the second hole of the direction finder, and pushed onto the bone through a second stab incision (Fig. 6).
– The trocar is removed and the 4.5 mm drill sleeve inserted. The 4.0 mm/4.5 mm drill bit is used to drill both cortices, passing through the nail (Fig. 7).
– After removal of the drill bit and drill sleeve, the length is measured with the depth gauge through the protection sleeve (Fig. 8).
– The chosen 4.9 mm locking bolt, 2 mm longer than measured, is inserted and firmly tightened using the large hexagonal screwdriver through the 11 mm/8 mm protection sleeve (Fig. 9). The sleeve is then left in this position.
– The fixation bolt is removed and the chosen locking bolt (2 mm longer than measured) inserted and firmly tightened in the first hole (Fig. 10).
– The distal aiming device assembly is then removed (Fig. 11).
– In universal tibial nails, the AP hole is prepared in similar manner.
– The C arm is turned 90° placing the leg between the X-ray source and aiming device.

6.12.5.5 Dynamisation of the Universal Nails

There may be indications to reduce the "stiffness" of the fixation, allowing increasing load to be transmitted through the bone. The progress of bone healing may thereby be stimulated. The removal of locking screws – some or all – is one technique for achieving such "dynamisation".

Dynamisation can be obtained by removing the locking bolt placed in the "static" hole. The locking bolt in the elongated hole may then "move" proximally allowing axial load at the fracture site, but still providing rotational stability of the fracture.

6.12.5.6 Instruments for the Insertion and Removal of Universal Femoral and Tibial Nails

Instruments for insertion universal femoral nails

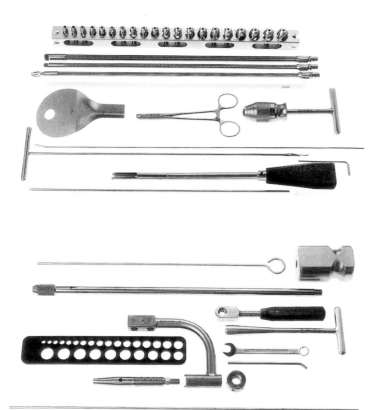

Instruments for insertion of universal tibial nails

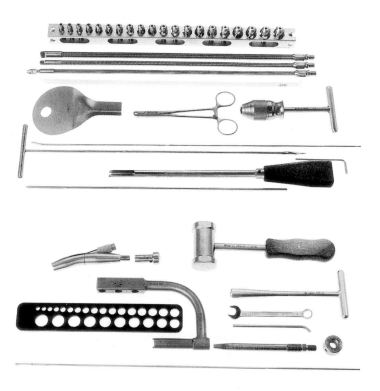

Instruments for locking of universal femoral and tibial nails using the radiolucent drive

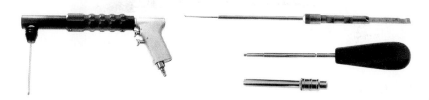

Instruments for locking of universal femoral nails using the aiming device

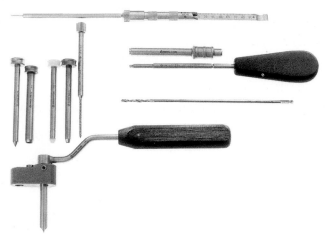

Instruments for locking of universal tibial nails using the aiming device

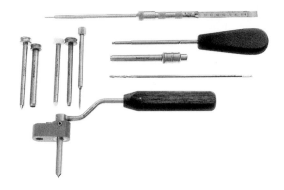

Instruments for removal of the universal femoral nails

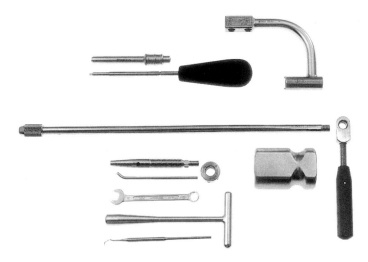

Instruments for removal of the universal tibial nails

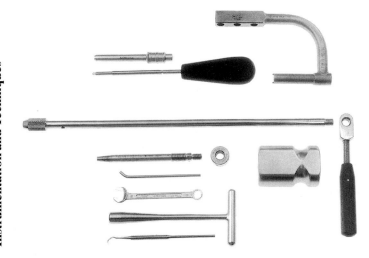

The universal nails are in general removed. Tibial nails are usually removed after 18–24 months, femoral nails after 24–36 months.

Step by step procedure:
- Locking bolts are first removed through stab incisions distally and proximally for tibial nails. For femoral nails the bolts are removed through the main distal incision. The proximal bolts are removed through incisions indicated by using the insertion handle and 11 mm/8 mm protection sleeve and trocar.
- After opening the site for the proximal nail end, the nail is carefully freed of ingrown soft tissue to clear the inner threads.
- The threaded conical bolt, insertion handle, and locking nut of correct size (corresponding to the nail type and size) is screwed in the nail end, and tightened firmly with the socket wrench or the combination wrench. The lugs of the insertion handle sleeve should engage the notches of the nail end. The insertion handle is necessary to prevent jamming of the threaded conical bolt in the nail end, when the nail is removed. It also serves to direct the screwdriver through appropriate stab incisions, using the 11 mm/8 mm protection sleeve when removing proximal femoral locking bolts.
- The ram guide is screwed onto the threaded conical bolt, the ram slid on, and the flexible grip attached. By means of strong blows against the flexible grip, the nail is driven out. Re-tightening the instruments after the first few blows prevents undesired loosening.

6.12.5.7 What If the Nail Cannot Be Removed by the Standard Method?

If the nail is firmly anchored by bony ingrowth, it may be dislodged by first driving the nail in a little further without damaging the joint, before trying to drive it out.

To remove strongly anchored femoral nails, another possibility is to use the extraction hook. The correct size hook (see markings) is screwed into the connector. The assembly is then pushed through the nail, and hooked on the distal end, avoiding the slot. The ram guide is screwed onto the proximal end of the connector, the ram slid on, and the flexible grip attached. With blows against the flexible grip the hook may force the nail out.

If none of the described attempts at removal has been successful, the only recourse may be the following: A longitudinal saw cut is made in the full thickness of the cortex down to the nail, throughout the whole length of the diaphysis. This will allow the bone to "spread" slightly, and reduce its grip on the nail.

6.12.6 The Unreamed Tibial Nailing System

Medullary nailing of shaft fractures of the lower extremity has long proven its value, especially with the introduction of reaming, and later interlocking. However, studies in recent years show that, embolisation of marrow into the major blood vessels in conjunction with reaming of the medullary canal may cause pulmonary compromise, especially in multiple system trauma. In fractures with extensive soft tissue damage and in open fractures grade I, II or, IIIA, the reaming procedure causes additional trauma to the already impaired blood supply,and nailing has not been the method of choice. The introduction of a solid nail with a small diameter has made it possible to treat these injuries with nailing but without reaming. The locking possibility ensures axial and rotational stability.

Current experience has also shown that treating open fractures with a solid nail is a good alternative to external fixation. A solid nail does not present the relatively large dead space of a hollow nail where bacteria may thrive and increase the risk of infection, The UTN finds application in fresh fractures of the diaphysis of the tibia; closed with extensive soft tissue damage, or open grade I, II, or IIIA. The unreamed nail is especially to be considered in multifragmentary/segmental fractures, if the bone is covered or can be covered with viable soft tissue within a few days of nailing. Furthermore, there must be no sign of infection already present at the fracture site.

Treatment with the unreamed nail may be temporary or definitive. The indication can be extended to some fresh fractures of the proximal and distal diaphysis if the locking bolts permit sufficient hold in the peripheral fragment, and do not compromise the proper internal fixation of any associated intra-articular extension.

Note: The UTN is designed for use with interlocking only. *Contraindications* are ongoing infections, poor bone stock, pathological fractures, malunions, and nonunions.

Because of the small diameter of both the nail and the locking bolts, excessive load on the implants must be avoided, or else they may undergo fatigue failure. Weight-bearing exceeding 15 kg must be avoided; in bony defects and segmental comminution, toe-touching is the limit. Increase of weight-bearing depends on clinical and radiological progress to healing.

In some cases, for example poor patient compliance, the unreamed nail may later be exchanged for a larger diameter reamed universal nail. This is done once soft tissue healing is assured, and limb vascularity is good.

Instrumentation and Techniques

■ 310

6.12.6.1 Instruments for the UTN

The instruments for the insertion of the UTN can be obtained in either a graphic case or a sterilising tray.

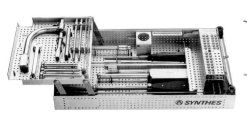
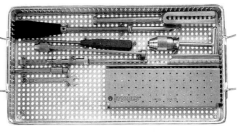
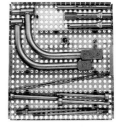

Centring Pin, 4 mm Diameter, 400 mm

This pin is connected with the universal chuck and introduced about 50 mm into the medullary canal at the point of insertion, and at the correct angle. It is used to guide the cannulated cutter.

Universal Chuck with T Handle

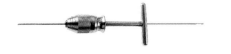

This chuck is used to insert the centring pin.

Cannulated Cutter, 11 mm Diameter, 350 mm

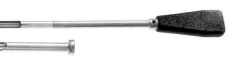

This cutter is used together with the centring pin to open the medullary canal. The centring pin can be fixed with the Allen screw. The cannulated cutter has a special sharpened tip to allow cutting/carving while rotating the instrument 180° by hand and then turning back. Some older instruments have a metal plate at the end of the handle, inviting use of the hammer, but this is *not recommended*, since damage to the cortex and to the delicate cutting edge may result. The cutting edge may be resharpened.

Protection Sleeve for the Cannulated Cutter

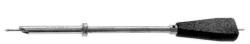

This sleeve is used to protect the soft tissue when opening the medullary canal.

Measuring Rod

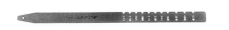

This measuring rod is 550 mm long and is used to determine the length of the UTN. A radiographic ruler has recently been developed.

Intramedullary Nailing Instruments and Implants

Coupling Block with Round Sleeve

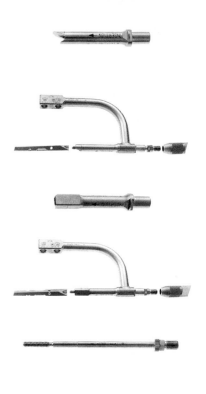

This block is used for insertion of the UTN, together with the insertion handle and the connecting bolt. The longer lip of the proximal end is positioned over the bevelled end of the nail. The marking indicates the end of the nail. The diameter of this end does not exceed the nail's cross-section in diameter, making insertion less critical. The notches of the distal end connect the insertion handle for either the left or the right leg.

Coupling Block with Square Sleeve

This block may also be used for insertion of the UTN together with the insertion handle and the connecting bolt. The proximal end is fitted over the nail end so that the marking corresponds to the contour of the nail end. The use of this coupling block for the insertion assembly permits use of greater transverse force on the nail end, which may facilitate reduction.

Connecting Bolt

This bolt is passed through the insertion handle and the coupling block before being screwed into the upper end of the nail using the combination wrench. It should be firmly but not excessively tightened. This assembly is then used for insertion of the nail.

Insertion Handle for UTN, 8 mm and 9 mm Diameter

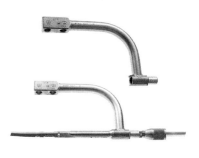

For insertion of the UTN, the handle is connected to the coupling block and secured in correct position before tightening the connecting bolt in the nail end. The handle is placed laterally for insertion if this gives better access, depending upon any soft tissue lesion. For locking, the insertion handle must be placed on the medial side The insertion handle is used for proximal static, or dynamic locking (see markings).

Insertion Handle, 45° for UTN

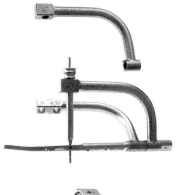

This handle is used if the fracture is in the proximal diaphysis, and locking of one of the diagonal holes is necessary. The handle is attached to the regular insertion handle with the lugs engaging the notches of the regular insertion handle. The connecting bolt is tightened in the nail end, and the knurled nut used to lock the handle.

Knurled Nut

This nut is used to fix the 45° insertion handle in position.

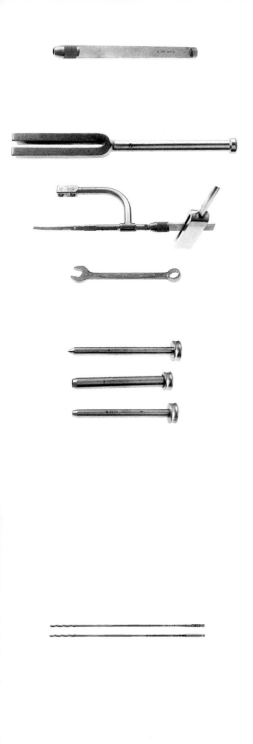

Inserter – Extractor for the UTN

This piece is screwed onto the distal end of the connecting bolt, and used with the slotted hammer for insertion and extraction of the UTN.

Slotted Hammer

This hammer is used over the inserter – extractor to insert the UTN by gentle blows.

Combination Wrench, 11 mm

This wrench is used to tighten the connecting bolt in the nail end.

Trocar, 8.0 mm Diameter

This trocar is inserted into the protection sleeve, 11 mm/8 mm, and the assembly positioned in the appropriate hole in the insertion handle to determine site for the proximal locking bolts.

Protection Sleeve, 11 mm/8.0 mm Diameter

This sleeve fits into the holes in the insertion handle, and is used to guide the drill sleeve 8.0 mm/3.2 mm, the depth gauge, and the screwdriver.

Drill Sleeve, 8.0 mm/3.2 mm Diameter

This sleeve fits in the protection sleeve 11 mm/8 mm, and is used when drilling for the proximal locking bolt with the 3.2 mm drill bit.

Drill Bit, 3.2 mm Diameter, Three-Fluted

This drill bit, 215 mm/190 mm, has a quick coupling end. It is used to pre-drill for the locking bolt 3.9 mm. The depth markings at 25–100 mm, in 5 mm increments, allow determination of the screw length, but only when the 8.0 mm/3.2 mm drill sleeve is used as its guide.

Hexagonal Screwdriver for 3.9 mm Diameter Locking Bolts

This screwdriver has a tip which is 2.5 mm wide across the flats to fit the 3.9 mm locking bolts. The shaft has a groove to accommodate the large screw-holding sleeve, and a small handle to prevent too much force from being exerted.

Intramedullary Nailing Instruments and Implants

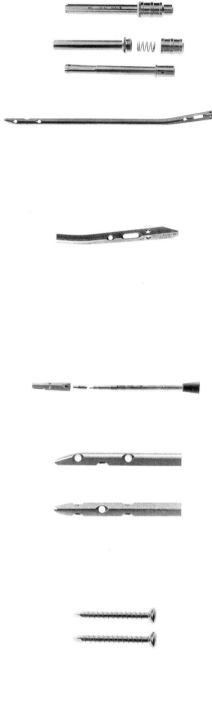

Large Holding Sleeve

This is a self-retaining screw-holding sleeve, necessary to hold and to allow traction when locking bolts are removed. It consists of three parts and must be disassembled for cleaning.

6.12.6.2 The UTN and Locking Bolt, 3.9 mm

The UTN is a solid nail made of cold-worked implant steel. Its surface has been roughened to enhance fatigue life (see Sect. 6.1.1). The slightly flared proximal end has a diamond-shaped cross-section, which at the anterior end is bevelled to prevent damage to the patellar ligament. The bend of the nail forms an angle of 9°, conforming to the anatomy of the tibia when correctly inserted.

The proximal end has two mediolateral locking holes; one round for static and one elongated for dynamic locking. Further, there are two holes for diagonal locking at 45° each to the frontal plane for additional anchoring of fractures in the proximal diaphysis. The round holes are 4 mm in diameter. Locking of the nail provides axial and rotational stability.

The threaded cannulation of the proximal end accepts a sealing screw, which can be inserted after locking, and left in place to prevent ingrowth of soft tissue.

The distal two thirds are straight, with a cross-section corresponding to a triangle with a semicircular posterior baseline. The posterior tapered tip of the distal end guides the nail along the posterior wall during insertion, reducing the risk of penetration of the cortex.

The distal end has two mediolateral locking holes, and one between them in an AP direction.

At present the UTN is available in 8 mm and 9 mm diameters, in lengths from 255 mm to 360 mm in 15 mm increments, and from 380 mm to 420 mm in 20 mm increments.

The Locking Bolt, 3.9 mm Diameter

This bolt has a core size of 3.2 mm and a shallow thread, which should engage both cortices to prevent backing out of the screw, and to facilitate removal of the bolt. The trocar tip is self-cutting, thus pre-tapping is not necessary. The low head profile is of advantage in areas with minimal soft tissue coverage. The 8.0 mm head diameter allows use of the large screw-holding sleeve, which fits on the special screwdriver for 3.9 mm locking screws.

The 3.9 mm locking bolt is available in lengths from 22 mm to 64 mm, in 2 mm increments, and from 68 mm to 80 mm, in 4 mm increments.

Instrumentation and Techniques

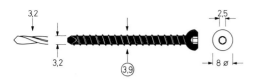

Important dimensions:
- Head diameter: 8.0 mm
- Head height: 2.5 mm
- Hexagonal socket width: 2.5 mm
- Thread diameter: 3.9 mm
- Core diameter: 3.2 mm
- Drill bit for pilot hole: 3.2 mm

6.12.6.3 Insertion and Locking of the UTN

Positioning of the Patient

Supine Position on a Traction Table

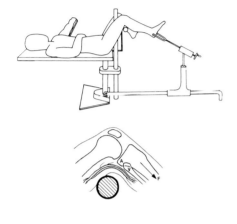

This position allows only limited treatment of soft tissue in-juries.

The knee of the injured leg is bent 90° over a well-padded popliteal support, and extended obliquely downwards. A pad is used to support also the distal femur at a sufficient distance from the popliteal artery and vein (*A* and *V*).

Extension can be applied by a padded boot or by calcaneal traction. If distal locking is planned skeletal traction has to be used, since the boot extends too far proximally and obstructs access to the locking area.

The uninjured leg is placed in abduction, flexion and external rotation at the hip to ensure free movement of the C arm of the image intensifier in AP and mediolateral directions. Reduction and correction of rotation must be carried out before sterile draping, since it is difficult to adjust during surgery.

Supine Position on a Standard Table

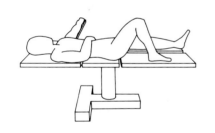

This position is recommended, especially for polytraumatised patients, and for grade II and III open fractures in order to ensure optimum soft tissue access. Reduction may be carried out using the large distractor. The Schanz screws are inserted in the frontal plane as close to both tibial ends as possible. A radiolucent table is necessary for image intensification. The knee is bent and held by an assistant during insertion of the nail.

Determining the Nail Length and Diameter

The length of the UTN can be determined by inserting the measuring rod into the medullary canal under image intensification control.

The required length can also be determined, also under image intensification, by holding a UTN next to the tibial shaft. The nail diameter is chosen by measuring the diameter of the medullary canal. Only 8 mm and 9 mm diameter nails are available. If the diameter is by any chance less than 8 mm the canal must be reamed before insertion.

Point of Insertion

The correct choice of the insertion point is essential for the success. As a general rule, the insertion point is in line with the long axis of the medullary canal, slightly medial to the tibial tubercle, and as proximal as possible without impinging on the anterior lip of the tibial plateau.

A longitudinal incision is made over the patellar ligament in the line with the medullary canal. The tendon is split. A step by step procedure is described below:

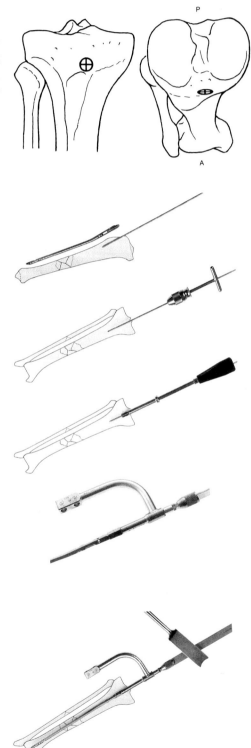

Opening the medullary canal:
- The 4 mm guide pin, held in the universal chuck with T handle, is placed at the point of insertion at an angle of 9° in the sagittal plane. The UTN can be held alongside the tibia to act as a guide. Its upper section indicates the correct angle. By simultaneously turning and pressing the universal chuck, the pin is inserted into the medullary canal.
- The cannulated cutter with protection sleeve is pushed over the guide pin and used to cut open the cortex and enter the medullary canal. The cutter is turned 180° by hand and then turned back. It should follow the direction of the guide pin, making a channel in the same axis as the upper end of the implant.
- The guide pin and cannulated cutter are removed.
- The coupling block, the insertion handle and the connecting bolt are assembled and tightened in the chosen nail, using the combination wrench. Excessive tightening must be avoided. The lugs of the handle must engage the notches of the coupling block. For insertion, the handle may be fixed either laterally or medially; for proximal locking the handle must be placed medially.

Insertion of the nail:
- The inserter – extractor is tightened on the connecting bolt, and the nail assembly inserted manually as far as possible.
- The slotted hammer is used to seat the nail gently. If any resistance is felt, the nail should never be forced into the medullary canal, but changed to a smaller size. The nail is inserted until the etched mark on the coupling block is flush with anterior surface of the tibia. The entire length of the nail is then in the tibia. If inserted beyond the mark the coupling block may jam or the bone may split.
- The slotted hammer and the inserter – extractor are removed.

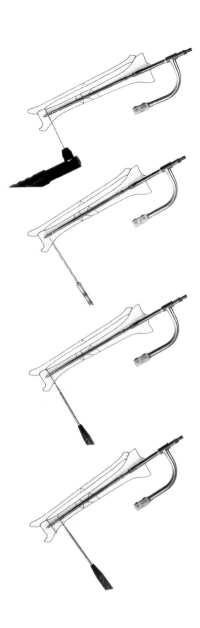

Distal Locking of the Nail Using Radiolucent Drive

In general, distal locking is performed first. If necessary, the distal fragment can then be manipulated using the insertion handle. The use of the radiolucent drive allows control of drilling under image intensification, and ensures that the surgeon's hands remain outside the main radiation field.

– The image intensifier is adjusted until the most distal hole is clearly visible and appears completely round.
– A stab incision is made.
– The tip of the 3.2 mm three-fluted drill bit, connected to the radiolucent drive, is positioned over the centre of the hole.
– The radiolucent drive is adjusted until the drill bit appears as a dot in the centre of the hole and of the centring ring.
– After centring the drill bit exactly, both cortices are drilled under image intensification. *Note:* Drilling must not start until position of drill bit is exact.
– The depth gauge is used to measure the length.
– A 3.9 mm locking bolt, 2 mm longer than measured, is inserted. This is necessary to ensure that the trocar tip is outside the bone, and the thread is engaging the entire far cortex.
– A second, and, if necessary, a third locking bolt is inserted using the same procedure.

Distal Locking Using the Distal Aiming Device

Distal locking can be performed using the distal aiming device employed for locking of the universal nails. A fixation bolt for the direction finder is not available, therefore the aiming procedure has to be repeated for the second locking bolt. The technique is the same as described for the universal nails, except that the 3.2 mm drill bit and 3.9 mm bolt are used; see p. 304.
Distal locking can also be performed using "free-hand technique".

Proximal Locking

Proximal locking is performed by using the insertion handle as a guide. The insertion handle must be placed medially for the locking procedure.

– The 11 mm/8 mm protection sleeve and trocar are inserted into the "static" hole of the handle and pushed through a stab incision in the soft tissue onto the bone (Fig. 1).
– After removing the trocar the 8 mm/3.2 mm drill sleeve is inserted. The 3.2 mm three-fluted drill bit is used to drill both cortices (Fig. 2).
– The length is measured with the depth gauge (Fig. 3).
– A 3.9 mm locking bolt, 2 mm longer than measured, is inserted. This is necessary to ensure that the tip is outside the bone, and the thread is fully engaging the far cortex (Fig. 4).
– The second locking bolt is inserted through the "dynamic" hole of the insertion handle, using the same technique as described above (Fig. 5).
– After loosening the connecting screw with the combination wrench, the insertion instruments are removed (Fig. 6).
– The sealing screw is inserted in the proximal end of the nail to prevent ingrowth of soft tissue, thereby facilitating nail removal (Fig. 7).

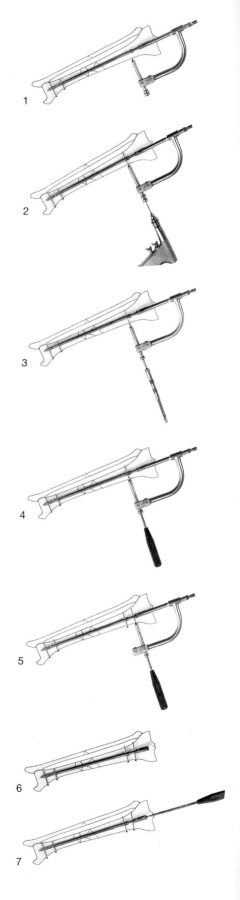

Dynamisation of the UTN

By inserting the locking bolt in the elongated hole using the insertion handle as a guide for correct placement, fractures of the types A1–3, B1–3, and C2 may be primarily dynamised. The main fragments must be in direct contact to prevent shortening. Secondary dynamisation within 6–10 weeks by removing the "static" locking bolt may be considered in certain fracture.

Proximal Locking Using the 45° Insertion Handle

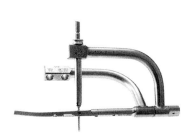

If the fracture is in the proximal diaphysis, it may be necessary to lock the nail by using one of the diagonal holes.
– The 45° insertion handle is attached to the regular handle and locked in the desired position with the locking nut.
– The diagonal locking bolt is inserted using the same technique as described above.

6.12.6.4 Instruments for Insertion and Locking of the UTN

See illustrations.

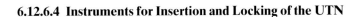

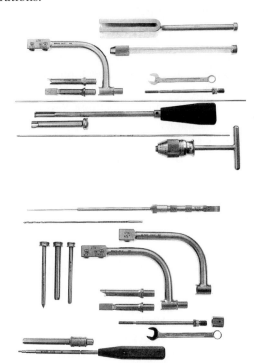

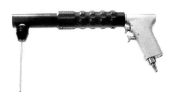

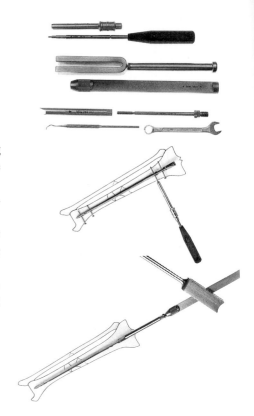

- The locking bolts are removed through stab incisions using the hexagonal screwdriver and the large screw-holding sleeve to exert traction.
- The nail end is cleared of tissue, and the sealing screw removed using the hexagonal screwdriver.
- The coupling block for extraction and the connecting screw are attached to the nail end using the combination wrench for tightening.
- The inserter – extractor is screwed onto the end of the connecting screw, and light blows from the slotted hammer used to extract the nail by gentle blows.

6.13 External Fixator Devices: Instruments and Implants

External fixation has been used since the last century to stabilise displaced fractures. Only with the development of mechanically sound devices has external fixation offered a reliable alternative to internal fixation in complex fractures. Several devices exist; some consisting of numerous components making them difficult to apply. Others are heavy in weight and cumbersome for the patient. The AO/ASIF tubular system is lightweight, consists of few components only and provides suffcient versatility and stability for successful treatment, also of most problem fractures where internal fixation is indicated.

Indications:
- Stabilisation and correction of extremity malalignment and length discrepancies in severe open fractures and infected nonunions
- Initial stabilisation of bony disruption and soft tissue injuries in polytraumatised patients
- Closed fractures with associated severe soft tissue damage
- Multifragmentary diaphyseal and periarticular lesions
- Certain pelvic ring disruptions
- Arthrodesis
- Compression fixation in osteotomies

Instrumentation and Techniques

6.13.1 The Large External Fixator – Tubular System

The large external fixator – tubular system can be obtained in sterilising trays or in aluminium cases. Graphic cases are being developed. Both stainless steel tubes and radiolucent carbon fibre rods are available.

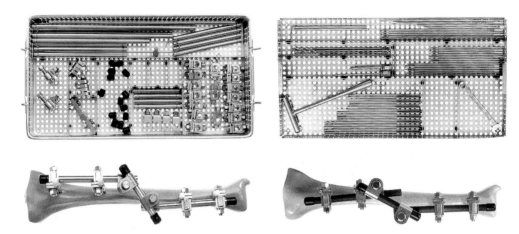

6.13.1.1 Standard Instruments, Implants, and Fixation Components

Drill Bit, 4.5 mm Diameter

This bit, two-fluted, 195 mm/170 mm, with a quick coupling end, is used to drill the pilot hole for the 5.0 mm Schanz screw with radial preload. It is also used to drill the near cortex if the 4.5 mm Schanz screw with the 18 mm thread is to be inserted and for both cortices when the Steinmann pin, 5.0 mm in diameter, is to be applied. The 4.5 mm drill bit is used with the drill sleeve 6.0 mm/5.0 mm.

Drill Bit, 3.5 mm Diameter

This drill bit, two-fluted, 195 mm/170 mm, with quick coupling end, is used to drill the pilot hole for the 5.0 mm Schanz screw with a core size of 3.5 mm. It is also used to drill the far cortex before inserting the 4.5 mm Schanz screw with 18 mm thread length, and to drill both cortices for the Steinmann pin, 4.5 mm in diameter. The 3.5 mm drill bit is used with the 5.0 mm/3.5 mm drill sleeve.

Triple Drill Sleeve Assembly, 110 mm

The triple drill sleeve assembly is employed as drill sleeve and tissue protector if the soft tissue is deep. It is also used if a double tube configuration is planned, where the drill sleeve assembly has to be long enough to pass through two sets of clamps and still reach the bone. The length of the drill bit may then have to be adapted.

– The *trocar,* 3.5 mm in diameter, 110 mm long, used together with the two drill sleeves, helps to penetrate the soft tissue after the incision has been made.
– The *drill sleeve,* 5.0 mm/3.5 mm in diameter, accepts the trocar, 3.5 mm in diameter, and the drill bit, 3.5 mm in diameter.
– The *drill sleeve,* 6.0 mm/5.0 mm, is the outermost drill sleeve of the assembly. It accepts the other two components and is used separately as drill sleeve for the 4.5 mm drill bit and for insertion of the Schanz screws, 4.5 mm and 5.0 mm in diameter. The sleeve fits the adjustable clamp and remains in the clamp until the Schanz screw has been inserted.

Triple Drill Sleeve Assembly, 80 mm

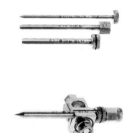

The 80 mm triple drill sleeve assembly is employed as drill sleeve and tissue protector where there is little depth of soft tissue (tibia). It can be inserted in the clamp and used as drill sleeve for single tube configurations, with short distances between clamp and bone.

– The *trocar,* 3.5 mm in diameter, 80 mm, used with the other two drill sleeves helps to penetrate the soft tissue after the stab incision has been made.
– The *drill sleeve,* 5.0 mm/3.5 mm, accepts the trocar, 3.5 mm, and the drill bit 3.5 mm in diameter.
– The *drill sleeve,* 6.0 mm/5.0 mm, is the outermost drill sleeve of the assembly. It accepts the other two components and is used separately as drill sleeve for the 4.5 mm drill bit and for insertion of the 4.5 mm and 5.0 mm Schanz screws. This sleeve fits the adjustable clamp and remains in the clamp until the Schanz screw has been inserted.

Depth Gauge for Schanz Screws

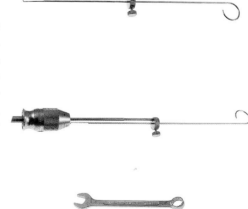

The depth gauge is used to determine the the length of insertion of the Schanz screws. After drilling both cortices the depth gauge is inserted through the 6.0 mm/5.0 mm drill sleeve and hooked on the far cortex. The knurled disc is moved onto the top of the drill sleeve, tightened with the screw, and the depth gauge removed. The Schanz screw which has been selected is tightened in the universal chuck with T handle at the distance indicated by the depth gauge, between the hook and the knurled disc.

Combination Wrench, 11 mm

The combination wrench is used to tighten the nuts on the clamps and the open compressor.

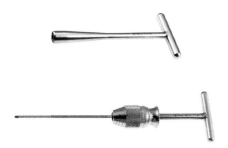

Socket Wrench

This wrench, 11 mm in width across flats, is also employed for tightening nuts on the clamps or the open compressor.

Universal Chuck with T Handle

The chuck is used to insert the Schanz screws or Steinmann pins. By turning the T handle clockwise the jaws close. For releasing the pin the upper part of the chuck is pulled back and the handle turned anticlockwise.

Implants for the Tubular System

Schanz Screw, 5.0 mm Diameter, for Radial Preload

The 5.0 mm Schanz screw for radial preload is a newly developed screw, which may be the implant of choice for the external fixator in the future. The blunted trocar tip is self-cutting. The core size of the screw, which is only slightly larger than the drill hole of 4.5 mm, allows the screw to exert radial preload. This has shown to significantly reduce pin loosening and pin track infection. The screw has demonstrated good strength in relation to a force acting perpendicular to the long axis.

Schanz Screw, 4.5 mm Diameter

The 4.5 mm Schanz screw has a 3.5 mm diameter core, 18 mm thread length, and a slightly rounded off trocar tip. This screw provides good purchase in cortical bone. The threaded portion engages the far cortex after pre-drilling with the 3.5 mm drill bit. The stiff 4.5 mm shaft has a tight interference fit in the near cortex in the 4.5 mm drill hole. This enhances the rigidity of the frame by placing the large diameter (4.5 mm) shaft within the near cortex where bending forces are the highest.
The 4.5 mm Schanz screw is available in lengths from 100 to 250 mm, in 25 mm increments.

Schanz Screw, 5.0 mm Diameter

The 5.0 mm Schanz screw, with a 3.8 mm core and 50 mm thread length, has a slightly rounded off trocar tip to prevent damage to the soft tissue. Since part of the threaded portion with the 3.8 mm core remains outside the bone, the screw is less stiff an implant than the screws presented above.
These screws, core size 3.8 mm diameter, thread length 50 mm, are inserted in the two main fragments, and connected to the distractor. They are used in lengths 150, 175, and 200 mm.

Fixation Components

Stainless Steel Tubes, 11 mm Diameter

These tubes are the longitudinal stress-bearing elements. The stainless steel tubes are highly corrosion resistant and provide a safe and strong frame. They are light and add little weight to a frame configuration. The grooves at each end were originally meant to keep the plugs in place, which were used formerly to prevent the clamps from slipping off the tube during initial assembly. These plugs have now been replaced by the protective caps.

The tubes are available in lengths from 100 to 450 mm, in 50 mm increments, and also lengths of 550 and 650 mm.

Carbon Fibre Rods, 11 mm Diameter

Carbon fibre rods are also used as longitudinal stress-bearing elements, and have the advantage of being radiolucent. They are approximately 30% stiffer and 40% lighter than the stainless steel tubes. The rods are manufactured from carbon fibre-reinforced epoxy. They have a special coating, which provides increased protection against fibre damage when clamps are tightened. The coating also improves the friction properties between the clamp and the rod, and eliminates moisture penetration during autoclaving.

The carbon fibre rods are available in lengths from 100 to 600 mm in 50 mm increments.

Connecting Bar, 5 mm Diameter

The connecting bar of stainless steel is used to connect two frames to increase the stiffness. It is connected by using two additional clamps, e. g. open clamps.

The bar is available in lengths from 100 to 300 mm, in 50 mm increments.

Adjustable Clamp

The adjustable clamp is the basic clamp connecting 4.5 mm or 5.0 mm Schanz screws or Steinmann pins to the tube or the carbon fibre rod. The clamp permits screw or pin insertion for angle adjustments over 15° in the frontal plane. The rectangular grooving of the vice plate assembly accepts the triple drill sleeve assembly, allowing drilling and insertion of a screw or pin through the clamp. The vice plate is identified by a ring and the number 6. Older vice plates had no markings and must be replaced before the triple drill sleeve assembly can be used.

The different parts of the adjustable clamp may be replaced as necessary.

Note: The clamp is not suitable for use with 6.0 mm screws or pins.

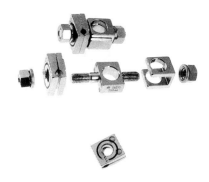

Instrumentation and Techniques

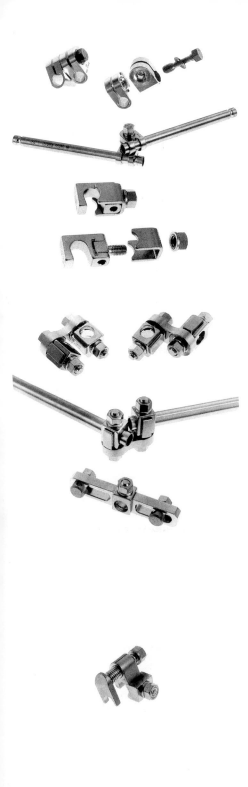

Tube-to-Tube Clamp

The tube-to-tube clamp is used to connect one tube or rod to another. It is tightened with one bolt only; the serration on the clamp bodies, however, provide a safe lock.

Open Clamp

The open clamp may be added to a frame configuration already built, to connect further Schanz screws to the tube or rod. It can also be used to connect two unilateral frames with a connecting bar. The open clamp does not permit any range of motion of the pins in the plane of the tube's long axis.

Universal Joint for Two Tubes

The universal joint can also be used to connect two tubes or rods. It consists of two clamp bodies and one intermediate piece and can be mounted with the bodies beside each other or in opposition.

The range of motion is limited and is less versatile than the tube-to-tube clamp.

Transverse Clamp

The transverse clamp, 90 mm long, connects the tube or rod with two Schanz screws placed in the transverse plane without limiting pin angulation or distance between pins. This results in greater control and improved stability of relatively short, metaphyseal fragments.

The clamp may be used in proximal and distal tibial fractures or in ankle arthrodesis. It is also used in segmental bone transport and bone lengthening procedures. See p. 334.

Open Compressor

The open compressor may be used for compression or distraction. It is placed on the tube with the plate in the closed position and adjacent to a clamp. Its attachment nut is tightened. The tube-holding nut on the clamp is loosened and the combination wrench or the socket wrench used to turn the nut on the open compressor. It then exerts pressure on the clamp causing movement on the Schanz screw. Before removing the open compressor the tube-holding nut on the clamp must be tightened.

Caps for Tubes and Rods

The caps, made of a sterilisable plastic material, fit on the ends of the tube and rod to prevent the clamps from slipping off during initial assembly and application.

6.13.1.2 Supplementary Instruments

Drill Bits, 3.5 mm and 4.5 mm, Three-Fluted

The 3.5 and 4.5 mm drill bits are of great advantage when drilling for the Schanz screws. The three cutting edges minimise the tendency for the drill bit to skid off the bone surface, even when drilling at an acute angle. The drill bits may be used with the oscillating attachment. These drill bits have quick coupling ends only. See Sect. 6.3.1.

Oscillating Attachment

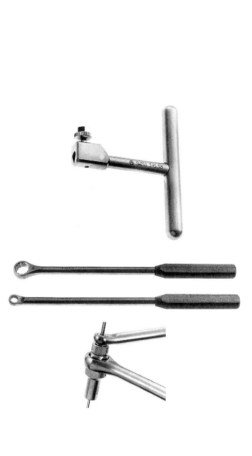

The oscillating attachment, which is used with the small air drill, converts the rotation of the drill bit into oscillating movements (270°). The oscillation prevents spooling of soft tissue around the drill bit, reducing the risk of neurovascular or other damage. The attachment is locked in place over the top trigger of the small air drill, preventing activation of the reverse gear. Only drill bits with a quick coupling end can be used. By pushing the collar forward the drill bit is inserted and turned until fully seated. The collar is then released.

Simple Handle

The handle is for insertion of Schanz screws and Steinmann pins. The locking screw may be tightened by hand or by the hexagonal Allen key.

Bolt Cutter Assembly

The handles for the bolt cutter, 13 mm and 24 mm, 460 mm long, are used together with the bolt cutter heads, 4.5 mm diameter and 5.0 mm diameter to shorten Schanz screws or Steinmann pins of corresponding diameters.

6.13.1.3 Additional Instruments for Segment Transport and Bone Lengthening

Threaded Rod, 8 mm Diameter

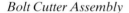

The rod is assembled with the components listed below, as well as with transverse and adjustable clamps and used for segmental bone transport and bone lengthening.
The threaded rod is available in lengths from 250 to 450 mm, in 50 mm increments.

Instrumentation and Techniques

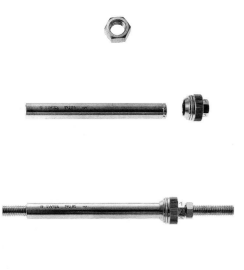

Nuts, 11 mm, for Threaded Rod 8 mm Diameter

These nuts are used to lock the transport tubes on the threaded rod.

Transport Tubes, 11 mm Diameter

These tubes are fixed on the threaded rod with a nut at each end, and accept the clamps connected to the Schanz screws in segment transport and bone lengthening procedures. Three lengths are provided: 60, 80, and 100 mm.

Transport Nut

The nut screwed on the threaded rod is used to move the transport tube. It has indentations, which when turned in increments, each accomplished by a "click", cause a segment displacement of 0.2 mm.

6.13.1.4 Additional Instruments and Implants for Bilateral Frame Configuration

A bilateral frame configuration may be applied, for example, in arthrodesis of the knee or ankle.

Aiming Device Assembly

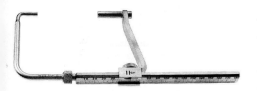

The aiming device is used for accurate placement of the third and fourth Steinmann pin in a bilateral frame configuration. The hook is fixed on the measuring bar by the locking screw. The locking sleeve is slid on the measuring bar in the direction indicated by the arrow on top of the carriage. The measuring bar holds the hook and the locking sleeve, forming a "C". The check tube is used to align the hook and sleeve.

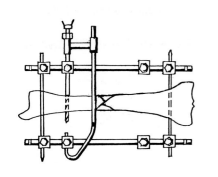

When drilling the pilot hole for the third Steinmann pin, the hook is first fitted in the clamp on the opposite side of the bone. The 110 mm long 5.0 mm/3.5 mm drill sleeve and the 110 mm trocar are tightened in the locking sleeve. The locking sleeve is then slid on the measuring bar and pushed onto the bone through the near clamp. The drill bit, 3.5 mm, can now be used to drill for the Steinmann pin. See also Sect. 6.20.

Steinmann Pins, 4.5 mm and 5.0 mm Diameter

The Steinmann pins, with trocar tip, slightly rounded off, are used for bilateral frame construction with the tubular system, when the pin has to be inserted through the bone. The pins are inserted by hand using the universal chuck or the simple handle, but *never* with a power maschine, since this would cause thermal damage and increase the risk of pin loosening and pin track infection.

The pilot hole is drilled with the 3.5 mm drill bit for the 4.5 mm pin and with the 4.5 mm drill bit for the 5.0 mm pin.

Steinmann pins are available in both stainless steel and titanium alloy in lengths from 125 to 300 mm (see SYNTHES catalogue for details).

Protective Caps, 4.5 mm and 5.0 mm Diameter

The protective caps are used if the Schanz screw or Steinmann pin is cut, to cover the sharp end.

6.13.1.5 Considerations When Applying the External Fixator

Depending on the indication for external fixation, different biomechanical, anatomical, and technical aspects have to be considered before deciding on the frame configuration. By using only a few elements a great number of different frames can be built to achieve the necessary stability.

Frame Stiffness and Fracture Stabilisation of Long Bones

Clinical and experimental evidence have shown that the stiffness of a tubular frame can be increased and motion at the fracture site diminished by the following:

– Placing the main frame in the sagittal plane.
– Increasing the distance between the Schanz screws in each main fragment (Fig. 1).
– Preloading the Schanz screws by pre-drilling 4.5 mm and using the 5.0 mm Schanz screws with 4.6 mm core size (radial preload). Other Schanz screws can be preloaded to a certain extent by applying tension to the screws. This may be done by the open compressor, a reduction forceps, or by hand (Fig. 2).
– Increasing the number of Schanz screws in each main fragment.
– Reducing the distance between the bone and tube.
– Using a "double tube" frame.
– Increasing the distance between the tubes.
– Applying a two-plane unilateral frame (Fig. 3).

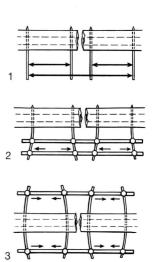

Preloading of Schanz Screws and Steinmann Pins

By applying preloading tension between pairs of screws and pins, micromovement between the cortical bone and the screw/pin is minimised. The risk of bone resorbtion around the screws, loosening and possible pin track infection is thereby reduced. See p. 27.

See p. 27.

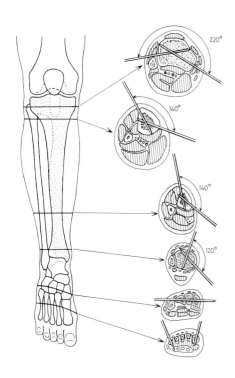

Schanz Screw Insertion in the Tibia

Taking the "safe corridor" into consideration when determining the site for Schanz screw insertion and using the oscillating attachment for pre-drilling help in avoiding injury to the main vessels, nerves, and musculotendinous units. The placement of the frame must also be planned such that it does not interfere with wound access. This may be necessary for initial debridment, or for secondary procedures, such as transfer of soft tissue flaps, sequestrectomies, or the placement of a bone graft.

6.13.1.6 Application Techniques of the Large External Fixator – Tubular System

Application of a Unilateral, One-Plane Frame – Single Tube Using Schanz Screws, 4.5 mm with an 18 mm Thread

A single tube unilateral frame may be applied for the stabilisation of open fractures grade II and III with minimal bone loss.

Note: The Schanz screws with radial preload can also be used. In this case only the 4.5 mm drill bit is used to drill the pilot hole.

Step by step procedure:
– The fracture is grossly reduced before applying the fixator.
– After stab incision, the triple drill sleeve assembly is pushed through the soft tissue onto the bone and positioned at right angles to the long axis. This first Schanz screw should be inserted close to the joint (Fig. 1).
– The trocar is removed, and the 3.5 mm drill bit used to drill both cortices (Fig. 2).

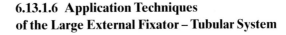

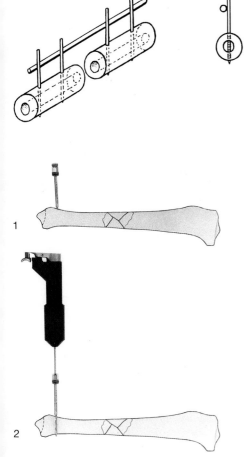

1

2

- The 3.5 mm drill sleeve is removed, and the 4.5 mm drill bit used to drill the near cortex (Fig. 3).
- The depth gauge is pushed through the 4.5 mm drill sleeve and hooked on the far cortex. The knurled disc is moved onto the top of the drill sleeve and its screw tightened (Fig. 4).
- The Schanz screw of appropriate length is tightened in the universal chuck with the T handle at the distance indicated with the depth gauge (p. 322). It is then inserted through the drill sleeve until the chuck abuts the top of the drill sleeve (Fig. 5).
- A long enough tube is prepared with at least four adjustable clamps and caps at each end. The most distal clamp is fixed on the Schanz screw (Fig. 6).

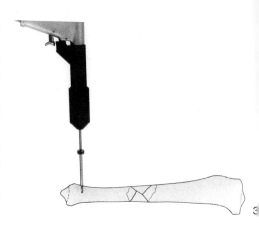

3

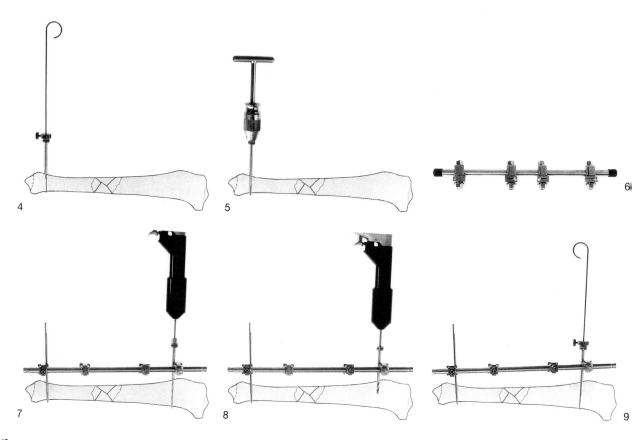

4

5

6

7

8

9

- Axial and rotational alignment of the fracture is checked. The triple trocar is pushed through the most proximal clamp and positioned at right angles to the long axis of the bone. The 3.5 mm drill bit is then used to drill through both cortices (Fig. 7).
- The 3.5 mm drill sleeve is removed and the 4.5 mm drill bit used to drill the near cortex (Fig. 8).
- The length is measured with the depth gauge (Fig. 9).
- The second Schanz screw is inserted (Fig. 10).
- Before tightening the clamps on the tube, proper length and rotational alignment must be secured. The clamps are tightened with the combination wrench or socket wrench.

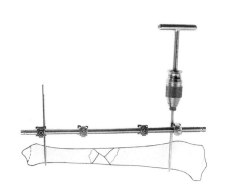

10

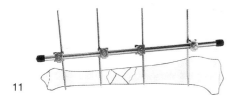

11

– The third and fourth Schanz screws are inserted through their respective clamps, one in each main fragment. They are placed near the fracture, but leaving at least 2 cm between the screws and the fracture area. The same technique of insertion as was described for the second screw is used (Fig. 11).

– The screws should be preloaded one by one by bending the pair of screws in each main fragment towards each other. Preload can be achieved by using the open compressor, a forceps, or by hand. The nut fixing the adjustable clamp on the tube is loosened and the clamp with the Schanz screw placed under tension. The nut is retightened.

Application of a Unilateral, One-Plane Frame – Short Tubes, and Tube-to-Tube Clamp

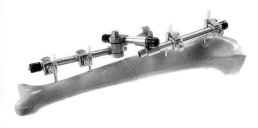

The application technique is similar to the one described above, but the Schanz screws may be applied in different planes before reduction. The screws in each main fragment are connected with short tubes. Each of these tubes is then connected by a tube-to-tube clamp to an intermediate connecting tube. Alignment changes are easily made after loosening the two joints connecting the intermediate tube to the other two tubes.

Application of a Unilateral, One-Plane Frame – Double Tubes, Using Schanz Screws, 5.0 mm, with Radial Preload

Two tubes stacked on top of each other for unilateral fixation increase the stiffness of the frame. This may be needed in fractures with large areas of comminution or bone loss.

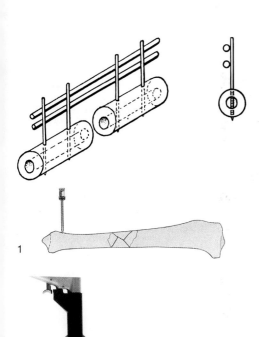

1

2

Step by step procedure:

– The fracture is grossly aligned.

– After stab incision, the long triple drill sleeve assembly is pushed through the soft tissue onto the bone at right angle to the long axis (Fig. 1).

– The trocar and the 3.5 mm sleeve are removed and the 4.5 mm drill bit used to drill through both cortices (Fig. 2).

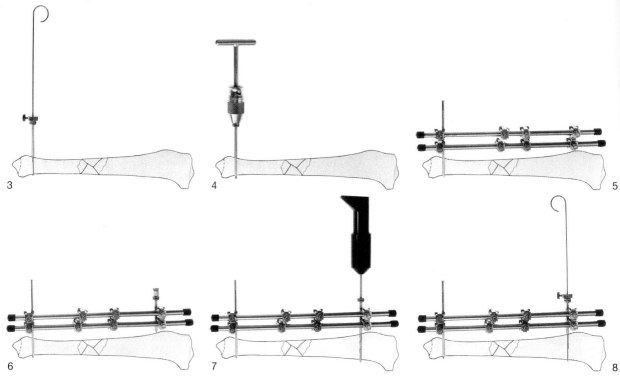

3   4   5

6   7   8

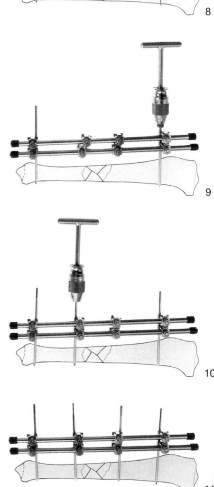

9

10

11

- The depth gauge is pushed through the 4.5 mm drill sleeve and hooked on the far cortex. The knurled disc is moved onto the top of the drill sleeve and its screw tightened (Fig. 3).
- The 5.0 mm Schanz screw, with radial preload and of appropriate length, is tightened in the universal chuck with T handle at the distance indicated by the depth gauge. It is inserted through the drill sleeve until the chuck abuts the drill sleeve (Fig. 4).
- Two tubes are prepared with at least four adjustable clamps on each and caps at the ends. The Schanz screw is fixed to the two tubes with adjustable clamps (Fig. 5).
- The fracture is reduced manually and axial and rotational alignment checked. In the most proximal pair of adjustable clamps the long triple drill sleeve assembly is inserted. It is pushed through the stab incision onto the bone (Fig. 6).
- After removal of the trocar and the 3.5 mm drill sleeve the 4.5 mm drill bit is used to drill through both cortices (Fig. 7).
- The length is measured (Fig. 8).
- The second 5.0 mm Schanz screw with radial preload is tightened in the universal chuck with T handle at the measured distance. It is inserted through the drill sleeve until the chuck abuts the top of the sleeve (Fig. 9).
- Before tightening the clamps on the tube, proper length and rotational alignment must be secured. The clamps are tightened with the combination wrench or socket wrench.
- The third and fourth Schanz screws are inserted through their respective pair of clamps, one in each main fragment. They

■ 332

should be placed near the fracture, but leaving at least 2 cm between the screws and the fracture area. The same technique is used as described for the second screw (Figs. 10, 11).

Application of a Unilateral, Two Plane Frame – V-Shaped Frame

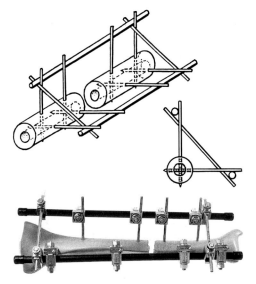

The stiffness of the frame can be increased by adding a second unilateral frame and then interconnecting the two frames. The technique of application is the same as described for the single tube frame (see above). The ventral frame is first applied in a nearly sagittal plane, slightly medially. The second unilateral frame is applied on the medial aspect at an angle between 60° and 100° with the first frame. Two or four Schanz screws are used for each frame. The two long tubes are then interconnected by adding connecting bars fixed with open clamps.

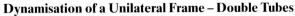

Dynamisation of a Unilateral Frame – Double Tubes

It appears that bone formation is stimulated by progressive force transmission at the site of the consolidated fracture. After soft tissue healing partial, and later full, weight-bearing induces the force transmission. This may also be achieved by gradually building down the rigidity of the fixator frame or through dynamisation.

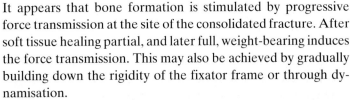

Dynamisation of a double-tube unilateral frame is obtained by crosswise release of the tube nuts. All Schanz screws must be in the same plane to permit longitudinal gliding.

Bone Segment Transport and Bone Lengthening

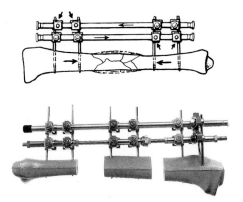

A technique for bone lengthening and segment transport after corticotomy has been introduced by Ilizarov. It is employed in segmental defects or length discrepancies of more than 3–4 cm. The elongation procedure starts 5–7 days after percutaneous corticotomy performed with an osteotome. Through gradual elongation over a period of time, the callus "stretches" to bridge the gap. The surrounding soft tissue, nerves, arteries, veins, and skin also lengthen during distraction. The elongation is accomplished by small frequent increments up to 1 mm per day, which causes the patients less pain and fewer neurological symptoms and circulatory problems than single-step increment.

The AO/ASIF double-tube frame combined with a few additional components can be applied to perform the elongation.

Step by step procedure (segment transport):

– A long enough tube is prepared with a transverse clamp (A), and at least five adjustable clamps. Protective caps are applied at each end. A threaded bar of corresponding length is prepared with three short tubes fixed with nuts (C). The proximal tube carries a transverse clamp and an adjustable clamp, locked in position with a nut at each end. The other two tubes are fitted with two adjustable clamps (E). The nut at one end of the central (transport) tube is the transport nut (D) (Fig. 1).

– A Schanz screw, 5.0 mm is inserted distally in the distal segment. A second 5.0 mm Schanz screw is inserted in the proximal segment about 2 cm proximal to the planned corticotomy site (A). In the metaphysis 5.0 mm Schanz screws are chosen. When a transverse clamp is used for the metaphyseal fragment the two Schanz screws are inserted later.

– The rod and tube prepared with the clamps are connected to the two Schanz screws. The clamps are stacked immediately on top of each other. Any deformities are corrected. The rod and tube must lie exactly parallel to the bone axis.

– Two 4.5 mm Schanz screws are inserted as far apart as possible into the planned transport segment distal to the corticotomy site. One 4.5 mm screw is inserted proximally in the distal segment. At least 2 cm must remain between the screws and the ends of the segments (B).

– Two 5.0 mm Schanz screws are inserted through the transverse clamp. For easy access the transverse clamp is positioned so that the pin-clamping nuts face proximally and the tube-clamping nut faces anteriorly.

– The corticotomy is performed in the metaphyseal – diaphyseal junction. Three-quarters of the circumference is cut with a sharp osteotome through a small skin incision. The cut is completed by twisting the segments in opposite directions to fracture the bone. It is verified by turning the transport nut with the combination wrench and advancing the segment 1 mm (five "clicks") (C) (Fig. 2).

– The Schanz screws are cut with the bolt cutter approximately 1 cm above the clamps, and the ends covered with protective caps.

– The progressive elongation starts after 5–7 days.

– The tube nuts of the two adjustable clamps on the outer (non-threaded) tube affixed to the transport segment Schanz screws are removed. The transport nut is turned with the combination wrench from one indentation to the next, which moves the segment in increments of 0.2 mm. Five turns daily give the desired 1 mm elongation (Fig. 3).

– Partial weight-bearing is recommended during the transport period.

– In segment transport procedures a cancellous onlay graft is placed over the "docking" area as soon as there is contact between the transport segment and the distal fragment.

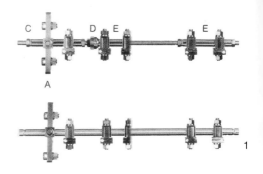

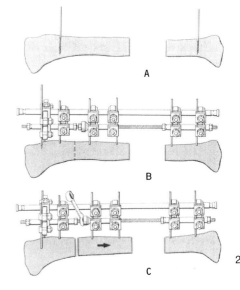

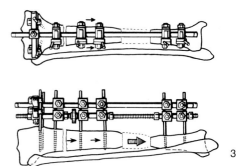

- The transport tube is now locked to the threaded rod by tightening the nuts at both its end.
- The nuts which were previously removed from the adjustable clamps on the outer tube are replaced and tightened. This "locks" the whole assembly to allow distraction regenerate to consolidate and the docking zone to unite. This process usually takes at least as long as the transport took.

Note: Close attention must be paid to the screw/pin sites during the course of lengthening. Signs of reddening must be carefully cleaned and covered and a short course of systemic antibiotics or an enlargement of the screw/pin entry site with a scalpel under local anaesthesia. A loose screw must be removed and a new one inserted at another site.

Leg lengthening is performed in similar manner, with only two Schanz screws in the distal fragment.

Application of a Bilateral Frame in Arthrodesis and Corrective Osteotomies

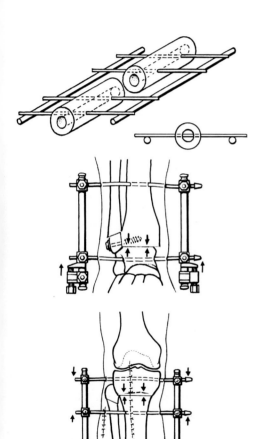

The tubular external fixator may be used for various arthrodeses and corrective osteotomies, where symmetrical compression at the osteotomy site is mandatory. This is best achieved by a bilateral frame. Depending upon the site and the compression needed, the stability of the one-plane bilateral frame is enhanced by a second plane frame. Compression by prestressing the pins, which also helps prevent pin loosening, is achieved by using open compressors. The size and number of pins in each fragment depends on the size of bone and type of fixator. Pre-planning by drawings of the planned osteotomy and insertion sites of the different pins is essential.

The technique of application differs from procedure to procedure and can not be described in detail. For further information see *Manual of Internal Fixation.* (Müller et al. 1991).

Step by step procedure for insertion of Steinmann pins and application of a bilateral frame:
- Through a stab incision the triple drill sleeve is pushed through the soft tissue onto the bone at the site of the first Steinmann pin.
- The trocar is removed and the drill bit, 3.5 mm (preferably three-fluted), used to drill through both cortices. A stab incision is made at the opposite side for the protruding drill bit.
- A 4.5 mm or 5.0 mm Steinmann pin is inserted with the universal chuck with T handle through the 5.0 mm drill sleeve.
- The second Steinamnn pin is inserted in similar manner in the opposite fragment, parallel to the first.
- Two tubes or rods are fitted with two or four adjustable clamps each and caps at the ends. The Steinmann pins are connected to the two tubes with the adjustable clamps and all nuts tightened slightly.

– If a second Steinmann pin in one or both main fragments is to be inserted, the aiming device is used. The hook of the assembled aiming device is inserted in the adjustable tube clamp on the far side of the bone, then the locking sleeve with the tightened 3.5 mm drill sleeve is pushed through the near clamp. This permits drilling a 3.5 mm hole into which the Steinmann pin can be inserted in correct alignment with the two clamps. To facilitate insertion of the pin, the hole may be overdrilled with the 4.5 mm drill bit (three-fluted) after the 3.5 mm sleeve has been removed.

Note: If Steinmann pins are inserted in the metaphyseal area, they may be better placed parallel in the horizontal plane and connected by a transverse clamp.

– After insertion of the Steinmann pins, compression at the osteotomy site is achieved by the use of open compressors. The pins in each fragment are prestressed one after the other. An open compressor in closed mode is attached at the end of the two tubes with the plate adjacent to the adjustable clamp.
– The tube nuts of the adjustable clamps are opened. Using the combination wrench or socket wrench the bolts of the open compressors are turned simultaneously, exerting pressure on the clamps and moving of the attached Schanz screws. The tube nuts of the clamps are retightened and the open compressors removed.
– The compression procedure is repeated for each Steinmann pin in the same manner.
– Protective caps are used to cover the sharp tips of the pins.

6.13.1.7 Instruments for the Application and Removal of External Fixators

Instruments for application of a tube to tube – unilateral external fixator

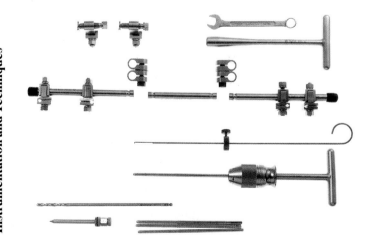

Instrumentation and Techniques

Instruments for application of a double tube or V-shaped unilateral external fixator

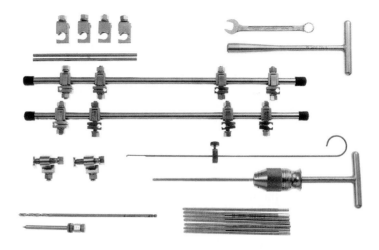

Instruments for application of an external fixator for segment transport and bone lengthening

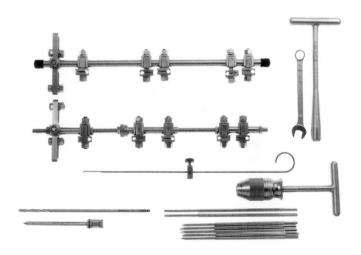

Instruments for removal of the large external fixator

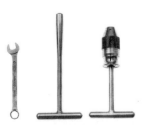

6.13.2 The Small External Fixator

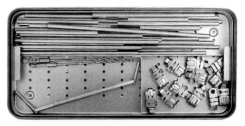

For the stabilisation of open fractures grade II and III, or of complex fractures with defects, in the distal forearm, the small external fixator may be applied instead of the large fixator. Distraction of the wrist joint is thus possible. Experience has shown that the length of the radius, restored by closed reduction, and, if possible, percutaneous pinning, can be maintained by distraction due to pull of the intact capsular ligamentous complex, so-called "ligamentotaxis". The small external fixator may also be applied to stabilise fractures in small bones, while treating soft tissue injuries.

Indications:
- Unstable fractures of the distal radius; wrist or hand
- Metaphyseal/epiphyseal comminution
- Metaphyseal comminution with loss of substance and marked dorsal tilt (Colles) or with radial shortening
- Fractures with volar tilt (Smith), or with volar intra-articular fragment (reversed Barton)
- Open fractures
- Multifragmentary fracture in combination with other fractures of the upper extremity, or injuries of the hand
- Fracture dislocation of the wrist joint
- Intra-articular comminuted fracture of the base of the first metacarpal
- Complex injuries of the hand where skeletal stabilisation is not otherwise possible

6.13.2.1 Instruments and Implants

A set of instruments and implants for the application of the small external fixator is obtainable in a sterilising tray or a small aluminium case.

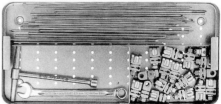

Instrumentation and Techniques

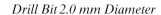

Drill Bit 2.0 mm Diameter

This bit, 100 mm/75 mm, two-fluted and for quick coupling, is used to drill for the 2.5 mm Kirschner wire with threaded tip in hard bone or for Kirschner wires used for fixation of fragments. The triple wire guide, 2.0 mm, is used as a drill guide.

Triple Wire Guide, 2.0 mm

The triple wire guide is used as a drill sleeve for the 2.0 mm drill bit or for parallel placement of Kirschner wires.

Double Drill Sleeve, 2.7 mm/2.0 mm

The double drill sleeve can be used as a guide when drilling with the 2.0 mm drill bit and to protect tissue when inserting the 2.5 mm Kirschner wire with thread.

Small Triple Drill Sleeve Assembly, 4.0 mm

Similar to the large triple drill sleeve assembly (see Sect. 6.13.1.1), a small drill sleeve assembly is being developed to be used with the clamps, 4.0 mm for the small external fixator. It consists of three parts:
– The *trocar,* 2.1 mm, is used with the two drill sleeves to penetrate soft tissue.
– The *drill sleeve,* 2.1 mm/2.7mm, accepts the trocar and the drill bit, 2.0 mm, necessary for pre-drilling for the Kirschner wire with threaded tip, 2.5 mm.
– The *drill sleeve,* 2.7 mm/4.0 mm, with handle is the outermost sleeve accepting the drill sleeve, 2.1 mm/2.7 mm, and the trocar, 2.1 mm. It fits in the 4.0 mm clamps and remains in the clamp until the Kirschner wire with threaded tip, 2.5 mm, has been inserted.

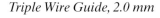

Kirschner Wires with Threaded Tip, 2.5 mm, 150 mm

The Kirschner wires are inserted in the index metacarpal in a very small radius, functioning as implants to connect the clamps with the bars. The wires may be inserted by power either straight-away or after pre-drilling with a 2.0 mm drill bit. The thread portion should rermain in the far cortex to ensure good purchase.

Kirschner Wires, 1.6 mm and 2.0 mm Diameter, 150 mm

The wires are used for percutaneous fixation of intra-articular fractures. Pre-drilling the hard cortex may sometimes be necessary. Kirschner wires are inserted with the small air drill equipped with Jacobs chuck using the triple wire guide.
Kirschner wires are available in other sizes, too. See SYNTHES catalogue.

External Fixators: Instruments and Implants

Schanz Screw, 4.0 mm Schaft and 3.0 mm Thread Diameter

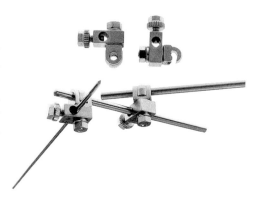

The Schanz screw, 80 mm long, may be used for insertion in the radius instead of the Kirschner wires. The 20 mm thread length ensures a good purchase in the bone. Pre-drilling with the 2.5 mm drill bit is necessary before inserting the Schanz screw by hand with the simple T handle or the universal chuck with T handle.

Clamp, with Pear-Shaped Hole, 4.0 mm

Recently developed, the clamp with the pear-shaped hole is used to connect both Schanz screws, 4.0 mm in diameter, and Kirschner wires with a threaded tip, 2.5 mm in diameter, to the 4.0 mm tube. Thanks to the pear-shaped hole, screws and wires with diameters between 2.5 mm and 4.0 mm can be used. They are fixed with the 7 mm nut. This clamp replaces the two clamps 4.0 mm/4.0 mm and 4.0 mm/2.5 mm.

Open Clamp with Pear-Shaped Hole, 4.0 mm

The open clamp can be added to the 4.0 mm bar to connect an additional screw or wire after the frame has been built. Thanks to its pear-shaped hole pins 2.5 mm – 4.0 mm in size can be connected. This clamp replaces the two open clamps described below.

Clamp, 4.0 mm/2.5 mm

The clamp is used to connect a 4.0 mm bar to the Kirschner wire with thread, 2.5 mm.

Clamp, 4.0 mm/4.0 mm

The clamp is similar to the 4.0 mm/2.5 mm clamp, but connects two 4.0 mm connecting bars or one bar to a Schanz screw, with 4.0 mm shaft.

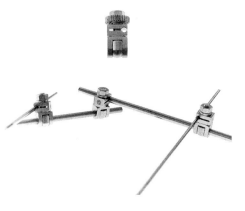

Open Clamp, 4.0 mm/4.0 mm

This clamp can be used to complete a 4.0 mm bar to bar connection after the frame has been built.

Open Clamp, 4.0 mm/2.5 mm

This clamp connects an additional 2.5 mm Kirschner wire with threaded tip to the 4.0 mm bar in a prebuilt frame.

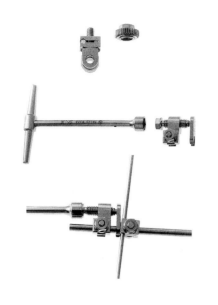

Spring-Loaded Nut

The spring-loaded nut is used for temporary tightening of the clamps but is not intended for use over a longer period of time, since the holding power decreases over time.

Small Open Compressor

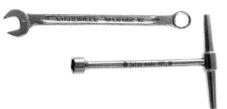

The compressor is used to prestress the screws or wires to prevent loosening and pin track infection. It is applied in closed mode on the 4.0 mm connecting bar or rod with the plate adjacent to the clamp. Tightening the screw with the socket wrench moves the clamp and its attached wire in the desired direction.

Combination Wrench, 7 mm, and Socket Wrench, 7 mm

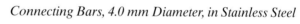

The combination and socket wrenches are used to tighten the nuts of the clamps.

Connecting Bars, 4.0 mm Diameter, in Stainless Steel

The connecting bars are used to build the frame of the small external fixator. They are available in lengths from 60 to 200 mm, in 20 mm increments.

Carbon Fibre Rods, 4.0 mm Diameter

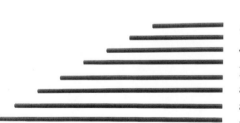

The carbon fibre rods are radiolucent and stiffer than the stainless steel rods. They are made of carbon fibre reinforced epoxy and have a special coating which provides increased protection against fibre damage when clamps are tightened. The coating also improves the friction properties between the clamp and the rod and eliminates moisture penetration during autoclaving.
The carbon fibre rods are available in lengths from 60 to 200 mm, in increments of 20 mm.

6.13.2.2 Application Technique of the Small External Fixator

Application of the small external fixator will obviously depend upon the type of fracture and the condition of the soft tissue. An unstable fracture of the distal radius is used as an example here.

Step by step procedure:
- The patient lies supine and the injured extremity is positioned horizontally on a radiolucent table. A tourniquet is generally applied.
- The fracture is manually reduced. Intra-articular fractures are fixed with percutaneous Kirschner wires using the small air drill with Jacobs chuck. Open reduction may be needed in severely displaced or impacted articular segments (Fig. 1).
- Two incisions are made over the index metacarpal, radial to the extensor tendons.
- Two 2.5 mm Kirschner wires with threaded tips are inserted, with or without pre-drilling with the 2.0 mm drill bit (Fig. 2). The wires should converge at an angle of 40° to 60° in the vertical plane (Fig. 3), without the points touching each other, and at 45° to the horizontal plane. The metacarpo-phalangeal joint is flexed to a right angle to avoid the extensor hood. The converging wires have a longer passage through the bone, and thereby a better hold.
- With the hand in pronation two incisions are made over the dorsoradial aspect of the radius, 1–2 cm long, and separated by a distance of 4–6 cm. The bone surface is exposed by blunt dissection, protecting the superficial branches of the radial nerve.
- The 2.5 mm drill bit is used to drill both cortices at 45° angles in the horizontal plane, and at 90° in the vertical plane. A corresponding drill sleeve is used to protect the soft tissue (Fig. 4).
- The 4.0 mm/3.0 mm Schanz screw is inserted with the universal chuck with T handle or the simple T handle. Two Schanz screws are inserted (Fig. 5). Image intensification is used to confirm that the thread of the screws or wires remain in the bone.
- If 2.5 mm Kirschner wires with threaded tips are used, they may be inserted directly using the small air drill with the Jacobs chuck or after pre-drilling with a 2.0 mm drill bit through the triple wire guide in the same direction as described above.
- The two Schanz screws are connected with the two 4.0 mm/4.0 mm clamps on the connecting bars. If double bars are used for increased stability of the frame, both bars have to be connected at the same time.
- Similarly, the two Kirschner wires are connected to the double bars with 4.0 mm/2.5 mm clamps. All nuts are tightened.

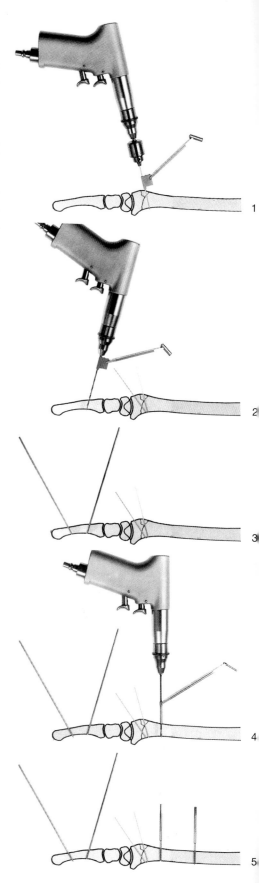

1

2

3

4

5

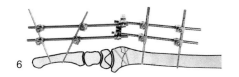

6

- The four bars may now be connected with two 4.0 mm/4.0 mm clamps (Fig. 6). These clamps are not fully tightened.
- Final reduction by distraction is performed and the interconnecting clamps tightened while the wrist is being held in the desired position.

The stability of the fixation may be increased by prestressing the screws or wires by hand towards each other in each fragment. The small open compressors may also be used.

Note: Four short bars may also be connected by two intermediate bars and four 4.0 mm/4.0 mm clamps.

Note: If one or two long bars are used, the two outer Kirschner wires or screws have to be connected to the clamps before drilling and inserting the two inner wires or screws through the corresponding clamps.

6.13.2.3 Instruments for Application of the Small External Fixator

Since different frame configurations are possible it is recommended that the complete sterilising tray or aluminium case be available for all applications. Additional Schanz screws may have to be added to the instrumentation.

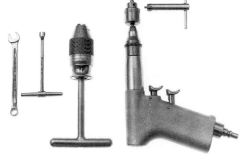

6.13.2.4 Instruments for the Removal of the Small External Fixator

The small external fixator frame is removed by disconnecting the clamps using the 7 mm socket wrench or combination wrench. The Kirschner wires may be removed by using the small air drill in reverse motion. Schanz screws are removed with the universal chuck with T handle.

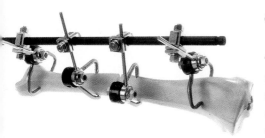

6.13.3 The Pinless Fixator

The large pinless fixator has recently been developed to provide temporary fixation in open or closed tibial fractures with major soft tissue injury. The fixation of the device to the bone is guaranteed by clamps inserted in the cortex only if the medullary cavity is not penetrated.

The risk of pin track infection with possible medullary contamination is excluded. The pinless fixator provides a reliable construct to protect the soft tissue in preparation for a secondary, final mode of fixation. A small size pinless fixator is being developed for use in forearm fractures.

Indications:
- Open or closed fractures with severe soft tissue damage in multiply injured patients whose prognosis for survival is uncertain
- Open tibial fractures (grade IIIc) with uncertain prognosis as to limb survival
- Open or closed tibia fractures, with or without soft tissue lesions, associated with severe cerebral damage
- Emergency fixation of tibia fractures in war surgery and mass casualties

The pinless fixator has also been used for skeletal traction.

6.13.3.1 Instruments

These instruments are:
- Pinless clamps with posts
- Handgrip
- Adjustable clamps (from external fixator tubular system)
- Stainless tube or carbon fibre rod (from tubular system)
- Combination wrench, 11 mm in width across flats

6.13.3.2 Application Technique

Step by step procedure:
- Provisional reduction of the fracture.
- Insertion of two pinless clamps in each main fragment. The trocar points of the clamps are pressed into the cortical surface by squeezing the handgrip and at the same time rotating backwards and forwards about the axis between the points.
- Attachment of the posts to the pinless clamps.
- Assembly of adjustable clamps to the posts.
- Connection of the four clamps by means of a tube or rod of appropriate length.
- Reduction of the fracture components with all the clamps in loosened positions.
- Tightening of all clamps to achieve the desired stability at the fracture site.

See also *Injury*, AO/ASIF Scientific Suppl 23 [Suppl 3].

6.13.4 The Lengthening Apparatus

The small and the large apparatus with their one-dimensional configuration and great stability were originally developed for gradual leg lengthening of the upper and, especially, the lower extremities. Lengthening may be indicated in juvenile patients with congenital or acquired shortening of a limb. Lengthening of more than 20 cm has been accomplished with the aid of this apparatus. The healing process requires many months; only very cooperative patients and a considerate, attentive and diligent surgeon should involve themselves in this type of surgical programme. The apparatus may also be used for fracture treatment, where unilateral fixation is desired.

The mini-lengthening apparatus is used in peripheral lengthening procedures.

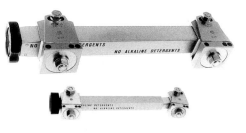

6.13.4.1 Large and Small Lengthening Apparatus, Instruments and Implants

Large and Small Lengthening Apparatus

The large apparatus is used in the lower extremity and the smaller one in the upper extremities. For femoral lengthening the apparatus is applied on the lateral aspect, for tibial lengthening on the antero-medial aspect.

The lengthening apparatus consists of two rectangular telescoping tubes made of anodised aluminium.

Relative movement of the tubes is produced by an internal threaded rod operated by a knob at one end. Notches on the knob indicate the distance of movement; one notch corresponds to 0.37 mm movement on the large apparatur and 0.33 mm on the small one.

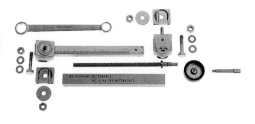

Each fixation head can hold two Schanz screws for fixing the apparatus to the bone. Both heads can be swiveled about each locking nut in the long axis, and the upper part can be rotated for angle correction in the frontal plane. The locking nuts are tightened with the 11 and 14 mm ring wrenches. The apparatus has to be disassembled for cleaning. See also Chap. 6.22.4.2.

Angled Piece, Large

By replacing the vice plate on the fixation head, the Schanz screws can be placed at 90° to the long axis of the large apparatus. It can then be used for rotational corrections.

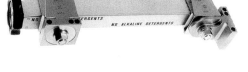

Angled Piece, Small

Similarly, the vice plate of the small apparatus can be used instead of the small angled piece to achieve the above mentioned screw placement.

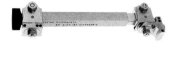

Drill Bit, 3.5 mm Diameter

The bit, 195 mm/170 mm, with a quick coupling end, is used to pre-drill the pilot hole for the Schanz screws, 6.0 mm. It is used with the drill sleeve, 6.0 mm/3.5 mm.

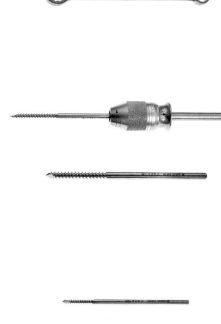

Drill Bit, 3.2 mm Diameter

The bit, 195 mm/170 mm, with quick coupling end, is used to pre-drill the pilot hole for the Schanz screws, 4.0 mm. It is used with the 4.0 mm/3.2 mm drill sleeve.

Drill Sleeve, 6.0 mm/3.5 mm

The sleeve, 110 mm, is used with the 3.5 mm trocar to advance through the soft tissue onto the bone surface. After removal of the trocar, the sleeve is used to guide the 3.5 mm drill bit.

Trocar, 3.5 mm Diameter

The trocar is inserted in the drill sleeve, 6.0 mm/3.5 mm, to penetrate the soft tissue before drilling for the 6.0 mm Schanz screw.

Drill Sleeve, 4.0 mm/3.2 mm

The drill sleeve, 60 mm, is used with the 3.2 mm trocar to advance through the soft tissue onto the bone surface. After removal of the trocar the sleeve is used to guide the drill bit, 3.2mm.

Trocar, 3.2 mm Diameter

The trocar is inserted in the drill sleeve, 4.0 mm/3.2 mm, to penetrate the soft tissue before drilling for the 4.0 mm Schanz screw.

Ring Wrench

The ring wrench, 11 mm or 14 mm in width across flats, is used to tighten the locking nuts of both the small and the large lengthening apparatus, respectively.

Universal Chuck with T Handle

The universal chuck is used to insert the Schanz screws.

Schanz Screws, 6.0 mm Diameter

The 6.0 mm Schanz screws with flat point are used for the application of the large apparatus. The thread length is 50 mm and the core size 4.0 mm. Pre-drilling 3.5 mm is necessary before inserting the screw with the universal chuck with T handle.The flat point facilitates insertion of the screw.

Schanz Screws, 4.0 mm Diameter

The 4.0 mm Schanz screws with flat point are used for the application of the small lengthening apparatus. The thread length is

25 mm and the core size 2.8 mm. The 3.2 mm drill bit is used for pre-drilling before inserting the screw with the universal chuck with T handle.

6.13.4.2 Application Technique of the Large Apparatus in the Femur

Step by step procedure:
- Through a stab incision, two to three fingerwidths above the lateral condyle, the drill sleeve, 6.0 mm/3.5 mm, with trocar, 3.5 mm, is pushed through the soft tissue onto the bone surface.
- After removal of the trocar the drill bit, 3.5 mm, is used to drill through both cortices parallel to the knee joint and centrally located in the AP plane.
- A 6.0 mm Schanz screw is inserted using the universal chuck with T handle.
- Using the same technique, a second Schanz screw is inserted in the proximal metaphysis, about 1.5 cm distal to the innominate lateral tubercle of the greater trochanter. The screw must be parallel to the first screw.
- The lengthening apparatus is placed on the anterior side of the screws to leave sufficient skin area for the subsequent postero-lateral approach to the femoral shaft.
- The drill sleeve with trocar is inserted through the second hole of the fixation head. It is then pushed through a stab incision and the soft tissue until it abuts the bone surface. This ensures that the Schanz screws in each fragment will be parallel. The procedure is repeated through the second fixation head. Two Schanz screws are then inserted in each fixation head.
- A postero-lateral insicion is made and a transverse osteotomy or corticotomy performed between the Schanz screws.
- The apparatus is lengthened until stabilisation is achieved by soft tissue tension. Drainage, wound dressing, and an elastic bandage is applied.
- Lengthening by turning the knob one revolution per day (1.5 mm), in increments, may be performed by the patient. Active motion of the knee joint and partial weight-bearing accompany the lengthening process. Careful attention must be paid to the site of the screws. Any soft tissue pressure against the screws must be avoided. Enlargement of the incisions may be necessary.
- In children, spontaneous regeneration of the bone may occur at the distraction site. When the desired length is reached, and sufficient bony integrity is radiographically confirmed, the knob of the lengthening device is turned in reverse and a compressive load applied. The device is left in place until the normal diameter of the bone has been reconstituted and the intramedullary canal becomes visible.

- In the majority of cases internal fixation and bone grafting are performed once the desired distraction has been achived. A long enough plate (broad lengthening plate) is contoured and applied on the postero-lateral aspect of the bone.
- If there is avascular scar tissue between the bone ends, bone grafting is necessary. Grafts are taken from the posterior iliac spine.
- After wound closure the apparatus is removed.

6.13.4.3 The Mini Lengthening Apparatus

For lengthening procedures in small bones, e.g. metacarpals, the mini lengthening apparatus is attached to the main fragments by 2.5 mm diameter Kirschner wires with 15 mm threaded tips or by 2.7 mm cortex screws. The end vice plate may be positioned longitudinally or transversely. Its position is adjusted with the small hexagonal screwdriver.

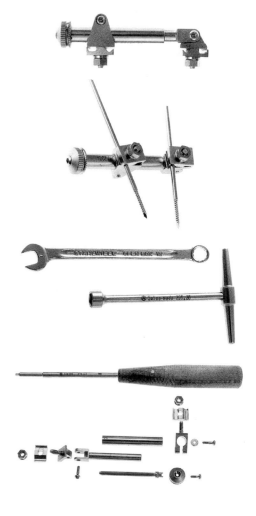

One spindle revolution is equivalent to 0.7 mm lengthening (from notch to notch approximately 0.23 mm). The combination wrench, or socket wrench, 7 mm is used for tighetening the nuts. The apparatus may also be used as a reduction aid or as an external fixator in small bones.

The apparatus must be disassembled for thorough cleaning. The telescoping sleeve is fully extended and the vice plate removed.

6.13.5 The Unifix

The Unifix is a unilateral external fixator which can be applied in tibial and femoral fractures. The body is made of titanium alloy and provides high strength at low weight. Compressible ball and socket joints permit a wide range of movement (25°) of the Schanz screws. The distance between the outermost holes is 225 mm, which is the limit for the application of the Schanz screws. Correction of axial, lateral, and rotational displacements are possible. Both compression and distraction can be achieved with the Unifix, as can dynamisation.

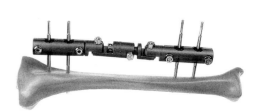

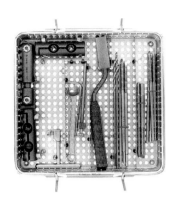

6.13.5.1 Instruments, Implants, and Fixation Components

The Unifix and the instruments and implants can be obtained in a sterilising tray.

Instruments

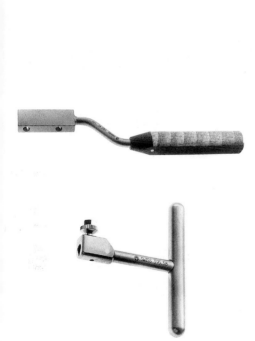

Drill Bit, 4.5 mm Diameter

This bit, 195 mm/170 mm, two-fluted, with quick coupling end, is used with the small air drill to drill the pilot hole for the Schanz screws.

Drill Bit ,4.5 mm Diameter

The 4.5 mm drill bit, 180 mm/165 mm, two-fluted, for Jacobs chuck, is used if a small air drill with quick coupling chuck is not available.

Drill Sleeve, 6.0 mm/4.5 mm

The drill sleeve is used when drilling for the two innermost Schanz screws.

Trocar, 4.5 mm Diameter

The trocar and the drill sleeve, 6.0 mm/4.5 mm, are inserted through the aiming device and the Unifix ball joint to determine the stab incision site.

Aiming Device

This device is used when drilling for the second parallel Schanz screw in each fragment. The holes in the aiming device match those of the clamp section.

Simple Handle

The simple handle is used to insert the Schanz screws. The Schanz screw is locked in place by the side screw.

Combination Wrench, 11 mm

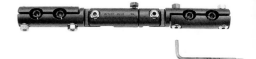

The combination wrench is used to tighten and loosen the nuts and the locking bolts.

Hexagonal Allen Key with Pin

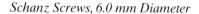

The hexagonal Allen key is used to tighten and loosen the internal hexagonal bolt of the Unifix.

Implants

Schanz Screw, 6.0 mm Diameter

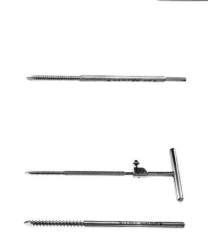

This 6.0 mm Schanz screw, for Unifix, has a roughened shaft surface to increase its durability. See Sect. 6.1.1. The screw has a core size of 4.8 mm, thread length of 50 mm, and a blunted trocar tip. The 4.5 mm drill bit is used for pre-drilling.
The screws are inserted with the simple handle. They are available in lengths of 125, 150, and 175 mm.

Schanz Screws, 6.0 mm Diameter

The 6.0 mm Schanz screws, with a core size of 4.1 mm, a thread length of 50 mm, and a flat point, may be applied in cancellous bone after pre-drilling with a 3.5 mm diameter drill bit. They are available in lengths of 130, 160, and 190 mm.

Fixation Components

Unifix

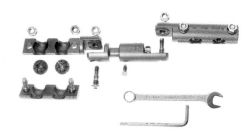

The Unifix consists of:
– Two clamp sections, with three 11 mm hexagonal nuts each
– Four Unifix ball clamps
– One central component with knurled compression bolt
– One locking bolt
– Six internal fixation bolts with nuts
High grade alloys are used in the manufacture of the individual parts and so they need no maintenance. Lubricants can even impair the stability of the Unifix.

6.13.5.2 Application Technique

Depending on the localisation the Unifix it is prepared with, or without, its central component. It is initially used in a straight position with tightened hinge joints so that it can act as a template.
If the central component is used, it should be in its middle position, allowing for either compression or distraction.

- The fracture is preliminarily reduced and the fixator position determined.
- The drill sleeve, 6.0 mm/4.5 mm, and trocar are inserted through the stab incision.
- The pilot hole for the Schanz screw is drilled perpendicular to the long axis of the bone using the 4.5 mm drill bit.
- The first 6.0 mm Schanz screw is inserted using the simple handle.
- The Unifix is placed onto the first screw and tightened *by hand.*
- The drill sleeve and trocar are pushed through the end ball joint on the other side of the fracture and a stab incision made.
- The 4.5 mm drill bit is used to drill for the second Schanz screw.
- The 6.0 mm Schanz screw is inserted with the simple handle.
- The aiming device is mounted on one of the screws. The drill sleeve with trocar are inserted through the second hole of the aiming device and the corresponding ball joint.
- After a stab incision and drilling 4.5 mm, the third Schanz screw is inserted.
- The second Schanz screw in the other main fragment is inserted using the same technique.

Note: Secondary correction of alignment is possible without disassembling the Unifix. All nuts have just to be loosened and retightened after correction. The following operations are possible:
- The locking bolt in the central component is loosened.
- Distraction with the central component is achieved by turning the knurled compression bolt.
- Axial, lateral and rotational displacements are corrected by loosening the six hexagonal nuts and retightening them after manipulation.
- Compression of the fracture is achieved by turning the knurled compression bolt. The Unifix then automatically adjusts from the initial straight position to a slightly angulated shape. Nuts are then all tightened.

Further Possibilities

Shortening:
- The central component can be removed by opening the two hinge joints.
- The two main components can then be fitted together directly.
- The shortened Unifix is secured by using one of the internal hexagonal bolts from the central components.
- The bolt is loosened in a clockwise direction and tightened in an anticlockwise direction as it is fitted with a *left hand thread.*

Additional Rotation

Further rotation than that which is possible with the ball and socket joints may be achieved by loosening the locking bolt in the central component. Rotation of another 35° is then possible. Note that longitudinal guidance of the locking bolt is only maintained when placed in the groove. If rotated, compression, distraction, or dynamisation is not possible.

6.13.5.3 Instruments for Removal of the Unifix

The Unifix is removed by loosening all the nuts with the 11 mm combination wrench. The Schanz screws are removed using the simple T handle, or even better the universal chuck with T handle.

6.14 The Distractor

The distractor is a reduction instrument for temporary use in simple or complex fractures. It offers the possibility of distraction or compression by controlled movement of the fragments. After insertion of the selected implant, the distractor is removed. A large and a small distractor are available.

6.14.1 The Large Distractor

The large distractor is of sufficient dimension to allow application of considerable force and is used for gentle open or closed reduction of fractures of femur and tibia, upper extremity, pelvis, and acetabulum. In many cases it serves as an alternative to positioning the patient on a fracture table. It may also be applied to facilitate reduction of complex intra-articular fractures, or even in arthroscopic surgery such as meniscus repair. It allows rotational control and correction in any plane about one or more axes. It is applied to the bone by Schanz screws.

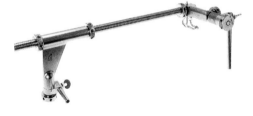

Its predecessor, a simple model, fixed to the bone by special connecting bolts, only allowed rotational correction up to 30°. Its versatility is therefore limited, but may still be useful in selected cases.

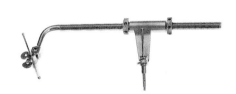

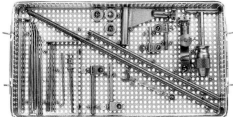

6.14.1.1 Instruments, Implants, and Distractor Components

The distractor components, the instruments and the implants can be obtained in a sterilising tray.

Standard Instruments

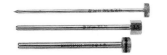

Drill Bit, 3.5 mm Diameter

This bit, 195 mm/170 mm, two-fluted, with quick coupling end, is used to drill the pilot hole for the 5.0 mm Schanz screws. The 110 mm triple drill sleeve assembly is used as drill sleeve.

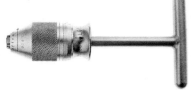
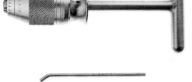

Triple Drill Sleeve Assembly, 110 mm

This sleeve is employed as the drill sleeve and tissue protector for the 3.5 mm drill bit. It consists of three parts:
- Trocar, 3.5 mm diameter, 110 mm, used together with the two drill sleeves, helps to penetrate the soft tissue after the incision has been made.
- Drill sleeve, 5.0 mm/3.5 mm, accepts the trocar, 3.5 mm diameter and the drill bit, 3.5 mm diameter.
- Drill sleeve, 6.0 mm/5.0 mm, is the outermost drill sleeve of the assembly. It accepts the other two components and is used separately for insertion of the 5.0 mm Schanz screw.

Universal Chuck with T Handle

This chuck is used to insert the Schanz screws manually.

Pin Wrench

This wrench can be employed to tighten the locking nuts.

Implants

Schanz Screws, 5.0 mm Diameter

These screws, core size 3.5 mm diameter, thread length 50 mm, are inserted in the two main fragments, and connected to the distractor. They are available in lengths 150, 175, and 200 mm.

Distractor

Distractor Components

Threaded Rod, 14 mm Diameter

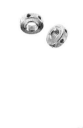

This rod is connected with the sleeve-holding bracket at one end and the hole and the carriage at the other end. These parts are locked in place with the locking nuts. Depending on the site for the distractor, the 440 mm or the 330 mm rod is used.

Locking Nut

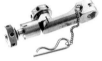

The locking nut is screwed on the rod and used to hold the carriage and the sleeve-holding bracket in place. The nuts on each side of the carriage are turned to achieve distraction or compression. The pin wrench can be used to tighten or loosen the nuts.

Sleeve-Holding Bracket

This bracket is screwed on the end of the threaded rod, which has a hole, and locked in its centre slot with the locking pin through the hole of the rod. The long screw-holding sleeve is attached after removal of the spring-loaded locking nut; the serrated surfaces of the bracket and the sleeve should engage. The nut is retightened. The sleeve-holding bracket allows connecting to Schanz screws in different planes.

Carriage

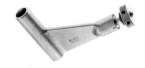

This carriage is placed at the other end of the threaded rod and locked in position by two locking nuts. After removal of the spring loaded locking nut, the short screw-holding sleeve is attached with the serrated surface engaging that of the carriage, and the nut retightened. The carriage is connected to the distal Schanz screw by this sleeve.

Screw-Holding Sleeve, 105 mm

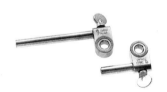

This sleeve is attached to the sleeve-holding bracket to hold the Schanz screw in the proximal fragment. The Schanz screw is fixed in the sleeve by the wing nut.

Screw-Holding Sleeve, 55 mm

This sleeve is attached to the carriage to hold the Schanz screw in the distal fragment. The Schanz screw is fixed in the sleeve by the wing nut.

Instrumentation and Techniques

6.14.1.2 Additional Components for Use with Universal Femoral Nailing System

See also p. 288.

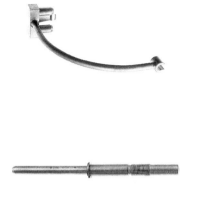

Curved Aiming Attachment

This piece is attached to the universal nail insertion handle. It allows proper placement of a 5.0 mm Schanz screw in the proximal femur in an antero-posterior direction, to which the upper end of the large distractor is connected. The curved aiming attachment accepts the 140 mm triple drill sleeve assembly and allows drilling and insertion of the Schanz screw perpendicular to the axis of the nail.

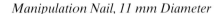

Manipulation Nail, 11 mm Diameter

This nail is connected with the universal nail insertion handle by the locking nut. It is inserted in the medullary canal and may be used for reduction or to indicate the nail axis, when placing the proximal Schanz screw for the distractor.

Drill Bit, 3.5 mm Diameter

This bit, 225 mm/200 mm, three-fluted, with quick coupling end, is used with the 140 mm long drill sleeve assembly fitted into the curved aiming attachment to drill for the proximal Schanz screw, 5.0 mm.

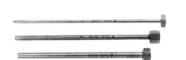

Triple Drill Sleeve Assembly, 140 mm

This assembly is employed as the drill sleeve and tissue protector for the 3.5 mm drill bit, when using the curved aiming attachment in the insertion handle It consists of three parts:
– Trocar, 3.5 mm diameter, 140 mm, used together with the two drill sleeves, helps to penetrate the soft tissue after the incision has been made.
– Drill sleeve, 5.0 mm/3.5 mm, accepts the trocar, 3.5 mm diameter and the drill bit, 3.5 mm diameter.
– Drill sleeve, 6.0 mm/5.0 mm, is the outermost drill sleeve of the assembly. It accepts the other two components and is used separately for insertion of the 5.0 mm Schanz screw.

6.14.1.3 Clinical Applications of the Distractor

Positioning of the patient:
– Any position on a standard operating table may be used.

Versatility in application:
– Schanz screws, 5.0 mm are inserted after pre-drilling 3.5 mm (three-fluted drill bit is recommended) in each main fragment perpendicular to the long axis of the bone.

Distractor

355 ∎

6.17 Wiring Instruments and Implants

Cerclage wires may be applied for temporary fixation or as figure-of-eight fixation in conjunction with Kirschner wires in fractures of the patella, olecranon, or of avulsion fractures of the malleoli.

Some of these instruments and implants are contained in a sterilising tray or in a graphic case. See SYNTHES catalogue.

6.17.1 Instruments and Implants

Drill Bit, 2.0 mm Diameter

This bit, 100 mm/75 mm, is used to pre-drill hard bone for insertion of cerclage wires, or occasionally before inserting Kirschner wires. The triple wire guide is used as tissue protector.

Triple Wire Guide, 2.0 mm

This wire guide is employed as tissue protector and guide when pre-drilling, or when inserting the Kirschner wires. The three holes permit parallel drilling and insertion of wires.

Wire Passers, 45 mm and 70 mm Diameter

The wire passer of appropriate size is passed around the bone, as close to its surface as possible. A cerclage wire is inserted into the tip of the instrument, which will be passed around the bone by withdrawing the instrument.

Wire Tightener

The wire tightener, with two pegs, 230 mm, is used to tighten cerclage wires with eye. The wire is inserted through the tip of the instrument and threaded through the peg, which is turned to fix the wire. The peg is then placed in the slot, and turned to tighten the wire. Two wires of sizes 1.2 mm diameter may be tightened simultaneously. If two wires are tightened, one peg is placed in the uppermost slot to prevent jamming.

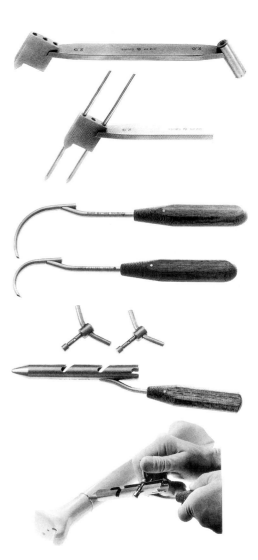

Instrumentation and Techniques

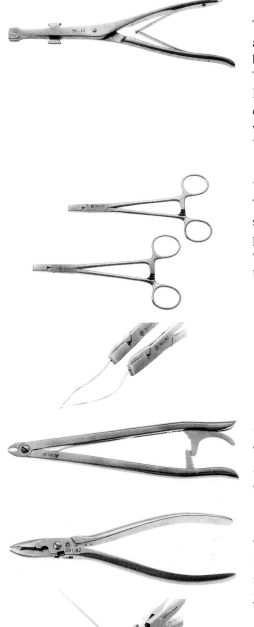

Wire Tightener, "Fastight"

This wire tightener, 260 mm, may be used temporarily to tighten and twist cerclage wires. After passing the wire around the bone, it is crossed in an X fashion and anchored on each side. The wire must first pass through the slot, then around the post. By squeezing the handles the wire is both gripped and tightened. To twist the wire, it must first be pulled then twisted. The wire should be centred between jaws so that the twist is equal. When the twist is completed, the wire is cut.

Holding Forceps for Cerclage Wires

These forceps, 170 mm, are special locking forceps, which ensure an absolutely secure grip on cerclage wires. The wire is passed through the hole in the tip of the forceps, which locks the wire when being closed. Two pairs of forceps are needed for twisting wires.

Long Wire Holding Forceps

These forceps, 212 mm, grip both wire ends for twisting, and areespecially useful when working in a deep wound. The handle can be easily locked and released by virtue of its special ratchet.

Wire-Bending Pliers

These pliers, 155 mm, are multi-purpose pliers. They can be used to grip Kirschner wires and cerclage wires with their fine, serrated tip. Wires up to 2.0 mm diameter can be bent in the jaws. Wires up to 1.6 mm diameter may even be cut.

Flat-Nosed Parallel Pliers

These pliers, 160 mm, are useful for different purposes in wiring techniques and for plate bending. The jaws open parallel owing to the double lever joint.

Vice Grip, Self-Locking

This vice grip, 180 mm, opens to a maximum of 34 mm. The screw at the end of one handle adjusts the distance between the closed jaws; the flap on the other handle is lifted to release the grip.

Wire Cutter, Small

This cutter, 165 mm, is used for cutting wires up to 2.0 mm.

Wire Cutter, Large

This cutter, 220 mm, has a double lever joint and can be used for cutting wires up to 2.5 mm diameter, as well as to shorten and to trim mini-plates.

Wire Cutter

This cutter, 230 mm, is used for cutting wires up to 1.25 mm diameter. The long handles facilitate cutting wires in areas with limited vision.

Wire Cutter

This cutter, 175 mm, is used for cutting wires up to 1.25 mm diameter, has a cutting edge that allows cutting at the very tip, which is especially useful when working with fine diameters and small bones.

Bending Iron for Kirschner Wires

This iron is 1.6–2.5 mm in diameter. The iron is passed over the shortened Kirschner wire end and bent over at the flat side. It may also be used as a bolt to hammer in the bent-back wire end.

Bending Iron for Kirschner Wires

This iron, 0.8–1.25 mm diameter, is double angled and used to bend the smaller diameter wires close to the bone or skin surface.

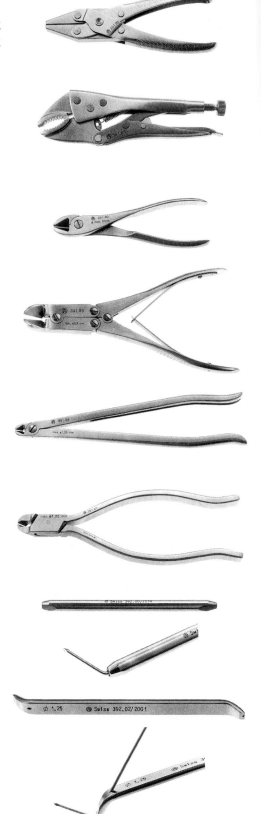

Implants

The cerclage wires and Kirschner wires are manufactured of the same stainless steel as are the screws and plate. The Kirschner wires are available also in titanium alloy.

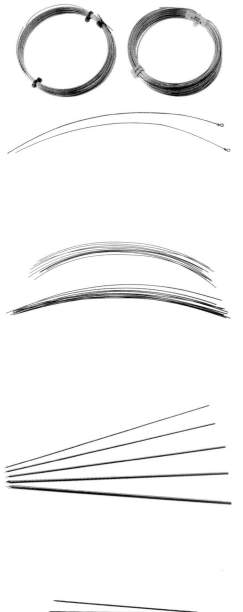

Cerclage Wire Coils

These coils are available 0.8, 1.0, 1.25, and 1.5 mm in diameter, and in 10 m lengths. The desired length is cut with a wire cutter.

Cerclage Wires with Eye

These wires are available 0.8, 1.0, 1.25, and 1.5 mm diameter and 180 mm long, and 1.0, 1.25, and 1.5 mm diameter and 600 mm long The cerclage wire with eye is used in the cerclage wiring technique, especially when the wire tightener with pegs is employed.

Cerclage Wires in Pre-Cut Lengths

These wires are available in the following sizes:
– 0.4 mm diameter and 150 mm long
– 0.6 mm diameter and 175 mm long
– 0.8 mm diameter and 200 mm long
– 1.0 mm diameter and 250 mm long
– 1.25 mm diameter and 300 mm long
The pre-cut length helps in identifying the diameter of the wire.

Kirschner Wires with Trocar Tip

These wires are available in the following sizes:
– 0.6 and 0.8 mm diameterand 70 mm long
– 1.0, 1.25, 1.6, 2.0, 2.5, and 3.0 mm diameter and 150 mm long
– 1.6, 2.0, 2.5, 2.5, and 3.0 mm diameter and 280 mm long
These are the standard Kirschner wires used for both temporary and definitive fixation. They may be inserted using the small air drill with Jacobs chuck, or the mini air machine (small diameter wires), In hard bone, however, pre-drilling the cortex with a drill bit of similar size is recommended.

Kirschner Wires with Threaded Tip

These wires are available in the following sizes:
– 1.6 mm diameter, 5 mm thread length, and 150 mm long
– 1.6, 2.0, 2.5 mm diameter, 15 mm thread length and 150 mm long
– 2.5 mm diameter, 15 mm thread length and 200 mm long
The Kirschner wires with threaded tip are used when the wire needs secure anchoring in the cortex.

Kirschner Wires with Double Trocar Tip

These wires are available in the following sizes:
– 0.6 mm and 0.8 mm diameter and 70 mm long
– 1.0, 1.25, 1.6, and 2.0 mm diameter and 150 mm long
The double-pointed Kirschner wires are used for retrograde insertion, for example, in the hand.

6.17.2 Supplementary Instruments

Telescoping Wire Guide

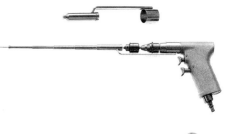

This wire guide is fitted on the small air drill for insertion of a long Kirschner wire, thereby preventing buckling of the wire.

Universal Chuck with T Handle

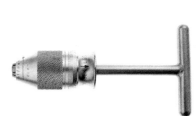

This chuck may be used to insert the large diameter Kirschner wires.

6.17.3 Tension Band Wiring Technique

Tension band wiring is mainly indicated in fractures of bones serving as ligament or muscle attachments. These includes fractures of the patella and the olecranon. Fractures (or osteotomies) of the greater trochanter and avulsion fractures of the malleolus may also be treated with tension band wiring.
If strong rotational forces act upon the fracture site, two parallel Kirschner wires are inserted before the tension band wire is applied.

Principle of Tension Band Wiring

The wire absorbs the tensile forces, the bone absorbs the compression forces. See also Sect. 4.1.

Tension Band Wiring of the Olecranon

Step by step procedure:
– The fracture is reduced and temporarily fixed with a pointed reduction forceps. The distal point may be introduced in a previously drilled cortical hole (Fig. 1).
– Using the triple wire guide for aiming and tissue protection, a

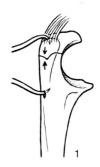

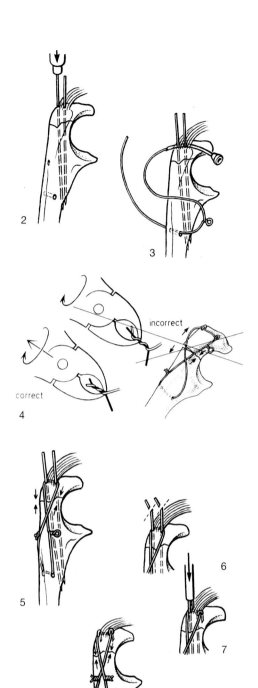

1.6 mm diameter Kirschner wire is inserted from proximal to distal. In hard bone, pre-drilling with the 2.0 mm drill may be necessary.

- The triple wire guide is placed over the inserted wire, and a second wire is inserted through the guide, parallel to the first (Fig. 2).
- A cerclage wire, 1.0 mm or 1.2 mm in diameter, about 500 mm long, is prepared with a small twisted loop placed eccentrically. The shorter end is inserted through the pre-drilled hole.
- The longer end is crossed over in a figure-of-eight fashion, and passed through a curved needle under the triceps tendon, and around the Kirschner wires (Fig. 3).
- The free ends of the cerclage wire are crossed at the same level as the prepared loop.
- Tightening of the wire loops to create symmetrical interfragmentary compression is done in several stages:
    - The loops are gripped with the wire bending or parallel pliers and tightened by pulling perpendicular to the axis of the bone.
    - The wire ends are then twisted whilst slightly diminishing the tension to take up the slack. This technique prevents one end being wound around the other (Fig. 4).
    - The procedure is repeated, alternating from one side to the other, until the figure-of-eight wire lies flat and taut on the bone surface (Fig. 5).
- The Kirschner wires are slightly pulled back and cut obliquely to create a sharp point. They are thereafter bent back through 180° to form a small hook (Fig. 6).
- Using the bending iron for Kirschner wires, 1.25–2.5 mm, as a punch the ends are tapped back into the bone over the wires (Fig. 7).
- The tension of the wire is examined, and the twists shortened and bent over to lie flat on the bone (Fig. 8).

Handle with Quick Coupling

This handle connects to the gouges, chisels, impactors, and rasps with quick coupling ends. The bolt on the handle is pressed down, and the selected instrument inserted and turned until locked in place.

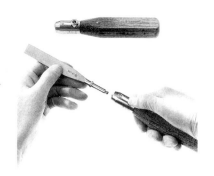

Gouges

These gouges are straight (in 5, 10, and 15 mm widths) and curved (in 5, 10, and 15 mm widths). The gouges are connected to the handle with quick coupling, and, for example, used to take strips of corticocancellous bone from the iliac fossa and the posterior part of the ilium.

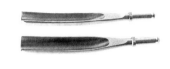

Chisels

The chisels are straight (in 4, 8, 16, and 20 mm widths) and curved (16 mm in width). The chisels are connected to the handle, and used to cut a window in the cortex to allow harvesting of pure cancellous bone.

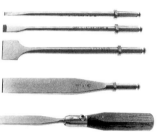

Cancellous Bone Impactors

The cancellous bone impactors are available in the following sizes:
– 6 mm and 8 mm, round, curved
– 6 mm, flat, curved,
– 6 × 16 mm, 10 × 20 mm, 10 × 30 mm, rectangular.
The impactors are used to pack the cancellous bone graft into a defect, or carefully to reconstruct an articular surface by pushing depressed fragments from within the bone.

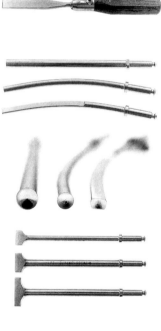

Rasps

The rasps are round and half-round, and may be used to "file" off sharp bony edges.

Instrumentation and Techniques

6.18.2 Donor Sites for Bone Grafts

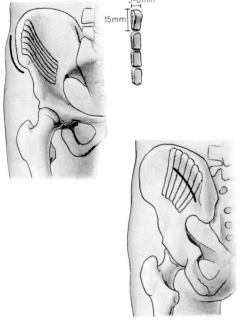

Corticocancellous bone is best obtained from the following sites:

– From the iliac fossa: A skin incision is made 20 mm lateral or medial to the iliac crest. The inner table of the iliac wing is exposed deep to the iliacus muscle. Long, parallel strips are taken with the gouge and are usually cut into smaller pieces about 15 mm long and 5 mm wide. Gelfoam is applied between the bone and iliacus muscle to stop bleeding. A vacuum drain is used.

– From the posterior portion of the os ilium: The patient is in the prone position, and the incision made just lateral to the posterior iliac spine. After incision of the fascia and retraction of the muscle, the grafts are taken with the gouge. The gouge with 10 mm wide blade, straight or curved is used in most cases. For small chips, the 5 mm gouge is chosen.

Pure cancellous bone is available in abundance in the greater trochanter and the head of tibia. If necessary, cancellous bone can be obtained from any accessible metaphysis:

– From the greater trochanter: A lateral oval opening is cut with the chisel, and pure cancellous bone is harvested with a curette. The trabeculae of the femoral neck should not be damaged.

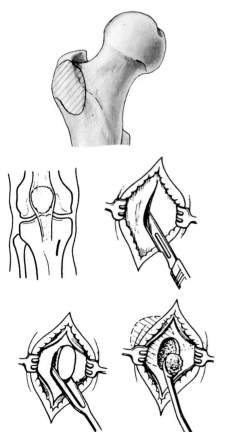

– From the head of the tibia: A skin incision is made about 30 mm below the tibial plateau. The periosteum is longitudinally split and retracted. An oval cortical opening is cut with the gouge, and cancellous bone is harvested with a large curette. Particularly in younger patients, large amounts of very high-quality cancellous bone can be obtained in this way.

Bone grafts should be kept in a sponge moistened with Ringers lactate solution or blood until used. Immersion in solutions should be avoided.

Bone Grafting Instruments

6.18.3 Application of Cancellous Bone Graft

When filling defects resulting from compression of the metaphysis or defects in the diaphysis, it is desirable to apply the cancellous bone graft with light pressure. This is done most effectively by packing the cancellous bone into the defect with the cancellous bone impactors. Note that the graft incorporates by the ingrowth of fine vessels into the pores of the graft. If it is too tightly impacted so as to abolish its spongy form, vascularisation may be delayed. The opposite cortex (for buttressing) can be grafted with pure cancellous bone (e. g. from the greater trochanter) or with small corticocancellous chips (taken from the inner surface of the upper ilium).

If bone infection is present, only pure cancellous grafts should be used.

6.19 Instruments for Removal of Damaged Screws

If a screw breaks or is otherwise damaged, removal may be impossible. If attempts to remove the damaged screw would lead to extensive bone damage, the screw should be left in.

Only if a free medullary cavity is required for intramedullary nailing, or the insertion of a prosthesis, must the screw be removed, also if problematical.

6.19.1 Instruments

The instruments are available as a set in a sterilising tray or in a small aluminium case.

Conical Extraction Screws

These screws, with left-hand thread, are used to remove screws with a damaged hexagonal socket. Connected to the T handle, the correct size conical extraction screw is screwed into the socket with left-hand turns. Three sizes are available: one for the 1.5 mm and 2.0 mm screws, one for 2.7, 3.5 mm and 4.0 mm screws, and a third for the 4.5 mm and 6.5 mm screws.

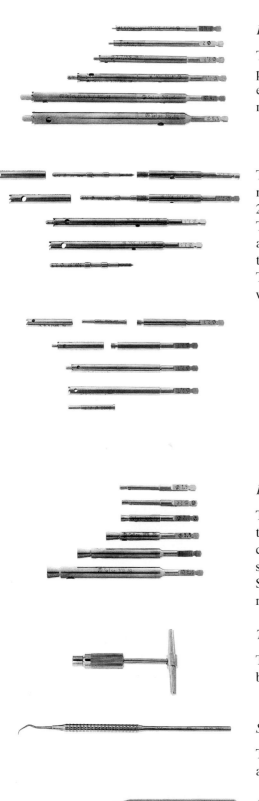

Hollow Reamers

The hollow reamer is an assembly of a shaft with a quick coupling end, a reamer tube, and a centring pin. Six different reamers are available: one each for screw sizes 1.5 mm, 2.0 mm, 2.7 mm, 3.5 and 4.0 mm, 4.5 mm, and 6.5 mm.

The method of assembly for the three larger sizes, 3.5 mm, 4.5 mm, and 6.5 mm and the three smaller sizes 1.5 mm, 2.0 mm and 2.7 mm are shown in the two sets of figures.

The reamers cut anticlockwise, and are used to ream to and around a screw fragment. It is connected to the T handle and turned anticlockwise

The small air drill may be used with the reverse trigger; but only with extreme care only since the reamer is easily damaged.

Extraction Bolts

These bolts have an internal conical left hand thread with which to engage and extract the exposed screw fragment. They are connected to the T handle and turned anticlockwise while pressure is exerted on the screw fragment.

Six different sizes are available: one each for screw sizes 1.5 mm, 2.0 mm, 2.7 mm, 3.5 and 4.0 mm, 4.5 mm, and 6.5 mm.

T Handle

The T handle, with quick coupling, is used to turn the extraction bolts and the hollow reamers.

Sharp Hook

This hook is useful in removing debris from the screw head or around the screw fragment.

Hollow Gouge

This gouge is used to expose the end of the screw fragment so that the hollow reamer can be centred over the remnant. The 500 g hammer is required.

Forceps for Screw Removal

These forceps is used to grasp and extract exposed screw fragments. The closure can easily be operated with one hand. It may be firmly locked on the screw fragment and turned for removal.

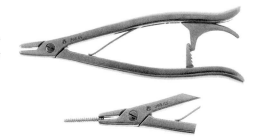

Spare Centring Pins for Hollow Reamer

These pins, available in six different sizes, are replacements for the centring pins assembled with the six sizes of hollow reamers. They are assembled in the proper size hollow reamer shaft by turning anticlockwise.

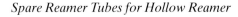

Spare Reamer Tubes for Hollow Reamer

These tubes, available in six different sizes, are replacements for the reamer tubes of the complete hollow reamers. They are assembled by turning them clockwise.

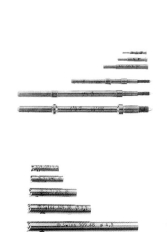

Application Diagram

This diagram, with schematic illustration of application, may be used as a guide during the a procedure. It is made of anodised aluminium and can be sterilised together with the instruments.

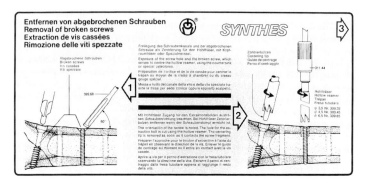

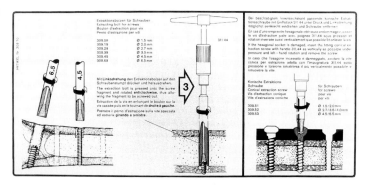

Instrumentation and Techniques

Additionally Necessary Instruments

A hammer, 500 g, is necessary for the use of the hollow gouge. Countersinks, 2.7–4.0 mm, and 4.5 mm, may be used to ream the cortex to expose the screw fragment.

6.19.2 Obsolete Instruments

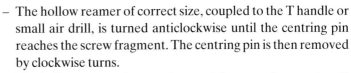

Drill Bit, 5.0 mm Diameter

This bit, of chrome-plated high-speed steel, was used to drill away the damaged large screw head. Its use is, however, not recommended since it creates heat and metal debris. The extraction bolts are used in its place.

6.19.3 Application Technique

See also the application diagram.

Removal of deep-seated screw fragments:
- A recess is produced in the cortex with the countersink of appropriate size, or with the hollow gouge.

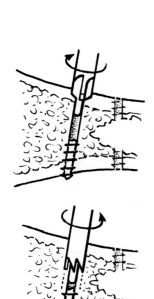

- The hollow reamer of correct size, coupled to the T handle or small air drill, is turned anticlockwise until the centring pin reaches the screw fragment. The centring pin is then removed by clockwise turns.
- The hollow reamer is turned around the screw fragment until approximately 5 mm length is exposed.

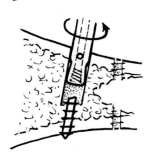

- The extraction bolt of correct size is coupled to the T handle. While applying pressure, the extraction bolt is screwed in an anticlockwise direction onto the screw fragment.

Instruments for Removal of Damaged Screws

375 ∎

– By continuing turning the extraction bolt, the screw fragment is unscrewed and removed.

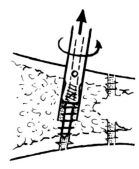

Removal of a screw with damaged hexagonal socket:
– The correct size conical extraction screw is selected, connected to the T handle and placed vertically in the damaged screw head. By applying pressure and turning anticlockwise the screw is removed.

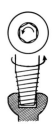

6.20 Aiming Device

The aiming device has various interchangeable attachments for different applications (see below). It can be obtained as a set in an insert tray for aluminium cases.

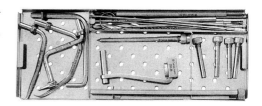

Measuring Bar

This bar is assembled with the locking sleeve, and one of the hooks. The scale allows measurements up to 180 mm.

Locking Sleeve

This sleeve is slid onto the measuring bar in the direction of the arrow on top, and fixed in the desired place with the screw. The sleeve has an inner diameter of 6.0 mm, and accepts the different drill sleeves with screw connection.

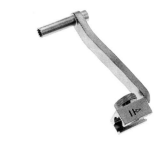

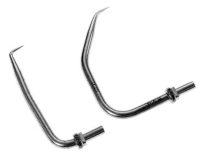

Small Hook and Large Hook for Knee

The large hook may be used for repair of the cruciate ligament. The small hook is applied for measuring. The distance between the inserted drill sleeve and the tip of the hook is read from the scale on the bar.

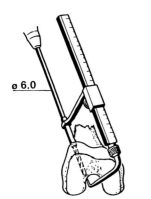

ø 6.0

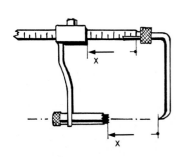

Hook for External Fixator

This hook is employed for the application of a bilateral external fixator. See also p. 327.

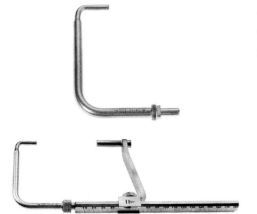

Offset Pointed Hook

This hook can be used as aiming device on the proximal femur. When the offset pointed hook is used, 40 mm must be added to the measurement read from the scale to compensate for the offset. Thus the distance $y = x + 40$ mm.

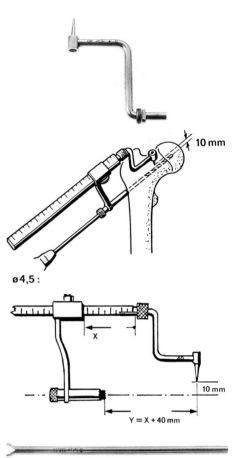

Forked Impactor

This impactor is used to position the offset pointed hook in the bone by tapping lightly with a hammer.

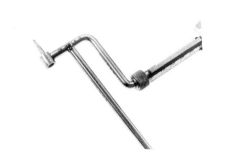

Check Tube

This tube is used to check the correct axis between the locking sleeve, and the hook for external fixation.

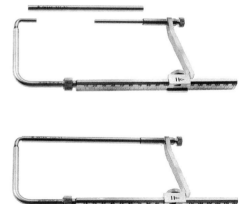

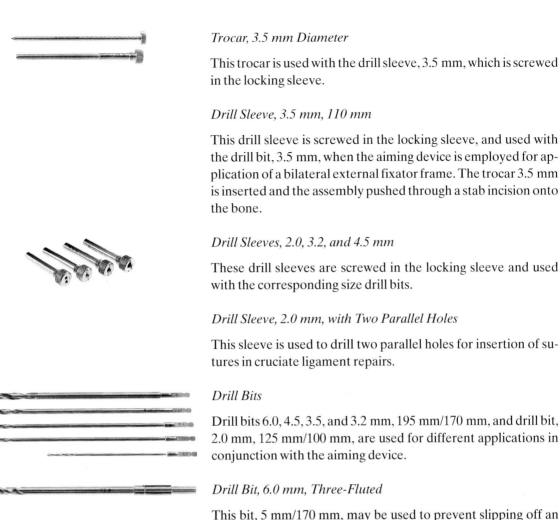

Trocar, 3.5 mm Diameter

This trocar is used with the drill sleeve, 3.5 mm, which is screwed in the locking sleeve.

Drill Sleeve, 3.5 mm, 110 mm

This drill sleeve is screwed in the locking sleeve, and used with the drill bit, 3.5 mm, when the aiming device is employed for application of a bilateral external fixator frame. The trocar 3.5 mm is inserted and the assembly pushed through a stab incision onto the bone.

Drill Sleeves, 2.0, 3.2, and 4.5 mm

These drill sleeves are screwed in the locking sleeve and used with the corresponding size drill bits.

Drill Sleeve, 2.0 mm, with Two Parallel Holes

This sleeve is used to drill two parallel holes for insertion of sutures in cruciate ligament repairs.

Drill Bits

Drill bits 6.0, 4.5, 3.5, and 3.2 mm, 195 mm/170 mm, and drill bit, 2.0 mm, 125 mm/100 mm, are used for different applications in conjunction with the aiming device.

Drill Bit, 6.0 mm, Three-Fluted

This bit, 5 mm/170 mm, may be used to prevent slipping off an oblique bone surface, for example in cruciate ligament repairs.

Suture Passer, 2.0 mm Diameter

This passer, for quick coupling, is used to drill two parallel holes for the sutures in cruciate ligament procedures.

Suture Pusher

This passer is used to push the suture through a pre-drilled hole in cruciate ligament repairs.

Aiming Device

6.21 Compressed Air Machines

6.21.1 Compressed Air as Power Source

The reason for choosing compressed air as power source for the AO/ASIF power equipment, was based on the following considerations:
– Easy availability of compressed air throughout the world
– Safe handling of compressed air
– Safe and easy sterilisation of air machines
– Variable and easy speed control
– Rapid stopping because of the machine's low inertia
– Relative light weight of air machines.

Compressed air as a power source has proved reliable and effective for more than three decades. It may be supplied either from a central supply system through pipes into the operating room, or from separate cylinders. Compressed nitrogen is a possible substitute.

Never Use Oxygen: There is a danger of fire and explosion!

6.21.1.1 Compressed Air (Nitrogen) from Cylinders in the Operating Room

Compressed air cylinders are available in various sizes, with filling pressures 150–200 bar (2200–3000 psi). The most commonly used size has a capacity of approximately 6 m³ (6000 l). The quantity of air remaining in the cylinder can be estimated from the pressure gauge. At 200 bar (3000 psi) the cylinder is full; at 100 bar (1500 psi) it is approximately half-full.

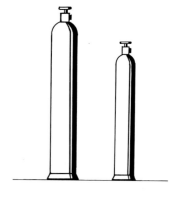

The air pressure (gauge A, also indicating the content) must be checked before each use, to ensure that enough air is available for the procedure. Approximately 3 m³ (3000 l) are needed for screw and plate fixation, about 5–6m³ (6000 l) for reaming of a medullary cavity. It is recommendable to have extra cylinders available, preferably with a reduction valve mounted and ready for replacement. The operating pressure for the machines (6 bar or 90 psi) is set on the pressure-regulating valve (gauge B), while the machine is running.

Pressure indicating and regulating valves may differ from country to country; the principle of function, however, remains the same. Compressed air, or nitrogen, from cylinders is generally clean, dry, and ready to use, but to ensure optimal function it is recommended always to use a filter system (see below).

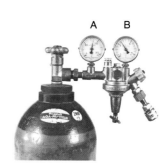

6.21.1.2 Compressed Air from a Central Supply System

In large hospitals air compressors, or a battery of air cylinders, are installed usually in the basement for the supply of compressed air. Through pipe lines the compressed air is carried to the operating theatre, where it is reduced to the required pressure and piped to wall outlets in the different rooms.

The pressure of the central supply system is normally adjusted to 10–12 bar (145–180 psi), which can be verified with an on-line pressure gauge. The critical pressure for triggering restarting of the compressor should not be below 8 bar (120 psi). The air reservoir and pipe lines to the operating theatre should be as large as possible to ensure that the pressure does not fall below the minimum required.

The necessary quantity of air is about 250–350 l/min per machine. The corresponding power requirement of the compressor motor is approximately 1.3–1.8 kW, depending on the distance to the operating room. The compressor should always be at lowest point of the compressed air circuit. Separators are necessary in the system to filter small particles of oil, dirt, and water that may be contained in the system.

The purity of the compressed air from a central supply system can only be ensured by continuous testing of the air at the wall outlet, or by installing a filter. Only then may the compressed air entering the machines be free of particles and microorganism.

6.21.1.3 Filters for Compressed Air

The filters described below are available for use in countries where special filter system do not already exist. The SYNTHES distributor can give further information about these installations.

Coarse Filter (A)

It is normal that rust, water, and condensation form in the pipe lines of a central supply system for compressed air. To retain this debris and condensation it is recommended that a coarse filter be installed. This should be upstream of the pressure regulating valve and connection point in the operating theatre. The risk of damaging the valves and the air machines is thereby reduced.

Microfilter (B)

This shock-resistant mechanical filter, is installed downstream of the pressure regulating valve (in the 6 bar or 90 psi area) to render the air free of particles as minute as 1 µm diameter. The protective glass of the microfilter has to be removed and cleaned every 2 weeks after shutting down the air supply. See

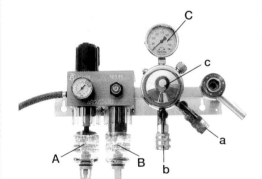

The small air drill is equipped with a double hose coupling (left). When used with a double hose the air exhaust away from the operating field. Old-style machines with single air hose couplings may still be in use (right). It must be noted that the air exhaust then causes turbulence near the operating field increasing the risk of cross-contamination. For care and maintenance see p. 424, 426.

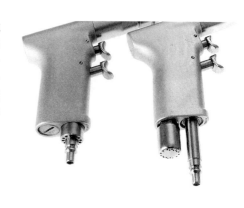

Technical Data

– Variable speed:	0–800 rpm (10%)
– Torque:	2.4 Nm (22 in./lb, approximately)
– Regulator pressure with running machine:	6 bar (90 psi)
– Compressed air consumption approximately:	250 l/min (9 cu.ft./min)
– Weight:	630 g (approximately 22 oz)

Quick Coupling of Instruments

Instruments with a quick-coupling end can be attached by pushing the coupling sleeve forward, inserting and turning the instrument until it clicks into place. The instrument is locked in place when the coupling is released. Detachment is possible by pushing the quick coupling forward.

Instruments that can be coupled are:
– Drill bits
– Taps (Caution)
– Screwdriver shafts
– Router
– Accessory instruments (see below)

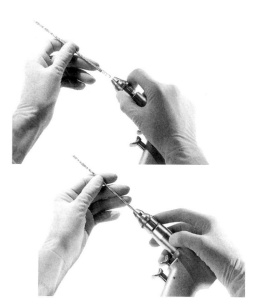

Operation

The lower trigger is depressed with the middle finger for forward motion, and regulates the speed up to approximately 800 rpm. By depressing both triggers simultaneously, the direction of motion can be immediately changed to reverse even when the drill is running.

Applications

Drilling and reaming for DHS/DCS is done by forward motion only, even when retrieving the drill. Bone debris may otherwise block the drill. It is recommended that the wound be irrigated with Ringer's lactate solution during drilling. Heat necrosis, and bacterial contamination of dry tissue can thereby be avoided.

In special situations it may be possible to tap with power. However, it is regarded as extremely dangerous and must be performed with greatest care. The machine must "follow" the tap, and no pressure be exerted. As soon as the tap protrudes from the opposite cortex it must be immediately reversed. If this is not done, great damage to viable soft tissue may be the result. When reversing the tap, it must not be pulled. The pre-cut thread in the bone may otherwise be damaged.

Insertion of screws may be performed with the screwdriver shafts. The screw must engage the pre-cut thread properly before running the machine, to avoid jamming. The screw is finally tightened by hand.

Removal of screws with the screwdriver shaft is possible; after cleaning the hexagonal socket, and loosening the screw manually, the machine is run in reverse.

Accessories

Jacobs Chuck with Key

This chuck is connected to the small air drill for insertion of Kirschner wires, and for use of instruments with round and triangular ends up to 4.0 mm and 4.5 mm respectively. The key is used to tighten and open the chuck.

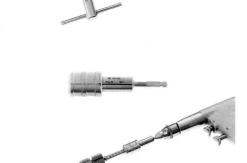

Quick Coupling for Small Air Drill

This is used to connect the DHS/DCS reamers, as well as large drill bits used for cruciate ligament repair. The outer sleeve is pushed forward to insert and couple the instrument.

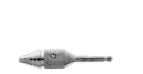

Mini Quick Coupling Chuck

This chuck connects drill bits and reamers that have mini quick coupling end. The outer sleeve is pushed back to couple the instruments.

Compressed Air Machines

Oscillating Attachment

This attachment converts the rotating motion of the small air drill to a back-and-forth motion over an arc of about 270°. The oscillating motion reduces the risk of damage to blood vessels and nerves by preventing spooling of soft tissue around the drill bit. The oscillating attachment is locked in place around the upper trigger of the small air drill. By pushing the outer sleeve of the attachment forward the drill bit is inserted and turned until it "clicks" into place. Releasing the sleeve locks the drill bit. The attachment is used preferably with a three-fluted drill bit, which prevents slipping on an oblique bone surface.

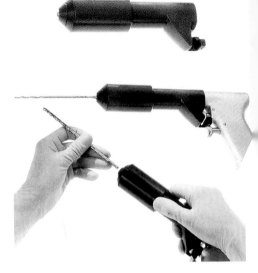

Radiolucent Drive

This drive is connected to the small air drill and allows accurate drilling of for example locking holes of medullary nails under image intensification. It is slid onto quick coupling of the small air drill, and the two parts pressed together until they engage. Additional locking is not necessary. The drill can be rotated around its own axis to the desired working position. While running the machine with one hand, the radiolucent drive is held with the other hand. The length of the drive places the surgeons hands at the periphery of the radiation zone (see p. 283). The radiolucent drive is used with three-fluted drill bits that have a special coupling end. The quick coupling of the drive is pushed forward and the drill bit inserted and turned to be properly seated. It is locked in this position by pulling back the quick coupling.

Three-fluted drill bits for radiolucent drive are available in sizes:

- 4.0 mm diameter, 150 mm/120 mm (total length/effective length) used for the 3.9 mm locking bolts for unreamed tibial nails.
- 3.2 mm diameter, 150 mm/120 mm (total length/effective length), used for the 4.9 mm locking bolts for universal femoral and tibial nails.

Further diameter drill bits for other applications are also available. See SYNTHES catalogue. See p. 427 for care and maintenance.

Telescoping Wire Guide

This guide may be fitted on the small air drill when inserting long Kirschner wires. It helps to avoid bending of the wire.

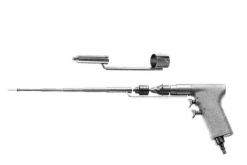

Instrumentation and Techniques

6.21.3.2 Universal Air Drill and Accessories

The Universal Drill

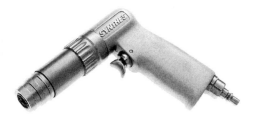

The universal air drill is a more powerful drill, used with the right-angle drive especially for medullary reaming. Different attachments allow the use of the universal air drill also for other applications, such as drilling, insertion of screws and Kirschner wires. The drill is designed for single-hand use, and for forward motion only.

Note: The universal air drill should not be connected directly with the flexible shafts, since the machine is not cannulated to accept the reaming rod. Acetabular reamers with correct coupling end for hip replacement can, however, be inserted directly. For care and maintenance see p. 424, 427.

Technical Data

Two-stage speed:

First stage	200 rpm
Second stage	450 rpm
– Regulator pressure with running machine:	6 bar (90 psi)
– Compressed air consumption approximately:	300 l/min (9 cu.ft./min)
– Weight:	800 g (approximately 28 oz)

Accessories

The following accessories can be attached to the universal air drill:

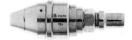

Small Quick Coupling

This allows use of all instruments which have a quick coupling end such as drill bits, taps, screwdriver shafts, router. By pushing the small quick coupling into the universal air drill's coupling, it is locked in position. It is disconnected by pulling back the outer sleeve of the coupling of the universal drill.

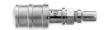

Quick Coupling

This is used to connect the DHS/DCS reamers, and the large drill bits used for cruciate ligament repair. The outer sleeve of the large quick coupling is pushed forward to insert and couple the instrument, the assembly then pushed into the universal drill.

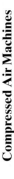

Compressed Air Machines

The blades are removed by reversing this technique. The teeth of the blades cannot be resharpened. Worn blades are discarded.

Mini Reciprocating Saw

This saw has a speed reduction gear that allows a maximum speed of 6000 rpm.

Saw Blade for Reciprocating Saw

This blade is 45 mm long. It is inserted into the slot at right angles to the machine axis. After rotating the blade about the carrier pin, it can be locked into place with the retaining ring. The reverse procedure is used for removal.

Drill Bits

These bits. in sizes 1.1, 1.5, 2.0, and 2.7 mm, in lengths from 28 mm to 67 mm, and with mini quick coupling end, are available for use with the mini compressed air machine. They may be used with a depth stop, or with a skull guard (for trephination). The small screwdriver is used for tightening.

A Lindemann reamer with spring guard is also available.

Burrs

Burrs, with mini quick coupling end, round, oval, egg-shaped, straight-edged, conical, and pear-shaped, are available with different diameters. Burrs up to 6.0 mm diameter may be used with a tissue protector.

Circular Saws

These saws, with 8, 10, 12, and 15 mm diameter, and 28 mm length can be used with the mini compressed air machine. A tissue protector is also available, which is fixed on the straight drill head attachment using the small screwdriver. See SYNTHES catalogue for details.

Double Air Hose

This is a flexible, 2 m long hose, which connects to the compressed air motor by a swivel coupling. The outer hose exhausts the air away from the operating area, and can be connected either to the diffuser, or to a exhaust air system.

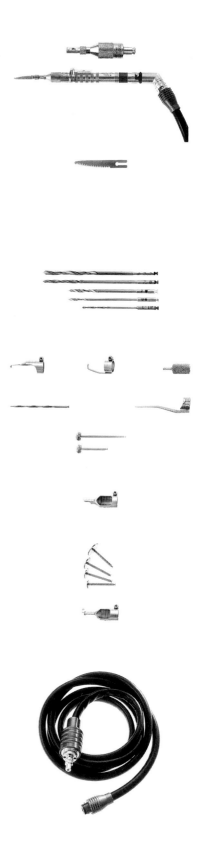

6.21.3.5 Hand Drill and Accessories

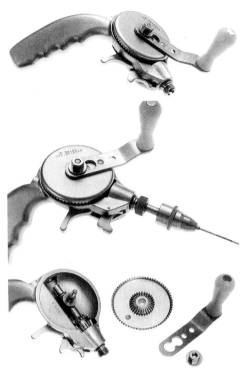

The hand drill is used as a reserve in emergency situations, for example if the compressed air machine, or air supply, fails during surgery. It can also serve in situations where compressed air and air machines are unavailable.

The drill has two speed settings. Pulling the lever near the handle engages the lower gear. If the lever is pushed forward, the drill is switched to a higher gear. The front lever is used to lock the low gear. The higher gear is used for drilling and inserting Kirschner wires. The lower gear is used for tapping, inserting and extracting screws. In emergency situations, the lower gear can be used for reaming the medullary canal.

The crank can be mounted into two positions with varying length. The long lever arm is used to obtain greater force, the short lever arm for greater speed.

By unscrewing the nut, the machine is easily dismantled into four parts for cleaning and lubrication.

The machine is sterilised as general instruments (see p. 417).

Accessories

Quick Coupling for Hand Drill

This is used to connect drill bits with quick coupling end.

Universal Chuck for Hand Drill

This chuck has an opening capacity of 1.0–6.0 mm diameter, and is cannulated to be used with Kirschner wires. It has an automatic locking mechanism.

Connector for Hand Drill

This connector has a quick coupling for flexible shafts. It is suitable only for reamers with a maximum diameter of 12.0 mm. It is cannulated to accept the reaming rod.

6.22 Care and Maintenance of AO/ASIF Instrumentation

By A. Murphy

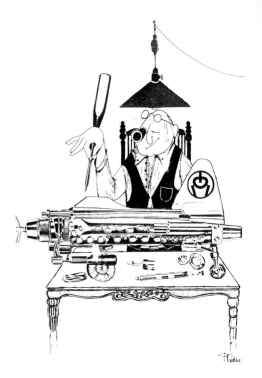

6.22.1 Definition

To define care and maintenance: it means to "look after" and "preserve".

Surgical instruments are a very large investment for any institution. Care and maintenance of these instruments is vital to ensure that they remain functional. AO/ASIF instruments and implants are made with great precision, and with vigilant upkeep they should endure use for many years.

Note: The following guidelines have been recommended by the AO/ASIF group. These may have to be adapted to suit regulations and practices in different countries or environments. The general principles for care of all surgical instruments also apply. Since most of the instruments are made from "stainless" steel how do they become stained, rusted or corroded? The following chapter outlines some of the reasons and describes measures taken to avoid such problems.

6.22.2 Causes of Corrosion

Corrosion is a gradual destruction, or wearing away, that may be caused by a chemical action. It can occur in poorly maintained instruments. To understand how to prevent instruments from becoming permanently damaged, it is essential to be aware of the sources of corrosion.

Damaged passive layer:
– If instruments or implants become scratched or dented this can damage the passivation or protective layer on the surface. Subsequent corrosion may develop.

Continuous exposure to surgical exudates:
– Blood, pus or other bodily secretions left on instruments for prolonged periods may also damage the surface.

Excessive exposure to certain solutions:
– Saline or solutions containing iodine or chloride can react with specific instruments. Also harmful would be, as well as certain disinfectants, if improperly used, strong acid or alkaline solutions. The water quality used for washing and rinsing instruments may be another influencing factor.

Rust transfer:
– Poorly maintained instruments may develop areas of rust. This can spread onto other instruments with which they come into contact.

Stress, strain and wear:
– Instruments used incorrectly, or for purposes for which they were not designed, will succumb to this abuse.
– If they are in constant use, natural wear is inevitable and the life cycle will be shortened (see also Sect. 6.1.2).

6.22.3 Care in Preparation For and During Surgery

The main objective is prevention of corrosion and permanent damage. The following procedures should be initiated to ensure maximum care of the instruments.

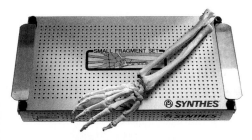

– Correctly stored, appropriate sterile instruments should be assembled for the operation. The surgery will determine what is required. The size of instruments should correspond to the size of the bone!

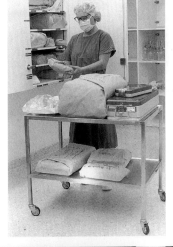

– The intact outer covering and expiry date on the pack should be noted.

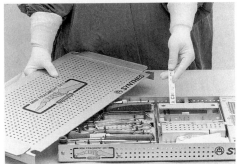

– A steriliser indicator inside the pack will confirm that the contents have been sterilised.

Care and Maintenance of Instrumentation

- Instruments should be arranged in sequential order on the instrument table. Only relevant instruments should be set out and the remaining ones placed in a convenient position until required.
- The sterile instruments should be prepared just prior to the procedure. Covering the instrument table and leaving it unattended is not an acceptable practice.

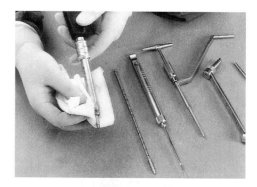

- Blood or other exudates should be wiped from instruments throughout the procedure. Ringer lactate solution or saline may be used, but the instruments should not be left to soak in these solutions.
- Once used each instrument should be returned to its allotted place on the instrument table.
- Each instrument is designed for a specific purpose and should be used only for that purpose. The user should be acquainted with its correct use and function.

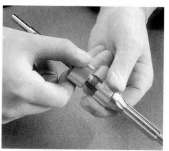

- To prevent damage during use it is important that instruments with multiple parts are assembled correctly. The assembly is verified before use on the patient.

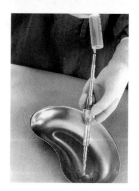

- Cannulated instruments are flushed to prevent bone debris and blood drying and adhering to the inside.

6.22.4 Management Following Surgery

Once surgery has been completed, the cleaning process must begin. Instruments should be cleaned as soon as possible. This consists of a number of stages, each one of equal importance.

Any instruments used during surgery are regarded as "contaminated". Those that have been used on a patient suspected of, or known to have, a transmissible infection may be processed in a similar manner.

At the end of the procedure, excess blood or debris should be wiped off to prevent it drying onto the surface.

A designated place away from the "clean area" of the operating suite is necessary for cleaning instruments. If they are going directly to a centralised area they must be covered to avoid contamination of personnel or surroundings en route.

Protective clothing should be worn when handling the contaminated instruments.

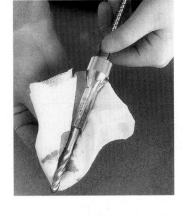

6.22.4.1 Dismantling

The following guidelines should be followed in disassembling instruments:
- Instruments that have removable parts should be disassembled. Any small pieces, e.g. screws, nuts or bolts, must be carefully gathered to prevent loss during cleaning.
- It is important to note that whoever takes an instrument apart should know how to reassemble it correctly!
- If blood or bone debris is not removed from all areas, it is "baked" onto the instrument during sterilisation and can cause irreparable damage.

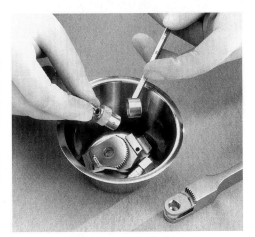

6.22.4.2 Disinfecting

This is a process necessary for the destruction of micro-organisms and is required following any surgical procedure. At present, with the ever-increasing risks to health care workers and patients, adequate decontamination of instruments is of even greater importance. This may be chemical or thermal:

Care and Maintenance of Instrumentation

Chemical: This involves soaking the open disassembled instruments in a disinfecting solution for the recommended time. Whatever solution is chosen it must be diluted and used according to the manufacturers' recommendations.

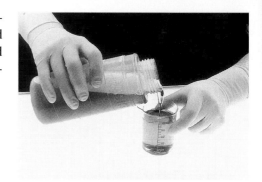

Thermal: Most instrument washing machines include a disinfecting phase. This is the preferred and safest method of decontamination.

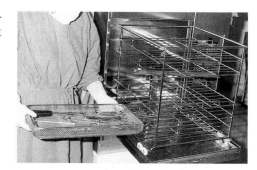

Note: Anodised aluminium, e.g. some instrument cases, templates, a few specific measuring devices and lengthening apparatus, should not come in contact with certain cleaning or disinfecting solutions. Therefore it is important to check the composition of the solution before subjecting the metal to a possible chemical reaction (see Sect. 6.1.2.2).

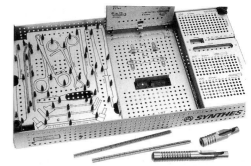

6.22.4.3 Cleaning

Two methods are available: mechanical or manual. Whatever detergent is used, in either method, it should be selected carefully. Instructions for use and dilution must be followed. Ideally the pH of the solution should be between 7.0 and 8.5 (see note in Sect. 6.22.4.2).

Mechanical Cleaning

This is the selected method available in many institutions. Several different washers/cleaners exist. Manufacturers instructions should always be adhered to.

Instrumentation and Techniques

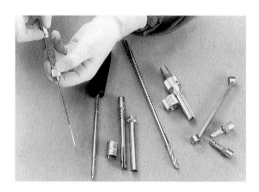

Some general guidelines:
– Firstly prepare and arrange the instruments by disassembling multi-component instruments and opening those with ratchets, box locks or hinges.

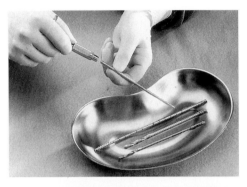

– Any sharp instruments should be removed for manual cleaning or put in a separate tray.
– Delicate instruments should not be washed in a machine.

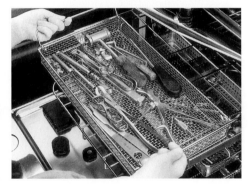

– Baskets must not be overloaded and heavy instruments should be placed on the bottom of the tray.
– Heavily soiled or cannulated instruments may need to be soaked or rinsed prior to machine washing to loosen any dried exudates.

Ultrasonic Cleaning

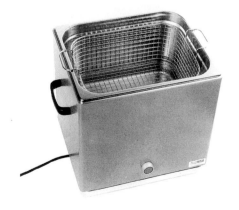

This is an alternative type of mechanical cleaning.
– Instruments must first be decontaminated.
– Once excess or dried exudates have been removed, the instruments can be placed in the machine.
– The ultrasonic waves passing through the water remove residual debris especially from threads and grooves which may be difficult to clean manually.
– Only instruments of similar metallic composition should be placed together in this machine.
– If there is any damage to the surface of chrome-plated instruments, ultrasonic cleaning may cause further damage.
– Normal rinsing must follow this process.

(Delicate and sharp instruments are withheld and should be cleaned manually.)

Once the mechanical cycle is complete, instruments are checked for cleanliness and should be rewashed if necessary. Mechanical cleaner units must be cleaned regularly on the inside and serviced as recommended by the manufacturer.

Note: Under no circumstances should any of the surgical power equipment be cleaned mechanically.

Manual Cleaning

Warm water with the appropriately diluted cleaning solution or detergent is used. The correct equipment should be available:
– A selection of soft nylon brushes.

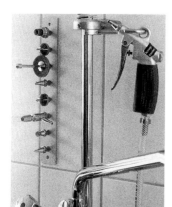 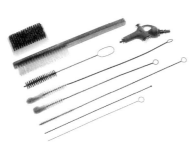

– Air jet and nozzle.
– Clean compressed air supply with a single hose or double hose and special connector.

Steel wool and abrasive cleansers must *never* be used. They would scratch the surface of the instruments causing permanent damage to the passivation layer.
If excessive blood or debris has coagulated on the instrument, it may need to be soaked before cleaning. The instruments should be placed in a blood-dissolving detergent for approximately 10 min (or according to instructions).

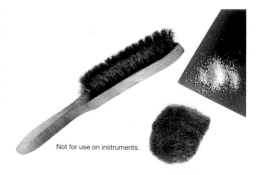

Not for use on instruments.

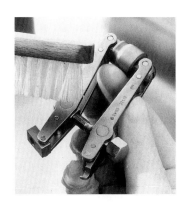

Special attention must be given to hinges, threads or hollow parts on instruments. Blood, water or other residue can lodge in these areas.

Instrument trays and cases must be cleaned following use. The manufacturing material of the case or tray will influence the cleaning procedure.

Stainless Steel Trays and Cases

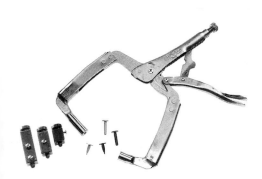

The pegs and brackets for holding instruments in position need not be removed for cleaning. The trays may be washed and dried in a similar manner to stainless steel instruments. Replacement pegs with a special inserter, as well as tray dividers, are available.

Aluminium Cases – Graphic Cases

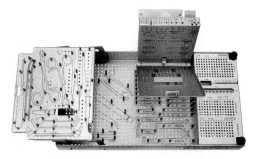

This anodised aluminium must be treated cautiously (see Sect. 6.22.4.2).

Cases with Removable Lids

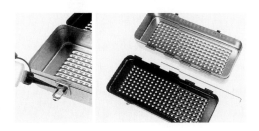

The pin holding the lid in position should be removed. Any removable tray in the case is washed separately. Once all areas have been dried thoroughly the case is reassembled, lid pin reinserted and hinges lubricated.

6.22.4.4 Rinsing After Cleaning

It is necessary to clear instruments of any residual cleaning solutions or debris.
- Instruments must be rinsed under flowing water paying particular attention to joints, threaded areas and hollow parts.
- The quality of the rinsing water is important. Excessive minerals may be contained in the water leaving a scum on the surface of the instrument. If neglected this can eventually lead to pitting corrosion.
- Distilled water can also be used for the final rinse to clear all remaining mineral residue.
- Rinsing is required following ultrasonic cleaning.

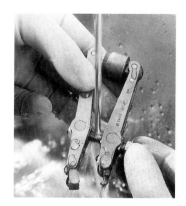

Note: If the water quality is suspected, it should be checked professionally. Special filters or detergents may be recommended to overcome this problem.

6.22.4.5 Drying

For drying instruments these guidelines should be followed:
- Each instrument must be dried thoroughly inside and out to prevent rusting and malfunction.
- A soft cloth should be used to avoid damage to the surface.
- Special attention must be paid to threads, ratchets and hinges or areas where fluid can accumulate.
- Open and close instruments so that all areas are reached.

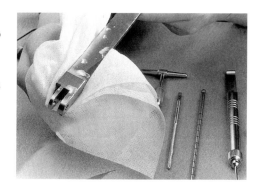

- Hollow parts should be dried using the air jet. Attached to a compressed air supply, this device allows air to be blown under pressure through the instrument drying the inside. High cleanliness of the air must be assured.
- A drying cycle is included in most mechanical washers. If not included the preceding instructions should be followed.

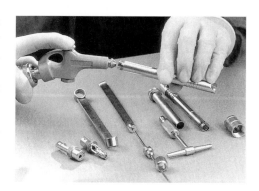

Note: If the instruments are to be used immediately and sterilised without packing then drying is unnecessary.

6.22.4.6 Lubrication

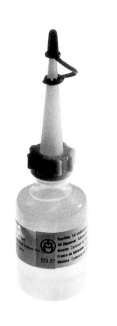

If an instrument has a movable part it must be oiled after each use to maintain its correct functional mobility. This also helps prevent rusting. Instrument lubricating solution is one method that can be used. The cleaned, rinsed instruments should be immersed for the recommended period in the solution. Rinsing is not required and once dried the instruments can be packed. This process may also be incorporated in the cycle of some instrument washing machines.

The manufacturers of AO/ASIF instruments also recommend the use of nonsilicone SYNTHES oil for lubrication. This specific antimicrobial oil allows steam penetration during autoclaving thus ensuring all areas will be sterilised.

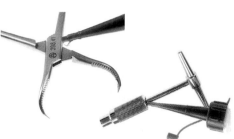

The following areas are oiled:
– Joints, hinges, box locks or any mobile parts on an instrument.

– Ball bearings present in instruments that have a rotating section. The instrument must be disassembled.

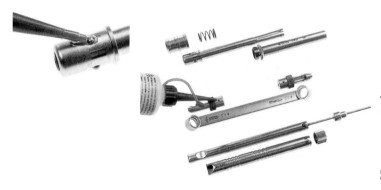

– Those with threaded parts that open and close.

One or two drops of oil are placed on the appropriate part. The instrument is assembled and tested for function. This movement also helps spread the oil and any excess oil should be removed using a soft cloth. Too much oil may cause seepage through the "wrapping" during autoclaving. This can lead to contamination of the sterile contents.

Note: In ultrasonic cleaning all lubricant is removed therefore particular emphasis must be placed on lubrication following this cleaning method.
Certain items in the AO instrumentation should not be lubricated, e. g. radiolucent drive or unifix. (Please see Sect. 6.22.5 for further information.)

The hinges on the pop-up rack for holding drill bits and taps should be lubricated using SYNTHES oil.

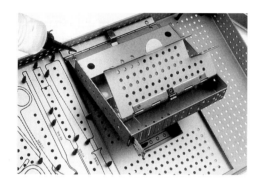

6.22.5 Complex Instruments

Outlined here are some frequently used, more complex instruments with specific reference to their care and maintenance.

6.22.5.1 DHS/DCS Triple Reamers

During surgery:
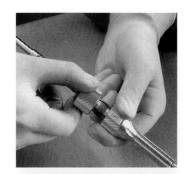
- Check that the sterile instrument is assembled correctly.
- The circle on the outside of the reaming segment follows the groove of the drill. It cannot be locked unless it has "clicked" into the correct position.
- The reamer is flushed immediately after use to prevent any debris coagulating on the inside.

- Care must be taken when handling the sharp reamer as gloves can easily be torn. Handle it correctly!

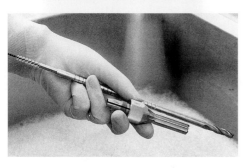

Following surgery:
- It must be dismantled before the normal cleaning procedure is followed. Particular attention is paid to the threads and cannulated parts. Ensure that a guide pin is not jammed inside the cannula.

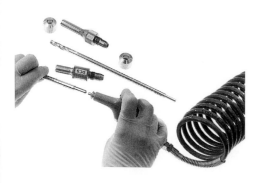

- All parts are dried using the air jet for hollow parts.
- One or two drops of oil are placed on the threaded area and the reamer is opened and closed to disperse the oil. Excess is gathered on a cloth.
- The drill is checked for sharpness and may be sent to the manufacturer for resharpening providing it is undamaged (see Sect. 6.22.10).

– For sterilising, the instrument can be left apart or loosely assembled.

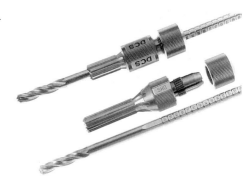

6.22.5.2 Flexible Shafts and Reamers

During surgery:
– To prevent damage to the patient and to the reamers it is important that they are used sequentially in 0.5 mm increments, changing the shafts when appropriate.
– Following use, the reamer head should be removed, wiped and returned to its allotted place. Turning it upside down on the peg will give an indication of the previous size used.

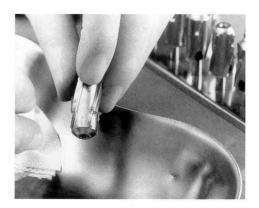

– The flexible shafts must be flushed using Ringer's lactate solution or saline. This prevents blood or bone debris coagulating on the inside of the shaft before the final cleaning can take place. The instruments must not be left to soak in these solutions. In certain countries sterile water is used as a rinsing solution. Care must be taken that this does not enter the wound.

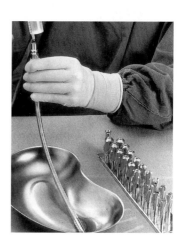

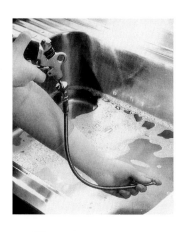

Following surgery:
- The flexible shafts should be cleaned manually using a water jet, nozzle and cleaning solution. The solution can be forced through the wire walls by putting a finger over the distal opening. This should be carried out under water to avoid spraying of personnel.
- By flexing the shaft back and forth it is possible to dislodge any residual debris.

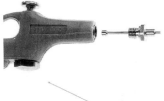

- The air jet should be used for drying the shaft using the compressed air supply.

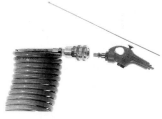

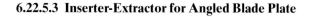

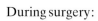

- Reamer heads are washed thoroughly, dried, checked for sharpness and replaced in their correct position.
- Reamer heads should not be resharpened, they must be replaced. With prolonged use or unauthorised sharpening the diameter of the reamer head may be diminished.

6.22.5.3 Inserter-Extractor for Angled Blade Plate

During surgery:
- To fix the plate to the inserter-extractor, it is laid flat on the instrument table.
- Tightening should be done using the combination wrench and not the hexagonal screwdriver.

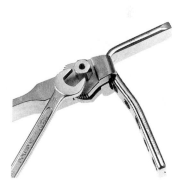

Following surgery:
– The instrument is disassembled for cleaning.

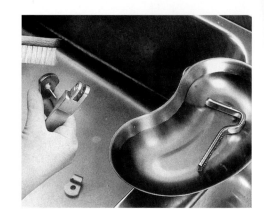

– Special attention is paid to the threaded part.
– Before replacing it in the set it is checked for wear. If the threads are damaged it will not grip the plate correctly.
– A light lubrication is needed on the mobile threaded part.

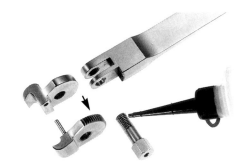

6.22.5.4 Cannulated Screw Instruments

During surgery:
– Once the cannulated instruments have been used residue should be cleared from the inside. A special stylet is available to help dislodge any debris.
– Flush the instruments with Ringers lactate solution or saline to keep them clear. In some countries sterile water is used as a rinsing solution. Care must be taken that this does not enter the wound.
– Excessive force should not be applied to the instruments.
– The appropriate uncannulated hexagonal screwdriver is used for the final tightening of screws once the guide wires have been removed.

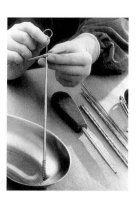

Following surgery:
– Cleaning is carried out directly following the procedure.
– The stylet is used to clear any debris. A special brush is also available to assist with cleaning. This is made from auto-clavable nylon and steel material.

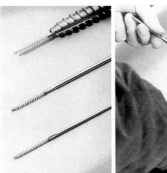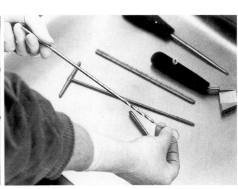

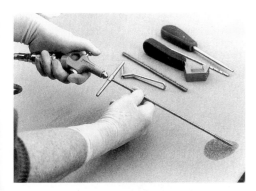

– Use of the air jet simplifies washing and drying of the instruments.
– Both inside and outside the instruments must be completely dry before checking, packing and autoclaving.
– The guide pin can be easily damaged so examine it carefully and replace if required. This is frequently necessary following each procedure. Since some are colour coded the appropriate pins should be assembled with the correct set.
– All other instruments are also checked.

6.22.5.5 External Fixators

During surgery:
– Check that all clamps are correctly assembled before mounting them onto the tubes.

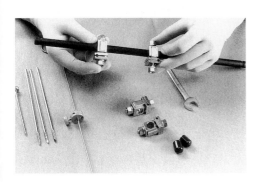

Following surgery:

– Once removed the clamps must be dismantled, decontaminated, cleaned and dried.
– They must be examined for possible damage. Damaged threads would prevent the clamp from maintaining stability while in use. They need to be replaced.

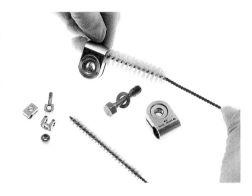

– Lubrication of the mobile parts is required.

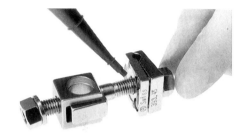

– Clamps are reassembled.

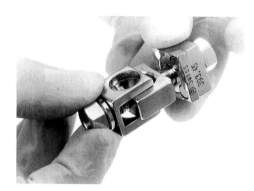

– The tubes are washed and dried in a similar manner before the set can be restocked and repacked.
– Caution is necessary when cleaning the case made of anodised aluminium (see Sect. 6.22.4.2).

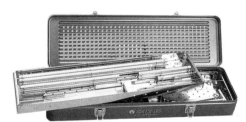

– Any Schanz screws that are removed from the patient are not to be reused and should be discarded. An adequate stock of new Schanz screws should be available to replace in the set.

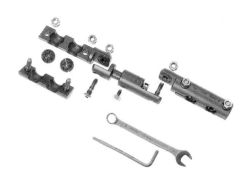

6.22.5.6 Unifix

During surgery:
- The ball clamps are tightened by hand initially.
- A position change should not be done forcefully.

Following surgery:
- Once the unifix has been removed from a patient, it must be completely dismantled for cleaning.
- A combination wrench and hexagonal spanner are necessary.
- The internal hexagonal bolts need not be removed for cleaning.
- This procedure is carefully observed to enable reassembly afterwards.

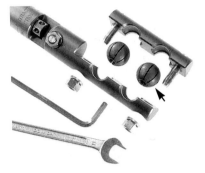

- As the surface of the ball clamps is sand-blasted, it can eventually become worn and the ball clamp should be replaced.

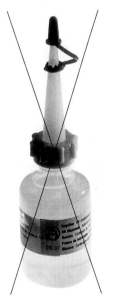

Note: No lubrication is required and might even impair its stability.

6.22.5.7 Bolt Cutter

During surgery:
– Before using the cutter, check its assembly. The teeth on the cutter head must engage fully.

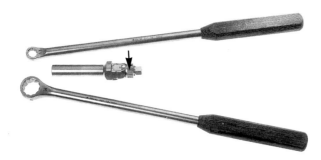

– The hole in the sleeve must be aligned with the hole in the cutter head. It may be necessary to rotate the sleeve until the holes are centred.

Following surgery:
– The cutter head must be disassembled completely for cleaning.
– The holes in the sleeve and body are aligned and the lock is retracted. This will allow the nut to be unscrewed.
– The sleeve is removed and the components should be washed, paying particular attention to the threads and hollow parts.

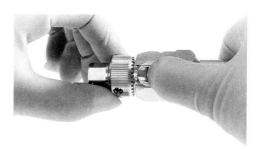

– Once dried, it is lubricated and the excess oil is wiped off. Adequate lubrication is essential to ensure smooth cutting.
– It can be reassembled before autoclaving leaving the nut loosely tightened.

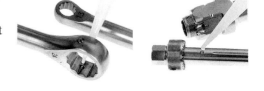

– The groove on the sleeve is aligned with the screw on the body of the bolt cutter head.
– The handles are cleaned in the usual manner.

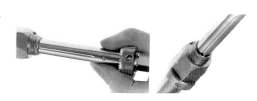

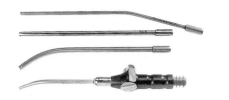

6.22.5.8 Suction Device

During surgery:
– The device should be flushed through to prevent coagulation of blood.
– The handpiece is made of anodised aluminium so the usual precautions are necessary (see Sect. 6.22.4.2).

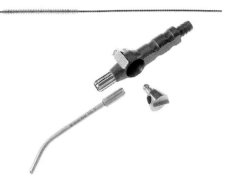

Following surgery:
– The valves should be removed for cleaning
– All metal suction nozzles and the suction tubing must be washed thoroughly. This is best done manually. A soft nylon brush is available for this purpose.

6.22.5.9 Plate Benders/Pliers

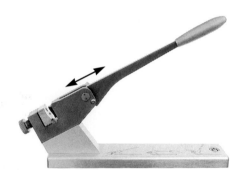

During surgery:
– Note the possible positions of the pliers and benders.
– The handle of the plate benders must be in the neutral position before commencement.

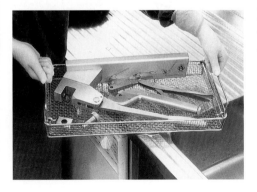

Following surgery:
– The plate benders and pliers are disassembled for cleaning.
– Particular areas that may harbour residual cleaning solutions need to be examined.
– The air jet can be used for drying these difficult areas once they have been rinsed.

- Lubrication is important to maintain optimum function.
- Open and close to disperse the oil.
- Collect any excess.

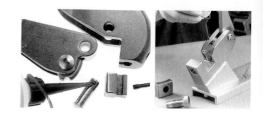

Reassembling:
- The block in the benders makes contact in one position only.
- The locking bar in the pliers must be inserted fully to allow it to function.

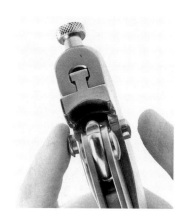

6.22.6 Preparation for and Sterilisation of AO/ASIF Instruments and Implants

Malfunctioning or damaged instruments may be hazardous to patients and personnel and should not be used., e. g. a blunt drill bit may cause bone necrosis or a damaged screwdriver could destroy the screw head making screw removal difficult if not impossible.

6.22.6.1 Inspection

Before packing, each instrument should be inspected.
- Sharp instruments need to be examined using some magnification otherwise it may not be possible to detect damage to the cutting edge. See also p. 61.

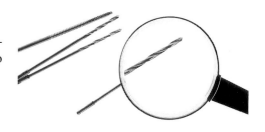

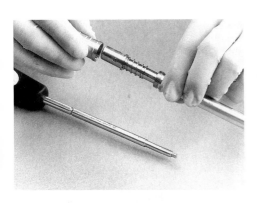

– Disassembled parts must be reassembled correctly with all components.

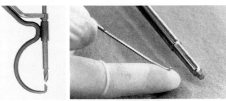

– Instruments should be checked for correct alignment and function. Open and close joints, ratchets, etc.

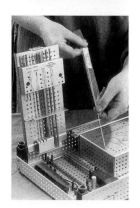

The surface is examined for any scratches which may lead to corrosion.
– Malfunctioning, broken, blunt or damaged instruments should be removed and replaced by a verified one.
– Screws, nuts or bolts may work themselves loose. Ensure that they are retightened or replaced.

6.22.6.2 Care of New Instruments

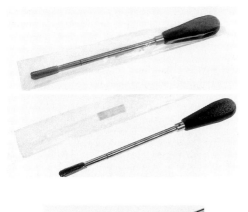

New instruments come individually wrapped. The label on the package provides the following information:
– The article number corresponding to the number in the catalogue.
– Material used, e. g. stainless steel.
– Lot number – each batch of metal used has a number for easy identification should a fault occur.
– On newer labels, a bar code is included for computerised hospital inventories.
Since new instruments do not come presterilised, they must be prepared for use. It is necessary to subject them to the same cleaning routine as for used instruments, i. e. dismantling, decontaminating, washing, rinsing, drying, lubricating, sterilising, packing and storing. Any plastic protective covers or plugs must be removed prior to cleaning and sterilising.

The handles on some of the instruments are light tan colour when new, e. g. hexagonal screwdriver or periosteal elevator. They will turn a darker colour with repeated sterilising but their function is not impaired.

6.22.6.3 Packing

An acceptable standard should be adhered to wherever items are prepared for sterilising:
– Instruments which belong in a set are replaced in the appropriate case. A checklist should be used to avoid error.
– The graphic case allows easy positioning of instruments and a quick check for completeness.

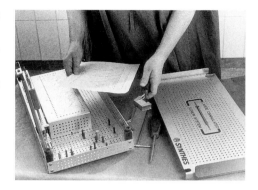

– Delicate or sharp instruments must be protected to avoid damage if they remain loose in the set. In newer cases, drill bits and taps can be held in a specially designed rack.
– Heavy instruments should not be put on top of delicate ones.
– Instruments with ratchets can be closed to first or second notch.
– Some multiple component instruments may be loosely reassembled.

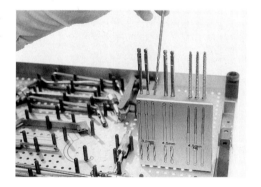

– Those with joints or screw closures remain slightly open to allow full steam penetration during sterilising.

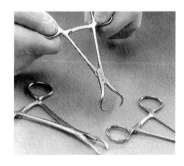

Instrumentation and Techniques

Material Used for Packing

A variety of different materials can be used depending on the availability in the area. Whatever is selected must comply with certain requirements.

– It must completely cover the instruments and allow easy removal when required.

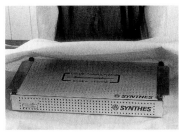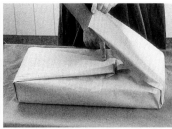

– It must allow penetration and release of sterilising agents to permit adequate sterilisation, aeration and drying of the contents.
– It must provide a protection against micro-organisms, dust and moisture during storage.

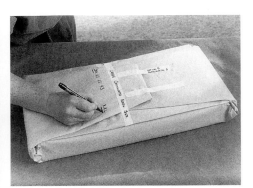

A sterility indicator placed inside each pack will confirm the sterilisation of the contents. Tapes or strips that change colour on the outside of the pack do not necessarily indicate sterility as they may automatically change colour at a certain temperature. The sterilising date and the contents must be noted clearly on the outside of the pack.

6.22.6.4 Sterilisation Methods Recommended for AO/ASIF Instruments and Implants

All AO/ASIF instruments or implants used in a surgical procedure must be sterile. Disinfection alone is inadequate and unacceptable in preventing infection during surgical interventions. Sterilisation is a process which destroys living micro-organisms including resistant spore-forming ones. It is not, however, a substitute for cleaning.

– Steam sterilisation was in use by the end of the nineteenth century and is still the most widely used method.
– Thermal sterilisation with steam under pressure (autoclave) can be used for all AO/ASIF instruments and implants with the exception of the air jet which does not require sterilisation.

Care and Maintenance of Instrumentation

– Different types of sterilisers exist. Manufacturers instructions for recommended use of the autoclave must be adhered to.

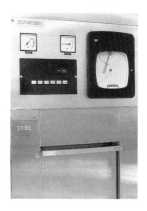

Gravity Displacement Steriliser

Steam entering the chamber under pressure displaces the air in the chamber downwards. The standard cycle for wrapped items: 121–123 °C at 15–17 psi, with an exposure time of 15–30 min. If the temperature is 131–133 °C at 15–17 psi, then exposure time is 15–20 min.

Prevacuum Steriliser

Air is first evacuated from the chamber before the steam is admitted. This takes place during the prevacuum phase. The standard cycle for wrapped items: 132–135 °C at 27–30 psi with a minimum exposure time of 4–10 min.

"Flash" Steriliser

This is a high-speed pressure steriliser most commonly with a gravity displacement cycle. The instruments for sterilisation are unwrapped. Its use is restricted to emergency situations, contaminated or forgotten items. The instruments are exposed to a temperature of 132 °C. for a period of 10 min.

Note: Implants that will remain in the body must not be sterilised in this manner as the sterility cannot be fully guaranteed.

It is advisable, and in some countries mandatory, to have a negative reading from the biological indicator used when sterilising implants. This is displayed 48 h after sterilisation, and implants may not be implanted unless this has been passed.
In an emergency situation if an implant is required it may be sterilised unwrapped following the normal time and temperature scale for prevacuum or gravity displacement sterilisers. It should not be used as a routine method of sterilising.

Instrumentation and Techniques

Table 1

Steriliser	Temperature	Pressure	Exposure Time	Wrapping
Gravity displacement steriliser	121°–123°C or 131°–133°C	15–17 psi 1–1.2 bar 15–17 p si	min. 30 min min. 20 min	wrapped wrapped
Prevacuum steriliser	132°–135 °C or up to 141 °C	27–32 psi 2–3 bar 27–30 psi	min. 4 min	wrapped
Flash steriliser (gravity displacement)	132°–134 °C	27–30 psi 2–3 bar	10 min	unwrapped

Hot Air Steriliser

Hot air sterilisation requires a longer exposure time and a higher temperature This prolonged exposure time may be hazardous to certain instruments, e. g. lubricated instruments or those with soldered parts:
– Temperature: 180–200 °C
– Exposure time: 30 min

Hot air sterilisation is not recommended for air-powered equipment as prolonged use may damage the sealings.

Chemical Sterilisation

Ethylene oxide gas and formaldehyde gas are just two examples. Since it is unnecessary and not recommended to use a chemical steriliser for AO/ASIF instruments, no further comment is necessary (it may be used according to guidelines, if no other method is available).

Sterilising

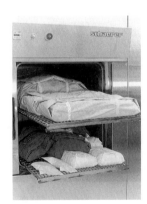

When loading the steriliser it is important to arrange the contents so that all items will be fully sterilised. The general recommendations for autoclaving should be followed.
Once the process is complete the packages are allowed to dry fully before being inspected and stored.
A specific test for sterility is recommended for each type of steriliser. This should be done on a daily basis, to monitor its function. Any positive reading from the sterility indicator should be reported and patients monitored for infection if items have been used from this load.
Regular cleaning and maintenance of the autoclave, according to manufacturers instructions, is essential to maintain optimum standards. A faulty autoclave may cause spotting or damage on the instrument surface.

- Couplings on air machines and hoses, when lubricated, should be moved back and forth to spread the oil.
- Triggers have to be depressed and released.
- A few drops of oil in each of these areas should be adequate and any excess oil can be wiped off.

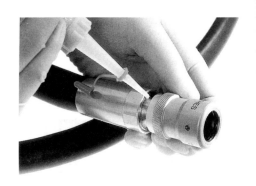

6.22.9.5 Small Air Drill

Clean as directed. The following parts should be lubricated:
- Air inlet.
- Triggers.
- Quick coupling

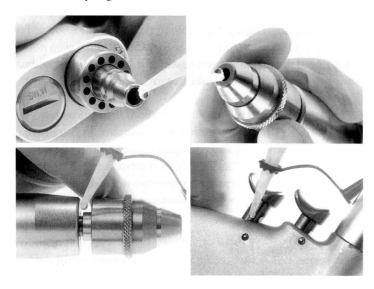

Adapters and Accessories

- Oscillating drill attachment:
  Clean as directed. Lubricate the ball bearing at connecting point.

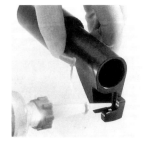

Instrumentation and Techniques

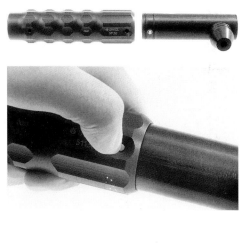

– Radiolucent drive:
  Clean as directed.
  It is important to clean *immediately* after use.
  It can be disassembled into two parts by depressing the button and pulling apart.
  Once it has been dried, it can be reassembled in reverse sequence ensuring the button has fully engaged in the hole.
  No lubrication is required.
  For sterilisation, autoclave up to 134 °C only.
  Do not use until fully cooled.

Note: Instructions for use should be carefully followed to avoid damage. When properly operated and cleaned the radiolucent drive does not need daily maintenance. A check-up by the manufacturers following use for 100–150 times or 1 year is recommended.

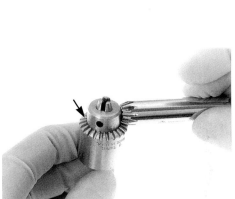

– Jacobs chuck and key and
– Small quick coupling chuck:
  Clean as directed, but particular attention must be paid to areas that could harbour debris.
  For lubrication, put a few drops of oil on the threaded portion. The chuck should be opened and closed to disperse the oil. Ensure that the teeth on the chuck and key are undamaged.

6.22.9.6 Universal Air Drill

Clean as directed. The following parts should be lubricated:
– Air inlet
– Trigger
– Quick coupling

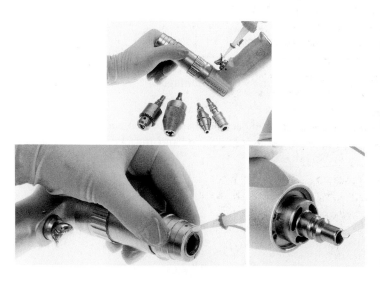

Adapters and Accessories

- Right-angled drive:
  Clean as directed, paying particular attention to cannulation for reaming rod.
  Lubricate the quick coupling and locking screw.
- Quick coupling chuck:
- Small quick coupling chuck:
- Universal chuck:
- Jacobs chuck and key:
  Clean and lubricate as directed.

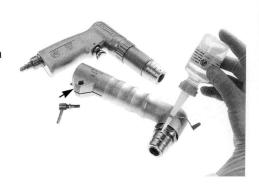

6.22.9.7 Oscillating Bone Saw

Clean as directed. The saw blade housing plate must be removed for cleaning. Using two Kirschner wires, the plate can be lifted and removed. It is washed and dried. If the pins are damaged they must be replaced by new ones. Under slight pressure they will click back in position. The following parts should be lubricated:
- Air inlet
- Operating lever
- Pin under lever
- Locking mechanism on lever

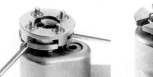 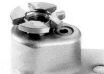

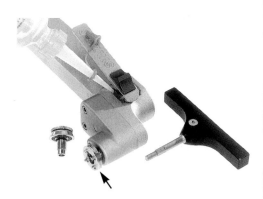

Adapters and Accessories

- Saw blades:
  Replace if they are worn or damaged.
- Locking key

All the adapters and accessories should be checked in the appropriate machine before packing and autoclaving.

Instrumentation and Techniques

6.22.9.8 Mini Compressed Air Machine

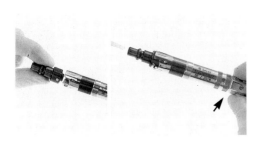

Clean the compressed air motor as directed. Lubrication should be carried out as follows:
– With the special oiling adapter attached to the drill put approximately 8–10 drops of oil into the air inlet.
– Connect the machine to an air hose and compressed air and use it to disperse the oil.
– Gather any excess oil on a cloth.
– The drive switch on the drill must also be lubricated.

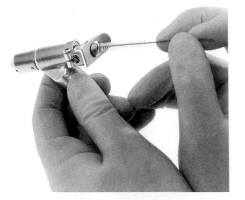

Accessories

– Mini oscillating saw
– Mini reciprocating saw
– Drill head attachment straight
– Drill head attachment 90°
– Drill head attachment 45°:
  This has a special cleaning brush.
– Angled hose connector
– Drill bits
– Burrs
– Saw blades:
  Tissue protectors and saw blades should be washed in the usual manner. Any worn or damaged blades must be replaced by new ones as they cannot be sharpened.

All attachments must be washed, dried and lubricated where necessary before being verified and replaced in the special case provided. The anodised aluminium case should be cleaned (see Sect. 6.22.4.2).

– Double air hose:
  This should be treated in the same way as all other hoses (see Sect. 6.22.92). When packing it into the set it should not be folded tightly. It is stored underneath the instrument tray and should not come in contact with the metal contents of the set.

6.22.9.9 Preparation and Packing of Air Equipment for Sterilisation

The standard guidelines for packing and sterilising also apply (see Sects. 6.226.3 and 6.22.6.4):

– The hose must not come into contact with metal. If a special tray is not available to separate the motor and hose, they should be wrapped individually.

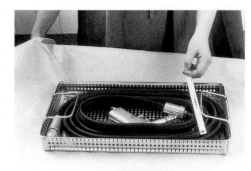

– Ensure that no material that may be affected by high temperatures is left on the machine, e. g. the plastic stopper in the air inlet of new machines.

– All accessories must be removed before packing.

– The hose ends should not be coupled for autoclaving. This may cause jamming of the couplings and bursting of the hose.

– A gentle coil for straight hoses is appropriate.
Spiral hoses can be held in place for autoclaving using a cloth bandage or nonadhesive tape.

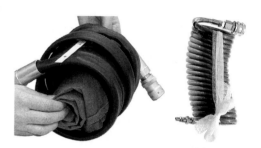

– The machines and hoses can be sterilised by thermal sterilisation (see Sect. 6.22.6.4). Radiolucent drive to 134 °C only.

– Hot air sterilisation is not recommended for the power equipment as it may damage the sealing on the machine. Also sterility cannot be fully guaranteed as the air may not fully penetrate all parts of machine.

– Flash sterilisation can be used provided the exposure time and temperature is adequate. (Independent testing was carried out in the USA which confirmed that under the correct conditions all areas of the air machine were sterilised.) (See Sect. 6.22.6.3).

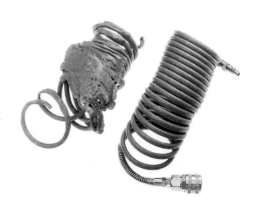

– No heavy weight or pressure should be placed on the hose especially during sterilisation or cooling. It may cause permanent deformity of the hose.

– The air-powered instruments should be used only when fully cooled. Hoses may otherwise deform or become brittle and leak and the sealing in the machine itself may be damaged if used while still hot.

6.22.9.10 Cleaning and Maintenance of Diffusor, Filters and Pressure Regulators

For details see Sect. 6.22.1.3.

– Exhaust air diffusor:
This is fitted between the single air hose from the supply and the double sterile "working" hose. It can be unscrewed to take apart for cleaning. As it is made of anodised aluminium, the usual precautions are necessary (see Sect. 6.22.4.2. and 3)

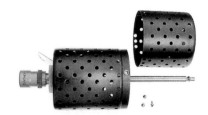

Instrumentation and Techniques

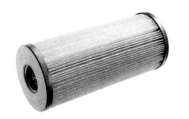

– Filter cartridge:
This is changed when the air drill is noticed to be losing power.

– Filters for air supply:
– Coarse filter and micro filter:
As both these filters render the air free from water, condensation, rust or other particles it is necessary to clean them regularly – every 2 weeks is the recommended practice.
The air supply must first be shut down and then the filter can be dismantled.
The outside and inside of the protective glass must be cleaned. The air filter element must also be cleaned with a long term anti-bactericidal spray.
Along with the cleaned connections the glass should also be sprayed with this antibactericidal spray.
Once a noticeable reduction occurs in the speed of the machine or following use for 1 year the filter element should be changed.

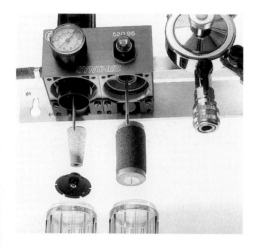

6.22.10 Repair Service

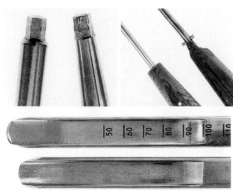

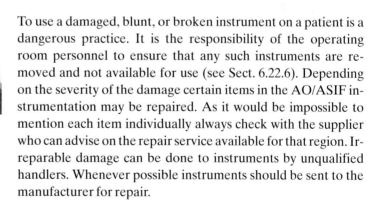

To use a damaged, blunt, or broken instrument on a patient is a dangerous practice. It is the responsibility of the operating room personnel to ensure that any such instruments are removed and not available for use (see Sect. 6.22.6). Depending on the severity of the damage certain items in the AO/ASIF instrumentation may be repaired. As it would be impossible to mention each item individually always check with the supplier who can advise on the repair service available for that region. Irreparable damage can be done to instruments by unqualified handlers. Whenever possible instruments should be sent to the manufacturer for repair.

As stated at the beginning of the chapter, misuse of instruments is one of the major causes of damage. Perhaps by studying the information carefully in this book along with the other literature which is available, the repair service can be diminished!

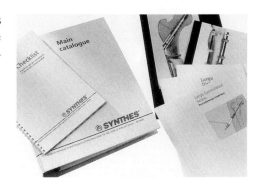

6.22.11 Handling of Retrieved Implants

There may be reasons for the return of retrieved implants for examination (for example breakage of an implant). Great care should be taken that the implant is not damaged during handling and shipping. Fracture surfaces of implants, or implant parts of special interest, should not rub against each other. In general retrieved implants should be handled as if they were contaminated by infectious micro-organisms.

Retrieved implants should be rinsed under flowing water to remove blood and exudates. Scrubbing, however, is not allowed, because areas of interest for investigation could be damaged. The rinsed implants may or may not be sterilised. Either condition should be declared with a label on the package. Nonsterilised retrieved implants should be packed in such a way that potential infection is prevented.

The retrieved implants, shipped for investigation, should be clearly identified: the hospital, the surgeon, the name and/or identification number and age of the patient, the implantation site, and the reason for return of the retrieved implant should be stated. In most instances it is highly desirable to obtain X-rays and the patient's history with such information as:

– Diagnosis
– Date of implantation
– Date of retrieval
– Complications
– Postoperative loading history
– Brief patient postoperative history

If tissues are excised and shipped with the implant they should be transferred immediately to a fixing agent like formalin or 80% ethanol. The tissues should be clearly identified with the location site and orientation described. The container and all wrapping should be secure and ensure that damage to the container and the specimen is prevented.

6.22.12 Handling of Damaged Instruments

The same rules in general apply to the handling of instruments to be returned for examination. However, sterilisation should always take place and should be indicated on the package. Clear identification is also important with instruments. The accompanying information should indicate:
– Reason for return
– If damaged, when, where and in which way did it occur
– Which surgical procedure was performed
– How long the instrument was in use

6.22.13 References

AORN standards and recommended practices for perioperative nursing (1992) Association of Operating Room Nurses, Denver

Deutschsprachiger Arbeitskreis für Krankenhaushygiene in Zusammenarbeit mit der AO-International (1992) Krankenhaushygiene. mhp Verlag, Wiesbaden

Gruendeman BJ, Meeker H (1987) Alexander's care of the patient in surgery. Mosby, St. Louis

ISSM (1990) Teaching and training manual for sterile service personnel. Working Group – Supplies Service, Northampton

Sequin F, Texhammar R (1981) AO/ASIF instrumentation. Springer, Berlin Heidelberg New York

7 Internal or External Fixation of Various Fractures

By R. Texhammar

In the following section some fractures and possible treatment using AO/ASIF technique will be discussed. This is meant to be used as a reference and a guide by the operating room personnel, once the surgical decision has been made to stabilise a fracture operatively. It may help the reader to perform her or his task with more confidence.

7.1 Fractures of the Scapula and the Shoulder Joint

Fractures of the scapula may be found in polytraumatised patients, although they may also be seen as isolated injuries. They are in most cases only minimally displaced and rarely require surgery. Severely displaced and unstable fractures of the neck, acromion or occasionally the coracoid process are indications for surgery. Often these fractures are associated with a fracture of the clavicle (see Sect. 7.2).

7.1.1 Anatomy

Left clavicle, scapula and humerus, from the front (Fig. 1a).
Left scapula and humerus, from behind (Fig. 1b).

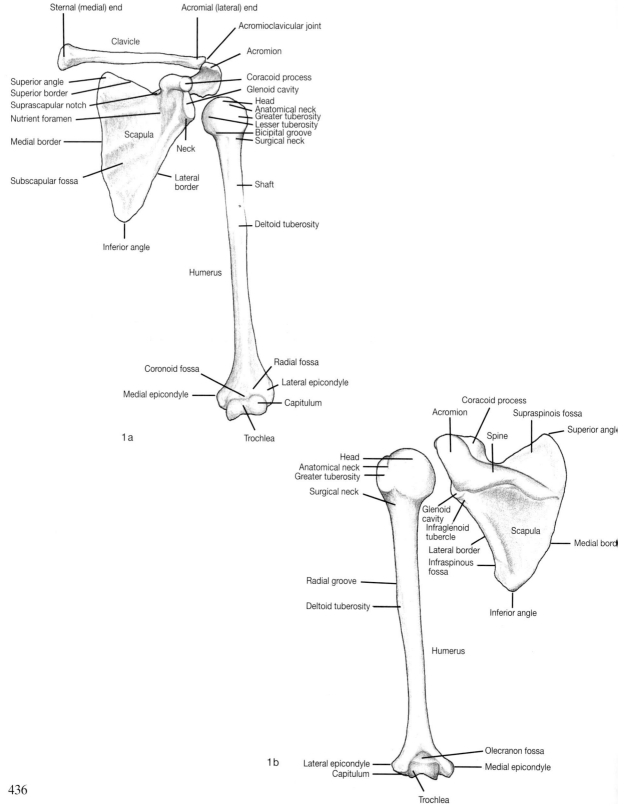

1a

1b

7.1.2 Assessment

Special examination:
– In multiply injured patients, check for thoracic and brachial plexus injuries.

Radiography:
– The antero-posterior (AP) view, angled perpendicular to the blade of the scapula, and the profile tangential views are standard.
– Acromio-clavicular joint: AP views of both joints are taken separately and the beam angled up 15° if necessary. Load-bearing views, with a weight in each hand, may reveal vertical instability.
– Shoulder: AP and axial views are standard. If the injury precludes the axial view, the Wallace and Heller view (Radiography 1990), with the patient seated, is the most helpful.

7.1.3 AO Classification

Scapular fractures are grouped with the clavicle, the mandible and the patella – bone group 9. The scapula is 9.1.3 – the subtypes and subgroups are not yet defined.

7.1.4 Indication for Osteosynthesis – Implants of Choice

Fracture:
– Displaced intra-articular fracture of the glenoid (Fig. 2).

Implants:
– 3.5 mm cortex screws or 4.0 mm cancellous bone screws as lag screws (Fig. 3). Some such fractures extend into the lateral border of the scapula and a small, infraglenoid, one-third tubular plate may be applied to the lateral border as a buttress.

Fracture:
– Markedly displaced extra-articular fracture of the glenoid neck (Fig. 4).

Implants:
– One-third tubular plate, 3.5 mm DCP, or LC-DCP (Fig. 5) for the fixation of the clavicle may suffice.

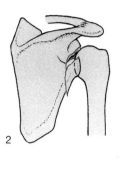

2

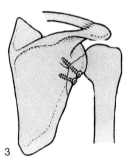

3

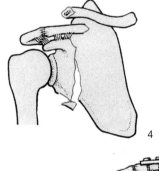

4

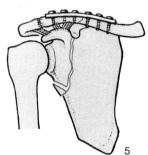

5

Scapula and Shoulder Joint

7.1.5 Preoperative Planning and Preparation

Timing:
– Rarely urgent. Determined by the need for other surgery and the patient's general condition.

Position:
– Prone or lateral with the arm supported. The arm is draped to be freely moved.

Incision:
– For fractures of the posterior aspect of the glenoid as well as of the lateral margin of the scapula, a curved skin incision starts at the palpable lateral prominence of the acromion, passes medially along the scapular spine and then caudally to end at the inferior angle of the scapula (Fig. 6).
– For fractures of the anterior and inferior margins of the glenoid, the delto-pectoral approach may be chosen. See Fig. 15 in Sect. 7.3.

Preparation of instruments:
– Instruments for insertion of 3.5 mm cortex screws as lag screws (p. 215).
– Instruments for insertion of 4.0 mm cancellous bone screws as lag screws (p. 214).
– Instruments for application of 3.5 mm DCP or LC-DCP (pp. 215, 216).
– Instruments for application of one-third tubular plate (p. 216).

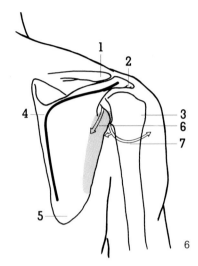

1 Clavicle
2 Acromion
3 Greater tubercule
4 "Spinal triangle" of spine of scapula
5 Inferior angle
6 Suprascapular nerve
7 Axillary nerve

7.1.6 Checklist for Operative Technique

Posterior approach in extra- or intra-articular fractures:
– Exposure and detachment of the deltoid muscle from the scapular spine and retraction laterally.
– The approach is deepened by developing the interval between infraspinatus and teres minor.
– Reduction can be achieved using pointed reduction forceps.
– Application of 3.5 mm DCP or LC-DCP (pp. 202, 208).
– Application of one-third tubular plate (p. 200).
– Application of 4.0 mm cancellous bone screws as lag screws (p. 195).

Anterior approach in fractures of the glenoid:
– Reduction of inferior glenoid fractures can be difficult.
– Osteotomy of the coracoid may be necessary for improved exposure. Later reattached with 4.5 mm cortex screw and polyacetate washer to prevent splitting of the coracoid tip.

Fixation of Various Fractures

7.1.7 Special Consideration – Escape Routes

Where access to the lateral border of the scapula is required, the more extensive Judet approach, where the belly of the infraspinatus muscle is reflected laterally to expose the whole infraspinous fossa, may be indicated.

7.1.8 Postoperative Care

- Suction drainage for 24–36 h.
- Temporary immobilisation in a Gilchrist or Desault bandage for 3–4 days followed by careful passive and active motion.

7.1.9 Implant Removal

Implant removal is difficult and rarely indicated.

7.1.10 Recommended Reading

Müller ME, Allgöwer M, Schneider R, Willenegger H (1991) Manual of internal fixation, 3rd edn. Springer, Berlin Heidelberg New York
Rüedi T, Hochstetter AHC, Schlumpf R (1984) Surgical Approaches for Internal Fixation. Springer, Berlin Heidelberg New York
Schatzker J, Tile M (1987) The rationale of operative fracture care. Springer, Berlin Heidelberg New York

7.2 Fractures of the Clavicle

Most clavicular shaft fractures usually heal without immobilisation and are therefore treated conservatively. Nevertheless, internal fixation may be chosen for the following indications:
– Open fractures
– Fractures associated with neuro-vascular lesions
– Fractures combined with scapular neck fractures – the imploded shoulder
– Fragment threatening to perforate skin
– Fractures associated with an apical pneumothorax or surgical emphysema
– Severely displaced fractures
– Pseudarthroses

7.2.1 Anatomy

Left clavicle and scapula from the front (Fig. 1).

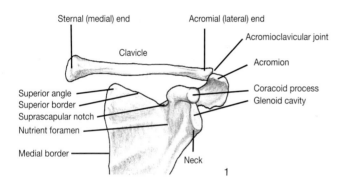

1

7.2.2 Assessment

Special examination:
– Inspection of skin.
– Palpation for surgical emphysema.

Radiography:
– Standard view, look for pneumothorax or surgical emphysema.
– With patient supine, two films at 90° to each other are taken with the overhead beam centred on the clavicle.

7.2.3 AO Classification

See Sect. 7.1.3. The 9.1.2 subtype groups are not yet defined.

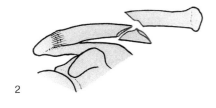

2

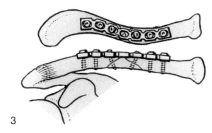

3

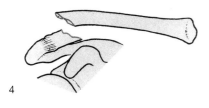

4

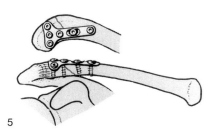

5

7.2.4 Indication for Osteosynthesis – Implants of Choice

Fracture:
– Midshaft fracture (Fig. 2).

Implants:
– 3.5 mm reconstruction plate (Fig. 3).
– 3.5 mm DCP or LC-DCP.

Fractures:
– Unstable displaced fracture – lateral end (Neer classification, type 2) (Fig. 4).

Implants:
– Small T plate (Fig. 5).
– Tension band figure-of-eight wire.

7.2.5 Preoperative Planning and Preparation

Timing:
– Urgent if pneumothorax or neuro-vascular compromise. Otherwise when the patient's condition is optimal.

Position:
– Supine with ample padding beneath the shoulder (vacuum mattress). The arm is draped free. The head is turned toward the opposite side.

Incision:
– A sabre cut incision running parallel to Lange's lines usually gives adequate access (Fig. 6).

Preparation of instruments:
– Instruments for application of 3.5 mm reconstruction plate (p. 216).
– Instruments for application of 3.5 mm DCP and LC-DCP (p. 215, 216).
– Instruments for application of small T plate (p. 216).
– Instruments for application of tension band wire (p. 369).

7.2.6 Checklist for Operative Technique

– Temporary reduction with a pointed reduction forceps.
– Aluminium template is contoured to the bone, the plate is shaped and then trial fit to bone. The plate may be placed on the anterior or superior aspect of the clavicle. A seven- to eight-hole reconstruction plate is chosen (p. 213).
– Fixation of a lateral clavicular fracture with a small T plate (p. 212).

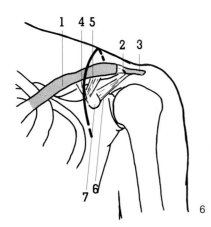

6

1 Clavicle
2 Acromio-clavicular joint
3 Acromion
4 Conoidal ligament
5 Trapezoidal ligament
6 Coraco-acromial ligament
7 Coracoid process

Clavicle

7.2.7 Special Consideration – Escape Routes

The oscillating drill is safer in this area. Because of the proximity of vital structures deep to the clavicle, overpenetration of the drill bit must be avoided; a bimanual hold on the drill, with the nondominant hand exerting counterpressure, is relatively safe.
If there should be any question of puncture of the lung, the wound should be filled with Hartmann's or Ringer's lactate solution and the anaesthetist asked to hyperinflate the lungs. If bubbles appear, a chest drain should be inserted and the patient nursed for about 48 h in the intensive care unit.

7.2.8 Postoperative Care

– Suction drainage for 24–36 h.
– If fixation is stable, a simple supportive sling until wound healing is assured.

7.2.9 Implant Removal

The plate and screws often cause symptoms and may be removed after sound bony healing at about 6–9 months.

7.2.10 Recommended Reading

Müller ME, Allgöwer M, Schneider R, Willenegger H (1991) Manual of internal fixation, 3rd edn. Springer, Berlin Heidelberg New York
Rüedi T, Hochstetter AHC, Schlumpf R (1984) Surgical Approaches for Internal Fixation. Springer, Berlin Heidelberg New York
Schatzker J, Tile M (1987) The rationale of operative fracture care. Springer, Berlin Heidelberg New York

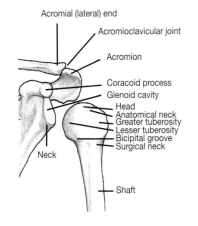

1a

Acromial (lateral) end
Acromioclavicular joint
Acromion
Coracoid process
Glenoid cavity
Head
Anatomical neck
Greater tuberosity
Lesser tuberosity
Bicipital groove
Surgical neck
Neck
Shaft

1b

Coracoid process
Acromion
Head
Anatomical neck
Greater tuberosity
Surgical neck
Glenoid cavity
Infraglenoid tubercle

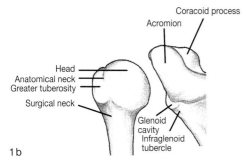

2

A1   A2   A3

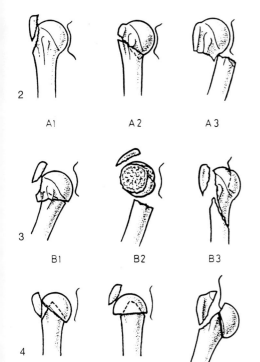

3

B1   B2   B3

4

C1   C2   C3

7.3 Fractures of the Proximal Humerus

Only a few fractures of the proximal humerus require osteosynthesis. Surgical treatment is chosen mainly to treat markedly displaced unstable fractures in young patients with good bone quality and in polytrauma patients. Internal fixation is often difficult and presents a challenge to the surgical team.

7.3.1 Anatomy

Proximal humerus and acromio-clavicular joint from the front (Fig. 1a).
Proximal humerus and shoulder joint from behind (Fig. 1b).

7.3.2 Assessment

Special examination:
– Neuro-vascular function of arm and hand.

Radiography:
– Standard AP view, axial view, and parasagittal view (posterior dislocation?)
– Tomography
– Computed tomography (CT) scan

7.3.3 AO Classification

See also Sect. 5.1

Type 11 A: Extra-articular fractures with one fragment (tuberosity or metaphyseal) (Fig. 2).
Type 11 B: Extra-articular fractures with two to three fragments (both tuberosity and metaphysis) (Fig. 3).
Type 11 C: Intra-articular fractures involving the anatomical neck (Fig. 4).

7.3.4 Indication for Osteosynthesis – Implants of Choice

Fractures type A:
– Fracture dislocation (Fig. 5).
– Displaced unstable fractures of the neck of greater tuberosity (collum chirurgicum) (Fig. 6).

Implants:
– Cancellous bone screws, 4.0 mm or 6.5 mm (displaced avulsion fragments) (Fig. 7).
– Tension band wiring (Fig. 8).
– T plate, three or four holes (large head fragment) (Fig. 9).

Fractures types B and C:
– Displaced fragments in young adults (Figs. 10, 11).

Implants:
– Tension band wiring and 4.0 mm or 6.5 mm cancellous bone screws (Figs. 12, 13).
– Kirschner wires percutaneously (Fig. 14).

7.3.5 Preoperative Planning and Preparation

Timing:
– Immediately, if skin and general condition allow.

Position:
– Supine with ample padding beneath the shoulder (e.g. vacuum mattress), arm abducted 45°, patient's head turned toward the opposite side. Arm draped free.

Incision:
– Anterior delto-pectoral approach in most cases. Posterior approach for irreducible posterior fracture dislocations (Fig. 15).

Preparation of instruments:
– Instruments for insertion of 4.0 mm cancellous bone screw (p. 214).
– Instruments for insertion of 6.5 mm cancellous bone screw (p. 82).
– Instruments for application of cerclage wires (p. 369).
– Instruments for application of a T plate (p. 112).

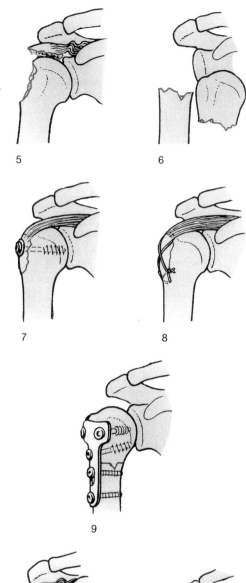

5   6

7   8

9

10   11

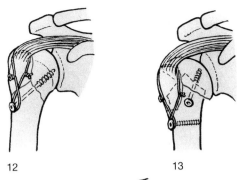

12   13

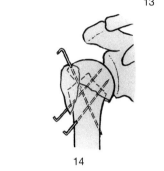

14

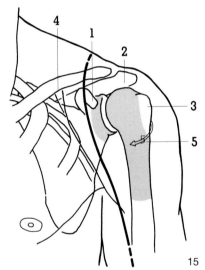

15

1 Coracoid process
2 Acromion
3 Greater tubercule
4 Clavicle
5 Axillary nerve

7.3.6 Checklist for Operative Technique

Fractures type A:
– Atraumatic anatomical reduction, temporary fixation with Kirschner wires.
– Insertion of 4.0 mm cancellous bone screws as lag screws (p. 195).
– Insertion of 6.5 mm cancellous bone screws as lag screws (p. 81).
– Application of tension band wire with a 1.25 mm diameter. cerclage wire (p. 366).

Fractures type B and C:
– Reflection of the deltoid muscle.
– For better exposure if necessary: anterior osteotomy of the acromion.

In good bone:
– Anatomical reduction.
– Fixation with 4.0 mm or 6.5 mm cancellous bone screws with washers as lag screws, combined with tension band wire (pp. 81, 195). Sometimes 4.5 mm cortex screw as lag screws (p. 77).

In poor bone:
– Impaction of the humeral shaft into the head fragment.
– Fixation with Kirschner wires 1.6 mm or 2.0 mm diameter, and tension band wire (p. 366).

In multifragmentary fractures:
– Provisional or definitive fixation of smaller fragments with Kirschner wires supplemented with a long T plate as a protection or buttress plate (p. 108).

7.3.7 Special Consideration – Escape Routes

Preservation of soft tissue attachment is mandatory. In poor bone, 6.5 mm cancellous bone screws may get a better hold. Fully threaded screws are used in the head of the T plate.

7.3.8 Postoperative Care

– Suction drainage for 24–36 h.
– Partially abducted position of the arm (pillows or skin traction).
– Active contraction of the deltoid muscle if suture allows.
– If there is concern about the fixation or the suture, abduction on splint until bone union occurs (4–6 weeks). Remove splint for pendulum exercise only.
– Careful clinical and radiological follow-up.
– If there is any sign of failure of implant or fixation, an abduction splint is used.

7.3.9 Implant Removal

In the upper limb metal implants can be left in place. Only in the case of inflammatory reaction, or if the implant disturbs the patient, e. g. impingement with the acromion on movement, especially abduction, is metal removal undertaken from 12–18 weeks.

7.3.10 Recommended Reading

Müller ME, Allgöwer M, Schneider R, Willenegger H (1991) Manual of internal fixation, 3rd edn. Springer, Berlin Heidelberg New York
Müller ME, Nazarian S, Koch P, Schatzker J (1990) The comprehensive AO classification of fractures of long bones. Springer, Berlin Heidelberg New York
Rüedi T, Hochstetter AHC, Schlumpf R (1984) Surgical Approaches for Internal Fixation. Springer, Berlin Heidelberg New York
Schatzker J, Tile M (1987) The rationale of operative fracture care. Springer, Berlin Heidelberg New York

7.4 Fractures of the Humeral Shaft

Most low-energy humeral shaft fractures can be treated conservatively and will unite rapidly. Osteosynthesis, however, will be considered for the following indications:
– Open fractures
– Radial nerve damage
– Polytrauma patients
– Pathological fractures
– Unstable transverse or short oblique fractures
– Nonunions or malunions
– Unstable transverse or short oblique fractures (relative indication), especially high-energy fractures.

7.4.1 Anatomy

Humerus from the front (Fig. 1a).
Humerus from behind (Fig. 1b).

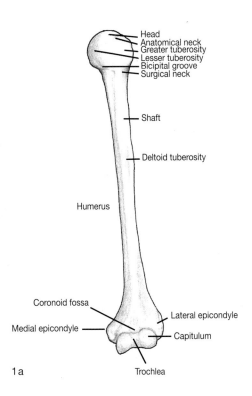

1a

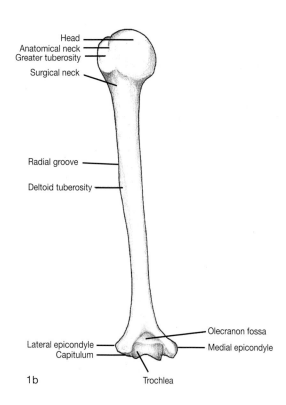

1b

7.4.2 Assessment

Special examination:
– Neuro-vascular damage (radial nerve injury is common).
– Chest injury.

Radiography:
– Standard AP view; shoulder and elbow to be seen.
– Lateral view; shoulder and elbow to be seen.

7.4.3 AO Classification

See also Sect. 5.1

Type 12 A: Simple fractures: transverse, spiral, or oblique (Fig. 2).
Type 12 B: One additional fragment: wedge or butterfly (Fig. 3).
Type 12 C: Complex fractures: spiral, two levels, or multifragmentary (Fig. 4).

7.4.4 Indications for Osteosynthesis – Implants of Choice

Fractures:
– Type A, B and C (Fig. 5).

Implants:
– Broad DCP or LC-DCP, 4.5 mm cortex screws as lag screws. For small individuals with very slender bone a narrow DCP or LC- DCP plate can be chosen.

7.4.5 Preoperative Planning and Preparation

Timing:
– Immediately for fractures of the mid- and distal third of the humerus, especially with lateral displacement of the distal fragment (radial nerve at risk). Immediately if radial nerve function is impaired or disappears during manipulation and closed reduction.

Position:
– Lateral (or prone) with the arm abducted 90° on an elbow support. The shoulder and the elbow are draped free.

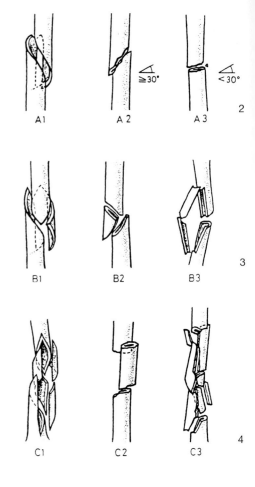

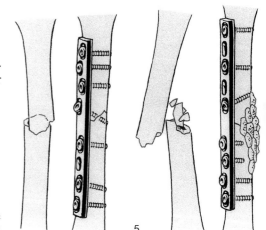

1 Coracoid process
2 Acromion
3 Lesser tubercule
4 Medial epicondyle
5 Axillary nerve
6 Musculo-cutaneous nerve
7 Radial nerve

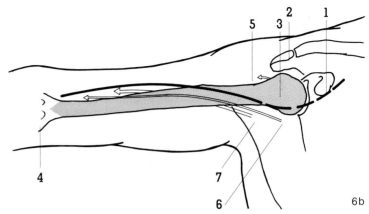

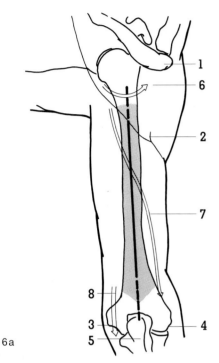

6a

1 Acromion
2 Deltoid muscle (dorsal border)
3 Medial epicondyle of humerus
4 Lateral epicondyle of humerus
5 Olecranon
6 Axillary nerve
7 Radial nerve
8 Ulnar nerve

6b

Incision:
- A posterior incision on a line joining the dorsal margin of the acromion with the olecranon for fractures of the distal two-thirds (Fig. 6a). For the upper third, the extended delto-pectoral and antero-lateral approach may be chosen (Fig. 6b).

Preparation of instruments:
- Instruments for application of a broad DCP or LC-DCP with 4.5 mm cortex screws as lag screws (p. 112).

7.4.6 Checklist for Operative Technique

Long spiral fractures:
- 4.5 mm cortex screws are inserted first as lag screws (p. 77), then a broad 4.5 mm DCP or LC-DCP is applied to protect the lag screw fixation (p. 97). Lag screws may also be placed through the plate.

Transverse or short oblique fractures:
- These fractures are stabilised with a broad 4.5 mm DCP or LC- DCP as a compression plate combined, in oblique fractures, with lag screws (4.5 mm} either separately or in the LC-DCP through the plate (p. 100). A broad plate is chosen because of its staggered holes. A narrow DCP or LC-DCP with the holes in line may fissure the bone, since the humeral cortex splinters easily.

Plate length:
- At least a six-hole plate which gives purchase in six cortices in each fragment. In osteoporotic bone a longer plate is used. In distal humeral shaft fractures approaching the metaphysis, two 3.5 mm reconstruction plates extending down the supracondylar ridges give good purchase on the short distal fragment.

Plate position:
- In the upper diaphysis the plate is most commonly placed on the antero-lateral surface of the bone. Fractures of the distal two-thirds of the humeral shaft should be plated posteriorly.

7.4.7 Special Consideration – Escape Routes

The radial nerve is often at risk in fractures at the junction of the mid- and distal third of the humeral shaft.

Lag screws alone do not give sufficient stability in long spiral fractures.

The plate can be slipped underneath the radial nerve and the vessels when applied to the posterior surface of the bone.

The position of the nerve where it crosses the plate in relation to the screw holes must be noted and documented, in case the plate should be removed later.

Autologous cancellous bone graft may be used in multifragmentary fractures.

In pathological fractures a combination of a long plate and methylmethacrylate cement may be the solution.

7.4.8 Postoperative Care

- To minimise postoperative swelling, the arm may be immobilised on a posterior plaster splint with the elbow in almost full extension and suspended for 24–48 h.
- Suction drains are removed after 24–36 h.
- Active mobilisation is started on the second or third day.

7.4.9 Implant Removal

Only if the plate gives symptoms should it be removed. The proximity of the radial nerve must be remembered. After plate removal the patient should abstain from heavy lifting or any sport for a period of 6–8 weeks.

7.4.10 Recommended Reading

Mast J, Jakob R, Ganz R (1989) Planning and reduction technique in fracture surgery. Springer, Berlin Heidelberg New York

Müller ME, Allgöwer M, Schneider R, Willenegger H (1991) Manual of internal fixation, 3rd edn. Springer, Berlin Heidelberg New York

Müller ME, Nazarian S, Koch P, Schatzker J (1990) The comprehensive AO classification of fractures of long bones. Springer, Berlin Heidelberg New York

Rüedi T, Hochstetter AHC, Schlumpf R (1984) Surgical Approaches for Internal Fixation. Springer, Berlin Heidelberg New York

Schatzker J, Tile M (1987) The rationale of operative fracture care. Springer, Berlin Heidelberg New York

Fixation of Various Fractures

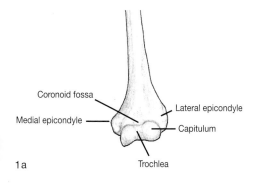

Coronoid fossa
Medial epicondyle
Lateral epicondyle
Capitulum
Trochlea

1a

7.5 Fractures of the Distal Humerus

Intra-articular fractures of the distal humerus, both simple and more complex, as well as open fractures constitute a positive indication for osteosynthesis. Extra-articular fractures are rare in adults, but because of a tendency to delayed union, internal fixation may be chosen.

7.5.1 Anatomy

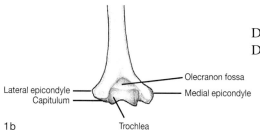

Olecranon fossa
Lateral epicondyle
Capitulum
Medial epicondyle
Trochlea

1b

Distal humerus from the front (Fig. 1a).
Distal humerus from behind (Fig. 1b).

7.5.2 Assessment

Special examination:
- Vascular and nerve injuries (brachial artery and radial nerve).
- Associated fractures of the humerus shaft, radius and ulna.
- Compartment syndrome.

Radiography:
- Standard views with traction and under anaesthesia (in the operating theatre if necessary).
- Angiography.
- Tomography (multifragmentary fractures).
- AP and lateral radiographs of the normal elbow (can be used as a template for preoperative planning if reversed).

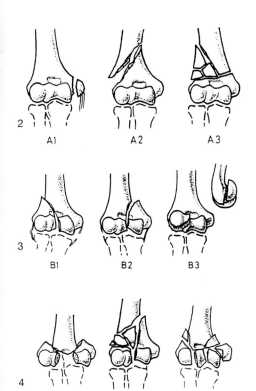

2
A1 A2 A3

3
B1 B2 B3

4
C1 C2 C3

7.5.3 AO Classification

See also Sect. 5.1

Type 13 A: Extra-articular fractures (Fig. 2).
Type 13 B: Intra-articular unicondylar fractures (Fig. 3).
Type 13 C: Intra-articular bicondylar fractures (Fig. 4).

Distal Humerus

7.5.4 Indication for Osteosynthesis – Implants of Choice

Fracture:
– Displaced fracture of the medial or lateral epicondyle or condyle (A1, B1, B2, B3).

Implants:
– 4.0 mm cancellous bone screws, 3.5 mm cortex screws, or 4.5 mm cannulated screws as lag screws (Figs. 5, 6).
– One-third tubular plate may be necessary for larger fragments.

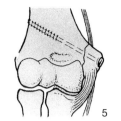

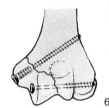

Fracture:
– Supracondylar fractures (A2, A3).

Implants:
– 3.5 mm DCP or LC-DCP (Fig. 7) sometimes combined with a one-third tubular plate.

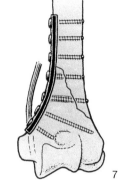

Fracture:
– Multifragmentary intra-articular fractures (C1–3).

Implants:
– 4.0 mm cancellous bone screws or 4.5 mm cortex screws, if possible as lag screws, for the reconstruction of the joint, or to lag other fragments (Fig. 8).
– Defects of the articular surface: 3.5 mm cortex screws as fixation screw in combination with bone grafting.
– 3.5 mm reconstruction plate and a one-third tubular plate (five to seven holes) or two 3.5 mm reconstruction plates (Fig. 9).

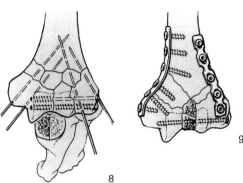

7.5.5 Preoperative Planning and Preparation

Timing:
– As soon as possible. Delay more than a few days is associated with myositis ossificans.

Position:
– Prone (if no vascular lesions) or lateral with arm abducted 90° on an elbow support. Forearm draped hanging free. Sterile tourniquet.

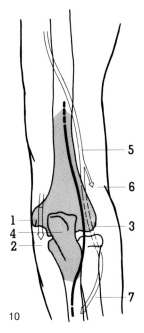

1 Medial epicondyle
2 Ulnar nerve
3 Lateral epicondyle
4 Olecranon
5 Radial nerve
6 Deep branch of radial nerve
7 Superficial branch of radial nerve

Incision:
– Posteriorly from the midline over the distal humerus, curving radially past and two finger widths from the olecranon to the posterior border of the ulna (Fig. 10).

Preparation of instruments:
– Instruments for insertion of 4.0 mm cancellous bone or 3.5 mm cortex screws (pp. 214, 215).
– Instruments for insertion of 4.5 mm cannulated screws (p. 128).
– Instruments for application of 3.5 mm reconstruction plate (p. 216).
– Instruments for application of one-third tubular plate (p. 216).
– Instruments for application of 3.5 mm DCP or LC-DCP (pp. 215, 216).

7.5.6 Checklist for Operative Technique

Fractures of the medial or lateral epicondyle or condyle (A1, B1–3):
– Medial or lateral approach.
– Identify ulnar nerve in medial approaches.
– Reduction with Kirschner wires, or small hook.
– Lag screw fixation with 4.0 mm cancellous bone screws (p. 195), 3.5 mm cortex screws (p. 196) or 4.5 mm cannulated screws (p. 126).
– Application of a one-third tubular plate for larger fragments (p. 201).

Supracondylar fractures (A2, A3):
  Posterior approach (Campbell, van Gorder approach, turning down tongue of triceps aponeurosis).
– The ulnar nerve is identified.
– Exposure of fracture using Hohmann style retractors medially and laterally, taking care not to damage the radial nerve on the lateral side.
– Reduction of the fracture with pointed reduction forceps and temporary fixation with Kirschner wires.
– Insertion of 3.5 mm cortex screws as lag screws if possible (p. 196).
– Application of 3.5 mm DCP or LC-DCP as compression or neutralisation plate (pp. 202, 208) Location of the plate depends on the fracture but most often it is placed on the posterior aspect of the bone. If distal purchase is not adequate in low fractures two 3.5 mm reconstruction plates (one medially and one laterally) are used (p. 213).

Distal Humerus

Incision:
– Starts in the middle of the supracondylar area of the humerus, curves radially to avoid the point of olecranon, continuing distally towards the posterior border of the ulna (Fig. 10).

Preparation of instruments
– Instruments for application of tension band wire (p. 369).
– Instruments for insertion of 4.0 mm cancellous bone screws (p. 214).
– Instruments for insertion of 3.5 mm cannulated screw (p. 134).
– Instruments for application of one-third tubular plate (p. 216).
– Instruments for application of 3.5 mm DCP or LC-DCP (pp. 215, 216).
– Instruments for application of 3.5 mm reconstruction plates (p. 216).

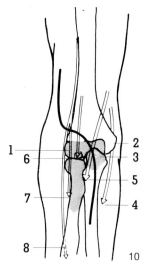

1 Capitulum of humerus
2 Medial epicondyle
3 Coronoid process
4 Ulnar nerve
5 Median nerve
6 Lateral cutaneous nerve of forearm
7 Deep branch of radial nerve
8 Superficial branch of radial nerve

7.6.6 Checklist for Operative Technique

Transverse or oblique fractures:
– The ulnar nerve is identified.
– Reduction with a small pointed reduction forceps. A 2.0 mm drill bit is used to pre-drill the distal transverse hole for the figure-of-eight wire.
– Insertion of the two parallel Kirschner wires.
– Insertion of the tension band wire deep to the triceps tendon, around the two Kirschner wires (p. 366).
– In oblique fractures a 4.0 mm cancellous bone screw may be inserted first as a lag screw (p. 195).

Multifragmentary fractures:
– The ulnar nerve is identified.
– Reduction first distally and then proceeding towards the joint using the small pointed forceps and Kirschner wires.
– An associated fracture of the coronoid process is reduced and fixed with a 4.0 mm cancellous bone screw or a 3.5 mm cannulated screw as a lag screw (pp. 126, 195).
– Insertion of further lag screws where necessary.
– Contouring of the selected plate.
– Protection of the lag screws with a one-third tubular plate, a 3.5 mm DCP or LC-DCP, or a 3.5 mm reconstruction plate (pp. 215, 216).
– In fractures proximal to the coronoid process, a tension band wire may suffice as long as the radial head is normal.
– Bone graft is necessary if there is a bone defect.

7.6.7 Special Consideration – Escape Routes

The Kirschner wires must not be crossed but placed parallel. They should not be angled too anteriorly near the coronoid process into the joint.

Before tightening the figure-of-eight wire, two loops should be made. This allows simultaneous tightening and twisting ensuring uniform tension in the wire. The wire loops are tightened by pulling, and the slack taken up by twisting. Trying to tighten the wire by twisting results in an asymmetrical spiral with the danger of wire breakage (p. 367).

Wires must be straightened first and then pulled and twisted at the same time to avoid failure.

Tension band wiring can be successfully employed also in osteoporotic bone.

7.6.8 Postoperative Care

- Suction drainage is used for 24–36 h.
- A well-padded posterior plaster splint is used for 2–3 days with the elbow in medium flexion.
- The arm is elevated so that the elbow is high and the forearm horizontal on a pillow.
- Active flexion – extension exercises are begun immediately.
- Continuous passive motion is advantageous, if available, when postoperative swelling has reduced.

7.6.9 Implant Removal

Implants should be removed only if they cause symptoms.

7.6.10 Recommended Reading

Heim U, Pfeiffer KM (1988) Internal fixation of small fragments, 3rd edn. Springer, Berlin Heidelberg New York

Müller ME, Allgöwer M, Schneider R, Willenegger H (1991) Manual of internal fixation, 3rd edn. Springer, Berlin Heidelberg New York

Müller ME, Nazarian S, Koch P, Schatzker J (1990) The comprehensive AO classification of fractures of long bones. Springer, Berlin Heidelberg New York

Rüedi T, Hochstetter AHC, Schlumpf R (1984) Surgical Approaches for Internal Fixation. Springer, Berlin Heidelberg New York

Schatzker J, Tile M (1987) The rationale of operative fracture care. Springer, Berlin Heidelberg New York

Sequin F, Texhammar R (1981) AO/ASIF instrumentation. Springer, Berlin Heidelberg New York

7.7 Fractures of the Radial Head

Displaced radial head fractures may result in loss of motion of the elbow and forearm rotation. They should be treated operatively, especially in younger patients. Radial head reconstruction is strongly indicated if there is associated instability of the humero-ulnar joint complex. A skilled, experienced surgeon is required for this difficult procedure.

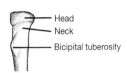

1a

7.7.1 Anatomy

Radial head from the front (Fig. 1a).
Radial head from behind (Fig. 1b).

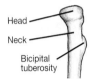

1b

7.7.2 Assessment

Special examination:
– Look for medial bruising to indicate associated humero-ulnar instability.
– Check for radial nerve function.

Radiography:
– AP and lateral views perpendicular to the radial head.
– Tomography.

7.7.3 AO Classification (Includes Proximal Ulna)

Type 21 A: Extra-articular fractures (see Fig. 7.6.2).
Type 21 B: Articular fractures of one bone (see Fig. 7.6.3).
Type 21 C: Articular fractures of both bones (see Fig. 7.6.4).

7.7.4 Indications for Osteosynthesis
– Implants of Choice

Fractures:
– Wedge fractures and depressed fractures multifragmentary fractures with intact segment of the radial head still in continuity with the shaft.

Implants:
– Depending of the size of fragment; 1.5 mm, 2.0 mm or 2.7 mm cortex screws as lag screws (Fig. 2).

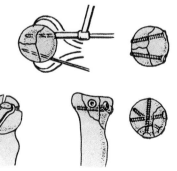

2

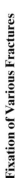

7.7.5 Preoperative Planning and Preparation

Timing:
– Earliest convenience. Not an emergency.

Position:
– Supine with the arm on an armboard in medium flexion, forearm in pronation.

Incision:
– Dorsolateral longitudinal incision. The exposure is enlarged with osteotomy of the lateral epicondyle and its reflection anteriorly with the extensor muscle origins (Fig. 3).

Preparation of instruments:
– Instruments for insertion of 1.5 mm cortex screw as lag screw (p. 269).
– Instruments for insertion of 2.0 mm cortex screw as lag screw (p. 268).
– Instruments for insertion of 2.7 mm cortex screw as lag screw (p. 267).

1 Lateral epicondyle
2 Head of radius
3 Olecranon
4 Deep branch of radial nerve
5 Superficial branch of radial nerve

7.7.6 Checklist for Operative Technique

– The radial nerve is identified in the substance of the supinator muscle. Pressure from retractors must be avoided.
– Reduction with fine pointed reduction forceps (termite or stag beetle reduction forceps).
– Provisional fixation with fine Kirschner wires (0.8 mm or 1.0 mm).
– Insertion of two or more screws as lag screws parallel to the joint and perpendicular to the fracture planes:
  1.5 mm cortex screw (p. 253).
  2.0 mm cortex screws (p. 251).
  2.7 mm cortex screws (p. 249).
– Bone graft is inserted in defect fractures.

7.7.7 Special Consideration – Escape Routes

If there is no continuity of the head and neck, reduction and fixation is impossible. The head is then excised. Prosthetic replacement is indicated when the elbow is dislocated and the medial collateral ligament ruptured and/or with associated fracture of the ulna.

Radial Head

461

7.7.8 Postoperative Care

– Suction drainage is used for 24–36 h.
– A well-padded posterior plaster splint is applied with the elbow at 90°.
– Active flexion – extension and pronation-supination exercises are begun early.

7.7.9 Implant Removal

Screw removal is only undertaken if the screw head causes discomfort to the patient.

7.7.10 Recommended Reading

Heim U, Pfeiffer KM (1988) Internal fixation of small fragments, 3rd edn. Springer, Berlin Heidelberg New York

Müller ME, Allgöwer M, Schneider R, Willenegger H (1991) Manual of internal fixation, 3rd edn. Springer, Berlin Heidelberg New York

Müller ME, Nazarian S, Koch P, Schatzker J (1990) The comprehensive AO classification of fractures of long bones. Springer, Berlin Heidelberg New York

Rüedi T, Hochstetter AHC, Schlumpf R (1984) Surgical Approaches for Internal Fixation. Springer, Berlin Heidelberg New York

Schatzker J, Tile M (1987) The rationale of operative fracture care. Springer, Berlin Heidelberg New York

7.8 Fractures of the Radius and the Ulna

Fractures of either one or both bones in the forearm constitute strong indications for operative stabilisation. It is the only way of achieving the early mobilisation necessary to ensure recovery of pronation and supination. Only undisplaced fractures of the distal third of the ulna may sometimes be treated by nonoperative means.

7.8.1 Anatomy

Ulna and radius from the front (Fig. 1 a).
Ulna and radius from behind (Fig. 1 b).

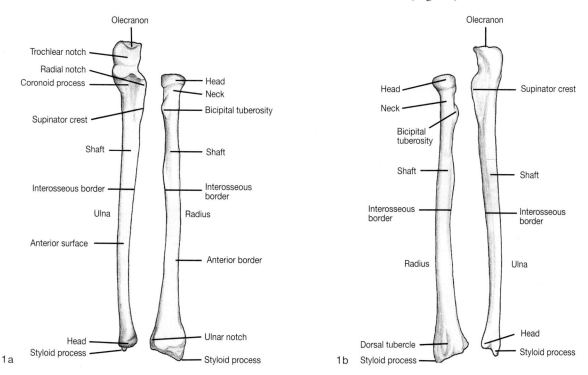

1 a

1 b

7.8.2 Assessment

Special examination:
– Compartment syndrome.

Radiography:
– Standard AP and lateral views.
– X-rays also of the distal and proximal ends of both bones.
– In ulnar fractures radial head displacement must be checked (Monteggia injury).

7.8.3 AO Classification

See also Sect. 5.1

Type 22 A: Simple fractures of one or both bones (Fig. 2)
Type 22 B: Wedge fractures of one or both bones (Fig. 3).
Type 22 C: Complex fractures of one or both bones (Fig. 4).

7.8.4 Indication for Osteosynthesis – Implants of Choice

Fractures:
– Fractures of the diaphysis.

Implants:
– 3.5 mm cortex screws as lag screws separate or through the plate.
– 3.5 mm DCP or LC-DCP seven, eight or more holes.
In the proximal or distal end a shorter plate may have to be chosen (Figs. 5, 6).
– 4.5 mm DCP or LC-DCP in tall patients.

7.8.5 Preoperative Planning and Preparation

Timing:
– As soon as possible. Urgently if evidence of compartment syndrome.

Position:
– Supine.
– Isolated ulnar fractures: arm pronated and laid across the chest.
– Isolated radial fractures: arm abducted and in neutral rotation.
– Both bones: arm maximally pronated and in abduction, elbow flexed.
– Tourniquet.

Incision:
– Ulnar shaft: Parallel and slightly volar to the subcutaneous crest of the ulna (Fig. 7a).
– Radial shaft: On a line joining the lateral epicondyle of humerus with radial styloid process.(Fig. 7b) An alternative is the Henry anterior approach to the radial shaft, through an incision starting at the flexor crease of the elbow and following the medial border of the brachioradialis belly distally toward the lower forearm: some surgeons prefer this for more proximal radial fractures.

Preparation of instruments:
– Instruments for the application of a 3.5 mm DCP or LC-DCP and 3.5 mm cortex screws as lag screws (pp. 215, 216).
– Instruments for the application of a 4.5 mm DCP or LC-DCP (p. 112).

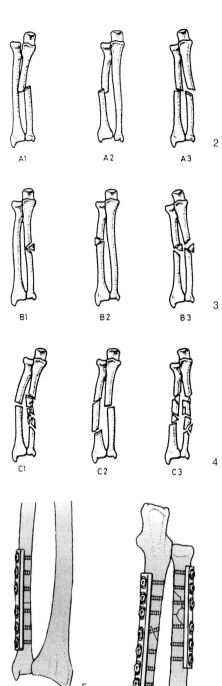

A1 A2 A3 2

B1 B2 B3 3

C1 C2 C3 4

5

6

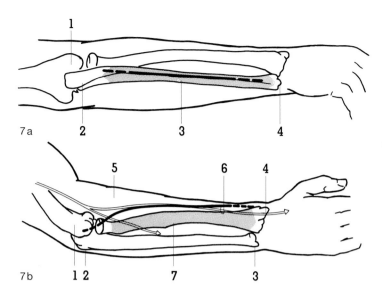

1 Lateral epicondyle of humerus
2 Olecranon
3 Posterior crest of ulna
4 Styloid process of ulna

1 Lateral epicondyle of humerus
2 Olecranon
3 Styloid process of ulna
4 Styloid process of radius
5 "Mobile wad" (radial extensor muscles)
6 Superficial branch of radial nerve
7 Deep branch of radial nerve

7.8.6 Checklist for Operative Technique (Both Bones)

– Approach and atraumatic reduction of the easiest fracture, usually the ulnar fracture. Both fractures should be exposed and provisionally reduced before either fixation is completed.
– The ulnar plate is applied to the medial border of the bone.
– The radial plate is most often placed on the anterior surface in the upper third and on the dorsolateral side in the distal two thirds. In distal fractures the flat anterior surface may be the best site.
– In oblique or wedge fractures 3.5 mm cortex screws are inserted as lag screws either separately first or through the plate.
– Contouring of the plates using the malleable templates.
– Fixation of the plate provisionally to one main fragment with a screw and to the other side with a small reduction forceps (or a screw).
– The second bone is approached and its fracture exposed.
– If reduction is impossible the plate on the other bone is loosened and the second bone reduced.
– After reduction and provisional fixation of both bones, pronation and supination are examined. If free, all the screws are inserted. The plate is applied either as a compression plate or as a neutralisation plate (pp. 202–211).
– Bone graft is applied when a defect or small devitalised fragments are present. The interosseous border must be avoided: radio-ulnar bridging callus may otherwise form.
– Closure of both incisions without tension may be difficult. The ulnar wound should preferably be closed, since it is located close to the subcutaneous border. The radial wound however, can be left open over a portion of its length, if the metal implant is safely placed under the muscle.

Radius and Ulna

465

7.8.7 Special Consideration – Escape Routes

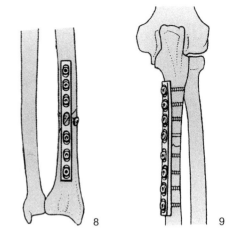

Fractures of the radius with distal radioulnar subluxation (Galeazzi fracture) (Fig. 8): The subluxation is most often reduced by anatomical reduction and stable fixation of the radial fracture. The stability of the joint must be checked by X-ray.

Fractures of the ulna with associated radial head dislocation (Monteggia injury) (Fig. 9): In most cases following anatomical reduction and stable fixation of the ulna, the radial head will reduce and remain stable in full supination. An X-ray is taken to confirm. If reduction is doubtful, the radial head is approached separately and inspected. Any soft tissue interposition (torn annular ligament or radial nerve) has to be removed and the ligament repaired. The radial head may now be stable.

If a single fragment of the radial head is present fixation with lag screws is necessary (see Sect. 7.7.6). In most cases, a long arm cast in supination is used for 6 weeks.

7.8.8 Postoperative Care

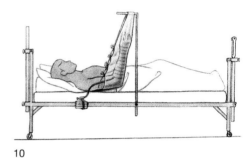

– Suction drainage is used for the first 24–36 h.
– A well-padded dressing is applied and the arm is kept elevated for the first 48 h (Fig. 10).
– Fingers, elbow and wrist are moved immediately. Functional mobilisation starts as soon as there is no pain.

10

7.8.9 Implant Removal

Plates in the diaphysis should not be removed earlier than 2 years after fixation. Plates in the proximal radius can be left in place.

7.8.10 Recommended Reading

Heim U, Pfeiffer KM (1988) Internal fixation of small fragments, 3rd edn. Springer, Berlin Heidelberg New York

Müller ME, Allgöwer M, Schneider R, Willenegger H (1991) Manual of internal fixation, 3rd edn. Springer, Berlin Heidelberg New York

Müller ME, Nazarian S, Koch P, Schatzker J (1990) The comprehensive AO classification of fractures of long bones. Springer, Berlin Heidelberg New York

Rüedi T, Hochstetter AHC, Schlumpf R (1984) Surgical Approaches for Internal Fixation. Springer, Berlin Heidelberg New York

Schatzker J, Tile M (1987) The rationale of operative fracture care. Springer, Berlin Heidelberg New York

7.9 Fractures of the Distal Radius

One of the most common fractures, the Colles fracture, is found in the distal radius region. As a fresh extra-articular fracture it is most often treated conservatively. Percutaneous Kirschner wires are sometimes used to maintain reduction. Open reduction and internal fixation has proved effective for:
– Fractures of the radial styloid, if displaced
– Flexion fractures, e. g. reversed Barton, Smith-Goyrand
– Multifragmentary articular fractures – Y-fractures

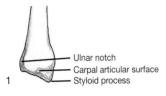

7.9.1 Anatomy

Ulnar notch
Carpal articular surface
Styloid process

Distal radius from the front (Fig. 1.)

7.9.2 Assessment

Special examination:
– Median nerve function.

Radiography:
– AP and lateral views are essential.
– Tomography for joint fractures.

7.9.3 AO Classification

See also Sect. 5.1

Type 23 A: Extra-articular fractures of the radius and/or the ulna (Fig. 2).
Type 23 B: Partial articular fracture of the radius (Fig. 3).
Type 23 C: Complete articular fracture of the radius (Fig. 4).

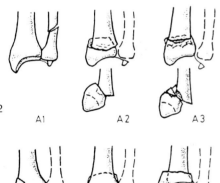

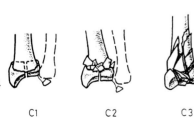

7.9.4 Indication for Osteosynthesis – Implants of Choice

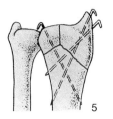
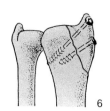

Fracture:
– Displaced Colles fracture (A2).

Implants:
– Kirschner wires (Fig. 5).

Fracture:
– Displaced unstable fracture of the styloid process (B1).

Implants:
– 4.0 mm cancellous bone screws, 3.5 mm cortex screws or 3.5 mm cannulated screws (Fig. 6).
– 2.7 mm condylar plate.

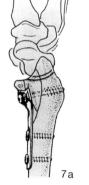
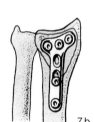

Fracture:
– Intra-articular fracture with proximal or volar displacement: reversed Barton (B3).

Implants:
– Small T plate on the volar aspect (Fig. 7).

Fracture:
– Y-fracture (C1).

Implants:
– Small T plate on the side of greater comminution.

Fracture:
– Multifragmentary articular fracture (C3).

Implants:
– Kirschner wires and small external fixator (Fig. 8).
– Small oblique T plate dorsally.
– Cancellous bone graft.

7.9.5 Preoperative Planning and Preparation

Timing:
– In fresh fractures as soon as possible, especially if evidence of median nerve compromise.

Position:
– Volar approach: Supine with the arm on an arm board abducted and supinated. The wrist is extended over a roll. Tourniquet
– Dorsal approach: Supine with the wrist slightly flexed and placed on an arm board. Tourniquet

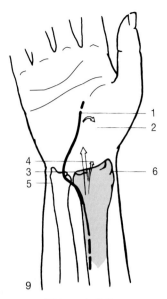

1 Thenar crease ("Linea vitalis")
2 Thenar branch of median nerve
3 Median nerve
4 Palmar branch of median nerve
5 Styloid process of ulna
6 Styloid process of radius

Incision:
– Volar approach: Starts at the thenar crease (linea vitalis) of the palm, curves toward the middle of the forearm, with a transverse segment as it crosses the volar flexion crease of the wrist (Fig. 9).
– Dorsal approach: A z- or s-shaped incision from the base of the second metacarpal over the wrist to the distal forearm is suggested for good healthy young skin. The safest incision is a straight midline longitudinal one in line with the third metacarpal and into the distal forearm. This passes safely between the dorsal sensory branches of the ulnar nerve medially, and of the radial nerve laterally.

Preparation of instruments:
– Instruments for application of the small external fixator (p. 338).
– Instruments for insertion of 4.0 mm cancellous bone screws or 3.5 mm cortex screws (pp. 214, 215).
– Instruments for insertion of 3.5 mm cannulated screws (p. 134).
– Instruments for application of small oblique or right angle T plates (p. 216).
– Instruments for harvesting cortical and cancellous bone grafts (p. 369).

7.9.6 Checklist for Operative Technique

Fractures of the radial styloid, multifragmentary fresh fractures and dorsally angulated metaphyseal fractures:
– Dorsal approach.
– Identification of ligaments, tendons, vessels, and the dorsal branch of the radial nerve.
– Exposure of the fracture using Hohmann-type retractors.
– Reduction with Kirschner wires and/or small reduction forceps.
– Lag screw fixation with 4.0 mm cancellous bone screws (p. 195) or 3.5 mm cortex screws (p. 196) or 3.5 mm cannulated screws (p. 133).
– Application of the small oblique or right angle T plate. First the plate is temporary fixed to the proximal fragment with a screw in the proximal oval hole. After final reduction and adjusting the plate, it is fixed definitively (p. 212).

Fractures with volar and proximal displacement (reversed Barton fracture):
– Identification of ligaments, tendons, vessels, and the median nerve for decompression.
– Reduction of volar fragment with small reduction forceps. Y-fractures are reduced by continuous traction of the thumb.

Distal Radius

– The small T plate is applied first with a screw in the proximal oval hole and after final reduction the remaining screws are inserted.

7.9.7 Special Consideration – Escape Routes

In conjunction with styloid fractures, a scaphoid fracture may exist as a result of a transscaphoid-perilunar fracture-dislocation. These fractures are fixed with 2.7 mm cortex screws.
In conjunction with a distal radius fracture a transverse or short oblique fracture of the distal narrow part of the ulna may occur. This is an absolute indication for a plate fixation with either a 3.5 mm or a 2.7 mm DCP or LC-DCP.

7.9.8 Postoperative Care

– Suction drainage for 24–36 h.
– A well-padded plaster splint is applied with the wrist slightly extended in a physiological position.
– The limb is elevated (see Fig. 10 in Sect. 7.8)
– Active mobilisation of the hand and the wrist is started at 24 h.

7.9.9 Implant Removal

In younger patients and if the implants cause discomfort of any kind they are removed after consolidation of the fracture (8 months or more).

7.9.10 Recommended Reading

Heim U, Pfeiffer KM (1988) Internal fixation of small fragments, 3rd edn. Springer, Berlin Heidelberg New York
Müller ME, Allgöwer M, Schneider R, Willenegger H (1991) Manual of internal fixation, 3rd edn. Springer, Berlin Heidelberg New York
Müller ME, Nazarian S, Koch P, Schatzker J (1990) The comprehensive AO classification of fractures of long bones. Springer, Berlin Heidelberg New York

7.10 Fractures in the Hand

Most fractures in the hand are treated conservatively. Open fractures with severe soft tissue damage may best be treated with Kirschner wires and cerclage or hemi-cerclage wiring. In multiple fractures with associated tendon, vascular,and/or nerve lesions, as well as in fractures involving the articular surface stable, internal fixation is necessary to achieve the best functional result. Internal fixation of hand fractures should be made as stable as possible with as little material as possible.

7.10.1 Anatomy

Hand, dorsal view (Fig. 1).

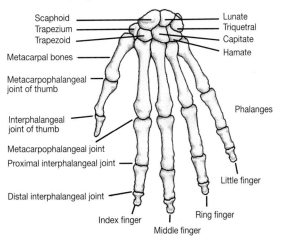

1

7.10.2 Assessment

Special examination:
– Clinical examination of tendon and neurological function to the extent that the injury permits.
– Examination also for rotational deformity of the fingers, especially in metacarpal fractures.

Radiography:
– AP, lateral and oblique views.
– Good views of the carpus as associated wrist injuries are common.

7.10.3 AO Classification

The hand and the carpal bones are in the anatomical zone 7. The subtypes and groups are not yet defined.

Hand

471 ■

7.10.4 Indication for Osteosynthesis – Implants of Choice

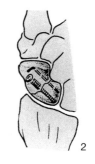

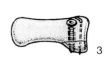

Fracture:
- Displaced, unstable scaphoid fracture, especially with lunate displacement.

Implants:
- 2.0 mm or 2.7 mm cortex screws as lag screws (Fig. 2).
- 3.5 mm cannulated screws as lag screws.

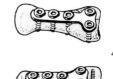

Fracture:
- Extra-and intra-articular fractures of the first metacarpal, e. g. Bennet's and Rolando's fractures.

Implants:
- Threaded or nonthreaded Kirschner wires (small-sized fragments).
- 2.0 mm or 2.7 mm cortex screws as lag screws (Fig. 3; Bennet's fracture).
- 2.7 mm T or L plates (Fig. 4. Rolando's fracture).
- 2.0 mm condylar plate.

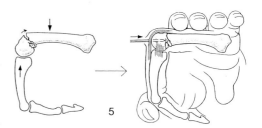

Fractures:
- Unstable, displaced fractures of the second to fifth metacarpals.

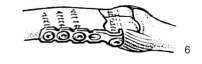

Implants:
- Percutaneous pinning with Kirschner wires 1.6 mm or 2.0 mm diameter in small fragments. Transosseous sutures (Fig. 5).
- 2.0 mm T plate or condylar plate in displaced basal fractures of second and fifth metacarpals (Fig. 6).
- Small external fixator in multifragmentary fractures.
- 2.0 mm or 2.7 mm cortex screws as lag screws in spiral fractures (see Fig. 7).
- Quarter-tubular plate or 2.7 mm DCP as neutralisation plate, especially in lag screw fixation of the second to fifth metacarpals, particularly spiral fractures with rotational displacement (see Fig. 7).

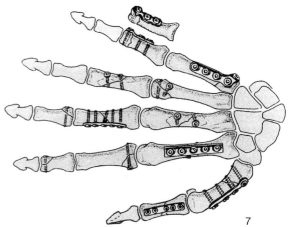

Fixation of Various Fractures

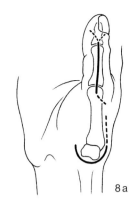

8a

Fracture:
- Articular fractures of the proximal interphalangeal (PIP) joints and the distal interphalangeal (DIP) joints.
- Phalangeal shaft fractures prone to secondary angular deformation in normal rotation.

Implants:
- Kirschner wires 1.0 mm or 1.25 mm in diameter.
- 1.5 mm or 2.0 mm cortex screws as lag screws (see Fig. 7).
- 1.5 mm or 2.0 mm condylar plates (see Fig. 7).

7.10.5 Preoperative Planning and Preparation

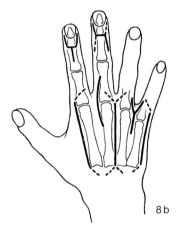

8b

Timing:
- As soon as possible in fresh fractures.

Position:
- Supine with the hand on a radiolucent armrest.

Incision:
- First metacarpal: dorso-ulnar or dorso-radial approach (Fig. 8a).
- Second to fifth metacarpals: longitudinal between the bones and with Y-extensions as necessary.
- Phalanges: longitudinal dorsolateral (Fig. 8b).

Preparation of instruments:
- Instruments for insertion of Kirschner wires (p. 234).
- Instruments for insertion of 1.5 mm or 2.0 mm cortex screws and mini-condylar plates (pp. 268, 269).
- Instruments for insertion of 2.7 mm cortex screws and 2.7 mm plates (p. 267).
- Instruments for insertion of 3.5 mm cannulated screws (p. 134).
- Instruments for application of the small external fixator (p. 338).

7.10.6 Checklist for Operative Technique

Scaphoid fractures:
- The superficial branch of the radial nerve is identified and retracted dorsally.
- The tendons and the radial artery retracted; direction depends on exact choice of surgical approach.
- The fracture is exposed and reduced with atraumatic elevators, fine forceps or small hook.
- A Kirschner wire, threaded or nonthreaded, is inserted from the tubercle across the fracture site.

Hand

- The length is determined.
- The 2.0 mm or the 2.7 mm cortex screws (pp. 249, 251), or the 3.5 mm cannulated screws are inserted as a lag screws (p. 133).

Fractures of the first metacarpal:
- Nerves and tendons are identified.
- The fracture is temporary reduced with fine Kirschner wires or fine reduction forceps.
- Lag screw fixation from the dorsal side with 2.7 mm or 2.0 mm cortex screws (pp. 249, 251).
- In intra-or extra articular fractures, a 2.7 mm T plate is applied after restoration of the articular surface with Kirschner wires (p. 259). A 2.0 mm condylar plate is an alternative (p. 264).

Fractures of the second to fifth metacarpals:
- Long spiral fractures of the shaft are fixed with 2.0 mm or 1.5 mm cortex screws as lag screws, sometimes combined with a 2.0 mm DCP as protection plate (p. 265).
- Transverse fractures of the shaft may be fixed with 2.0 mm DCP or H-plate (p. 266).
- Distal transverse fractures are fixed with a dorsal 2.7 mm or 2.0 mm T plate.
- Oblique fractures close to the joint are fixed with a lateral 2.0 mm or 1.5 mm mini-condylar plate.
- Basal, unstable fractures are fixed with a dorsal 2.0 mm T plate or 2.0 mm condylar plate (p. 264).

Articular phalangeal fractures:
- Condylar fractures are in general fixed with mini lag screws or mini-condylar plates. Devascularisation must be avoided.

Large dorsal fragments and volar avulsion fractures:
- These fractures may be fixed with minilag screws. Comminution of the fragment is quite common.

Multifragmentary fractures:
- Secondary arthrodesis is suggested, especially if the soft tissue condition is poor. Screw fixation (2.0 mm) in combination with corticocancellous grafting is recommended for large bony defects.

Fractures of the phalangeal shaft:
- Displaced shaft fractures of the middle phalanx may be best fixed with a laterally placed 1.5 mm straight plate or a 1.5 mm condylar plate (p. 266).
- Plating is rarely indicated, but may be advantageous in combination injuries and transverse fractures.
- Percutaneous Kirschner wires are used as intramedullary splints for basal transverse fractures and certain spiral fractures. The wires are inserted across the joint of the middle phalanx (MP).

■ 474

7.10.7 Special Consideration – Escape Routes

Temporary transarticular Kirschner wires across the PIP and DIP joints may be necessary if there is a danger that the fixation is not rigid enough or that fragments tend to dislocate in extension. Fixation with Kirschner wires is still the commonest method in phalangeal fractures despite the tendency for distraction to occur. Care must be taken to avoid concomitant fixation of neighbouring joints.

7.10.8 Postoperative Care

- Suction drainage for 24–36 h.
- Internal fixation of hand fractures is supplemented by a carefully shaped external plaster splint for 4–6 weeks, with judicious removal for carefully supervised active movements from an early stage.
- Elevation of the arm. See Fig. 10 in Sect. 7.8.

7.10.9 Implant Removal

Kirschner wires and external fixators are removed after fracture healing (4–6 weeks). Other implants are removed on request after 8–12 months.

7.10.10 Recommended Reading

Heim U, Pfeiffer KM (1988) Internal fixation of small fragments, 3rd edn. Springer, Berlin Heidelberg New York

Müller ME, Allgöwer M, Schneider R, Willenegger H (1991) Manual of internal fixation, 3rd edn. Springer, Berlin Heidelberg New York

Müller ME, Nazarian S, Koch P, Schatzker J (1990) The comprehensive AO classification of fractures of long bones. Springer, Berlin Heidelberg New York

Rüedi T, Hochstetter AHC, Schlumpf R (1984) Surgical Approaches for Internal Fixation. Springer, Berlin Heidelberg New York

Schatzker J, Tile M (1987) The rationale of operative fracture care. Springer, Berlin Heidelberg New York

7.11 Fractures of the Pelvis

Fractures of the pelvis have become a focus of increasing interest in recent years and numerous studies have been done with regard to different types of injury, treatment, and late results. These studies have shown that approximately 65 % of pelvic fractures are stable injuries, rarely requiring internal fixation. Unstable pelvic injuries may have rotational instability or linear instability. Rotationally unstable injuries are mostly of the "open book" type and become stable if closed. External fixation may well achieve this. In linear instability, the sacroiliac complex is totally disrupted and the hemipelvis migrates proximally and posteriorly. In this instance, internal fixation is usually required. The polytraumatised patient with a disruption of the pelvic ring has a very serious injury which carries a high mortality.

The essential management of polytrauma should include the stabilisation of musculo-skeletal injuries as early as possible. Sometimes the immediate stabilisation of the pelvis with a pelvic C-clamp, or an external fixator, may be lifesaving and the definitive stabilisation undertaken only when the patient's condition allows.

7.11.1 Anatomy

Male pelvis, from above and in front (Fig. 1 a).
Lateral (external) surface of the right pelvis from the front (Fig. 1 b).
Lateral (external) surface of the pelvis from behind (Fig. 1 c).

The pelvis is a ring structure. Its function is:
1. To transmit forces from the legs to the spine, and
2. To protect vital organs and major blood vessels within its cavity.

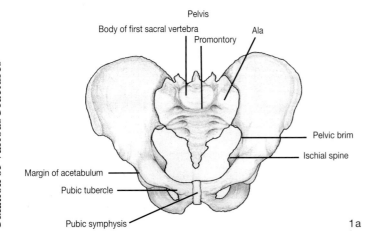

Pelvis
Body of first sacral vertebra
Ala
Promontory
Pelvic brim
Ischial spine
Margin of acetabulum
Pubic tubercle
Pubic symphysis
1a

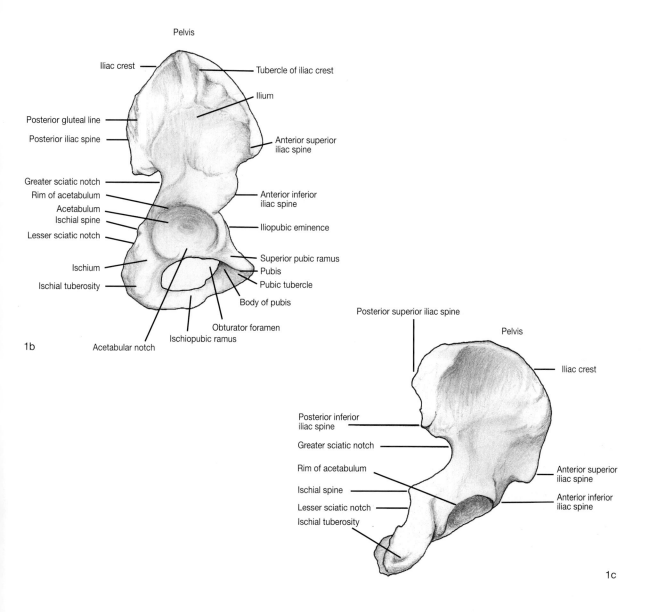

Pelvis

Iliac crest — — Tubercle of iliac crest

Ilium

Posterior gluteal line —

Posterior iliac spine —

— Anterior superior
iliac spine

Greater sciatic notch —
Rim of acetabulum —
Acetabulum —
Ischial spine —
Lesser sciatic notch —

— Anterior inferior
iliac spine

— Iliopubic eminence

Ischium —

— Superior pubic ramus
— Pubis
— Pubic tubercle
Body of pubis

Ischial tuberosity —

1b

Acetabular notch
Ischiopubic ramus
Obturator foramen

Posterior superior iliac spine

Pelvis

— Iliac crest

Posterior inferior
iliac spine —

Greater sciatic notch —

Rim of acetabulum —

— Anterior superior
iliac spine

Ischial spine —

— Anterior inferior
iliac spine

Lesser sciatic notch —

Ischial tuberosity —

1c

7.11.2 Assessment

Special examination:
– Mechanism of injury. Skin damage gives a clue to the likelihood of major injury, e. g. tyre marks on lower abdomen.
– General assessment of the polytraumatised patient (airway,
  bleeding, CNS).
– The lower urinary tract (urethra or bladder) may be injured –
  assessment by an appropriate surgeon should be made before
  catheterisation.
– Inspection for major bleeding, or wounding in the ano-genital
  area.

Pelvis

– Careful peripheral neurological examination of the lower limbs.
– Determination of pelvic stability.

Radiography:
– AP view in the acute phase
– Inlet view; X-ray beam directed 60° from the head to the mid-pelvis (posterior displacement).
– Outlet view; X-ray beam directed 45° from the foot to the symphysis (vertical migration of the hemipelvis).
– CT scan

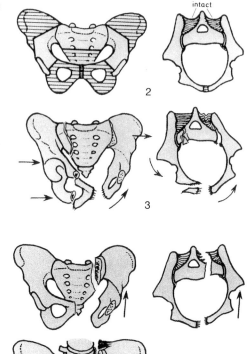

7.11.3 AO Classification (Tile)

Type A: Stable, minimally displaced. Pelvic ring is intact or not displaced (Fig. 2).
Type B: Rotationally unstable, vertically stable, including "open book" injury, lateral compression injury (Fig. 3).
Type C: Rotationally and vertically unstable, vertical shear. Rupture of the entire pelvic floor, including the sacroiliac complex (Fig. 4).

7.11.4 Indication for Osteosynthesis – Implants of Choice

Fracture:
– Open book fracture, more than 2.5 cm (Type B 1) without posterior instability.

Implants:
– External fixation, anteriorly
– Two- or three-hole 4.5 mm DCP, LC-DCP or reconstruction plate, on the superior aspect pelvis symphysis. Two plates in large patients (Fig. 5).

Fracture:
– Open book injury as part of a vertically unstable type C injury.

Implants:
– Two- or three-hole 4.5 mm DCP, LC-DCP, or reconstruction plate superiorly, and 3.5 mm (or 4.5 mm) reconstruction plate anteriorly (Fig. 6).

Fracture:
– Sacroiliac dislocation or fracture dislocation.

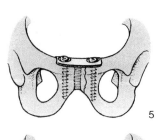

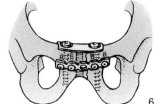

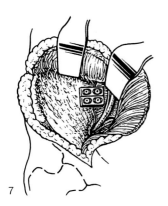

7

Implants:
- Two- or three-hole 3.5 mm DCP, placed across the anterior aspect of the sacroiliac joint. Usually two plates side to side (Fig. 7).
- 7.0 mm cannulated screws or 6.5 mm cancellous bone screws as lag screws inserted from the posterior aspect into sacrum with image intensification control in two planes (according to Matta) (Fig. 8).

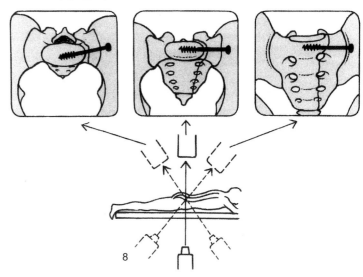

8

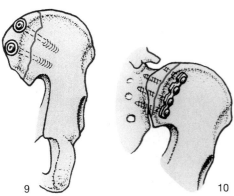

9

10

Fracture:
- Iliac fractures.

Implant:
- 7.0 mm cannulated screws or 6.5 mm cancellous bone screws as lag screws (Fig. 9).
- 3.5 mm or 4.5 mm DCP or reconstruction plates (Fig. 10).

Fracture:
- Sacral fracture, vertically unstable.

Implant:
- Sacral bars[1] (Fig. 11).
- 7.0 mm cannulated screws, especially in nonunions.

11

7.11.5 Preoperative Planning and Preparation

Timing:
- Early pelvic stabilisation with the pelvic C-clamp or with a simple anterior external frame is performed in patients with wide open book injury or unstable pelvic fractures. This reduces the intrapelvic venous and bony bleeding.

---

[1] Sacral bars in lengths from 100 mm to 200 mm in 20 mm increments are presently being developed. Contact SYNTHES for information.

Pelvis

– Definitive fixation is performed when the patient's general state has improved, usually after 5–7 days.

Positioning:
– Ruptures of the symphysis pubis: Supine with both anterior superior iliac spines freely accessible.
– Posterior fixation of the sacroiliac joint or the gluteal aspect of the ilium: Lateral or prone so that the entire wing of the ilium freely accessible.
– Anterior sacroiliac fixation: Supine with roll or pad beneath buttock, the whole wing of ilium accessible for ilio-inguinal approach.

Incision:
– Ruptures of the symphysis pubis: Horizontal incision about 15–20 cm one to two finger widths above the symphysis (Fig. 12).
– Posterior fixation of the sacroiliac joint or the gluteal aspect of the ilium: Starts one to two finger widths distally and laterally to the posterior superior iliac spine, extends upward parallel to the iliac crest, and terminates two to three finger widths past the highest point of the crest. The superior clunial nerves must be divided (Fig. 13).
– Anterior sacroiliac fixations: Incision starts at mid-inguinal point and follows the anterior 3/4 of iliac crest backwards (Fig. 14).

Preparation of instruments:
– Instruments for application of external fixation (p. 321).
– Instruments for application of 4.5 mm DCP or LC-DCP (p. 112).
– Instruments for application of 4.5 mm reconstruction plates (p. 112).
– Instruments for application of 3.5 mm reconstruction plates (p. 216).
– Instruments for inserting of 7.0 mm cannulated screws (p. 121).

7.11.6 Checklist for Operative Technique

Unstable injuries of the pelvic girdle:
– Acute stabilisation with the pelvic C-clamp (p. 222).

"Open book" injuries – external fixation:
– Application of a simple anterior rectangular frame. Two pins are placed percutaneously in each ilium at approximately 45° to each other, one in the anterior superior spine and one in the iliac tubercle, and joined by an anterior rectangular configuration.

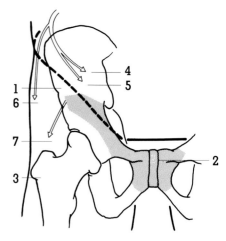

12

1 Anterior superior iliac spine
2 Symphysis pubis
3 Greater trochanter
4 Ilio-hypogastric nerve
5 Ilio-inguinal nerve
6 Lateral cutaneous branch of ilio-hypogastric nerve
7 Lateral cutaneous nerve of thigh

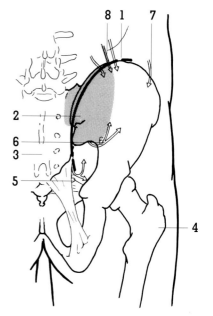

13

1 "Supracristal point" (highest point of iliac crest)
2 Posterior superior iliac spine
3 Medial sacral crest
4 Greater trochanter
5 Inferior gluteal nerve
6 Superior gluteal nerve
7 Lateral cutaneous branch of ilio-hypogastric nerve
8 Superior clunial nerves

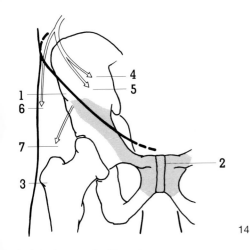

1 Anterior superior iliac spine
2 Symphysis pubis
3 Greater trochanter
4 Ilio-hypogastric nerve
5 Ilio-inguinal nerve
6 Lateral cutaneous branch
  of ilio-hypogastric nerve
7 Lateral cutaneous nerve of thigh

"Open book" injuries – plate fixation:
– Exposure of the obturator foramen and application of the pelvic reduction forceps through the foramen.
– Anatomical reduction. Care must be taken to avoid trapping the bladder or the urethra in the symphysis when closing the clamp.
– Application of a two- or three-hole DCP or LC-DCP fixed with fully threaded 6.5 mm cancellous bone screws on the superior aspect of the symphysis pubis (p. 94).
– In unstable pelvic disruption, application of an additional 3.5 mm reconstruction plate on the anterior aspect to avoid displacement in the vertical plane (p. 213).

14 Sacroiliac dislocation or fractures of the ilium, anterior ilio-inguinal approach:
– Exposure of the iliac crest and the sacroiliac joint including the ala of the sacrum.
– Anatomical reduction with pointed reduction forceps in the anterior superior spine of the ilium pulling forwards. The reduction is checked anteriorly at the greater sciatic notch. Care must be taken not to damage any nerves, especially the L5 root in front of the sacroiliac (SI) joint.
– Application of two two- or three-hole 3.5 mm DCP or LC-DCP (p. 202) fixed across the anterior surface of the sacroiliac joint with 4.0 mm fully threaded cancellous bone screws. Only one screw can be inserted into the sacrum to avoid the L5 nerve root, and only one or two into the adjacent ilium since the bone rapidly becomes very thin.
– In iliac fractures lag screw fixation with 7.0 mm cannulated screws (p. 117), or 6.5 mm cancellous bone screw (p. 81) may suffice or be complemented with a plate near the iliac crest.

Sacroiliac dislocation or fracture dislocation, posterior approach
– Exposure of the posterior superior spine, iliac crest and the sciatic notch. (Beware of the sciatic nerve.)
– Anatomical reduction, checked by placing the finger through the sciatic notch exploring the anterior aspect of the sacrum.
– A guide wire is inserted in the ala of the sacrum, across into the body of S1 and its position verified with image intensification.
– Insertion of one or two 7.0 mm cannulated screws with caution. Penetration of the neural canal or the S1 foramen is a serious complication. Image intensification is essential. The second screw is inserted distally to the S1 foramen where, however, the bone is extremely thin. Percutaneous insertion of the cannulated screws is possible in the most experienced hands.

Pelvis

Sacral fractures, posterior approach
- Exposure of the posterior spine
- A gliding hole is made through the posterior superior spine and a threaded bar driven through until it hits the opposite posterior iliac spine and emerges on the outer table of the iliac crest. Washers and nuts are applied and tightened and the bar cut off flush at the nut (Fig. 15).
- A second bar is placed distally and parallel to the first. The bars must be placed posterior to the sacrum to avoid the sacral spinal canal. The anterior sacral foramina may be palpated by placing a finger through the greater sciatic notch to the anterior surface of the sacrum and the posterior foramina may be visualised directly.

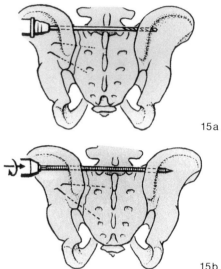

15a

15b

7.11.7 Special Consideration – Escape Routes

The posterior approach may be considered safe and straightforward, but there is a great risk of wound breakdown and nerve damage. Traction is used temporarily before surgery and often as postoperative care. Pelvic fractures may be associated with fractures of the acetabulum (See Sect. 7.12).

7.11.8 Postoperative Care

- Extensive multiple drainage for 24–48 h.
- The postoperative care is dependent on the quality of the fixation and the bone.
- If stability is secure both anteriorly and posteriorly, early mobilisation on crutches may start.
- To avoid asymmetrical load on the healing pelvis, swing-through (mermaid) walking with two crutches is advisable.

7.11.9 Implant Removal

Implants may be left in. Only in case of complaints are implants removed after 10 months. This usually applies only to sacral bars and screws in the iliac crest.

7.11.10 Recommended Reading

Müller ME, Allgöwer M, Schneider R, Willenegger H (1991) Manual of internal fixation, 3rd edn. Springer, Berlin Heidelberg New York
Rüedi T, Hochstetter AHC, Schlumpf R (1984) Surgical Approaches for Internal Fixation. Springer, Berlin Heidelberg New York
Schatzker J, Tile M (1987) The rationale of operative fracture care. Springer, Berlin Heidelberg New York

7.12 Fractures of the Acetabulum

Acetabular fractures are joint fractures and as such they require exact anatomical reduction to ensure a good long-term function of the hip joint. Closed reduction may be possible in a few cases, but more often open reduction and stable internal fixation are required. A satisfactory result may only be expected if the joint is congruous and stable following reduction, and if complications are avoided. This surgery is extremely demanding. It requires a skilful, experienced team and the best material resources. The age and the general state of the patient, as well as the assessment of other major injuries in the polytraumatised will determine the treatment. Traction may be the best option in elderly patients with poor bone quality.

Late complications such as avascular necrosis of the femoral head, heterotopic ossification, chondrolysis, and sciatic or femoral nerve injury may jeopardise the result.

7.12.1 Anatomy

Lateral (external) surface of the right pelvis from the front (see Fig. 1 b, p. 477).
Lateral (external) surface of the pelvis from behind (see Fig. 1 c, p. 477).

7.12.2 Assessment

Special examination:
– Detailed respiratory and hemodynamic appraisal in polytrauma.
– Monitoring of pulse, blood pressure, and urinary output.
– Urological and neurological injuries.

Radiography:
– AP view.
– A 45° oblique view of the pelvis with the hip rotated toward the X-ray tube (the obturator oblique).
– A 45° oblique view of the pelvis with the hip rotated away from the X-ray tube (the iliac oblique).
– CT scan of the pelvis.

7.12.3 AO Classification

Type A: Only one column of the acetabulum involved; posterior wall, posterior column, anterior wall fracture and variations (Fig. 1).

Type B: Transverse fracture component, where a portion of the roof remains attached to the intact ilium. (Fig. 2).

Type C: Fractures in both columns; fractures involving the anterior as well as the posterior column. All articular segments, including the roof, are detached from the remaining posterior segment of the intact ilium. (Fig. 3).

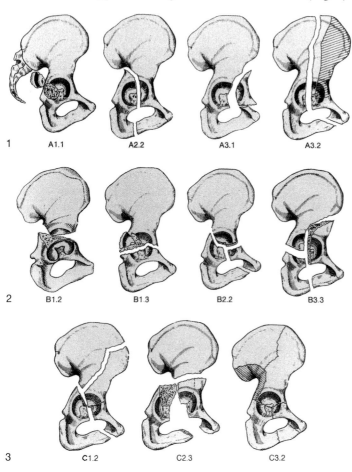

1   A1.1   A2.2   A3.1   A3.2

2   B1.2   B1.3   B2.2   B3.3

3   C1.2   C2.3   C3.2

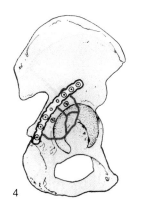

4

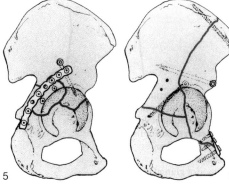

5   6

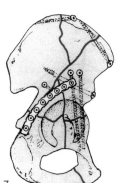

7

7.12.4 Indication for Osteosynthesis – Implants of Choice

Fracture:
– Posterior wall fracture (type A) (Fig. 4).

Implants:
– 6.5 mm cancellous bone screws as lag screws.
– 7.0 mm cannulated screws as lag screws.
– 4.0 mm cancellous bone screws.
– 3.5 mm reconstruction plate, curved.

Fracture:
– Anterior column and hemitransverse fractures (type B) (Figs. 5, 6).

Implants:
– 6.5 mm cancellous bone screws as lag screws.
– 7.0 mm cannulated screws.
– 4.0 mm cancellous bone screws.
– 3.5 mm reconstruction plate, straight.

Fracture:
– Fractures of both columns (type C) (Fig. 7).

Implants:
– 6.5 mm cancellous bone screws as lag screws.
– 7.0 mm cannulated screws as lag screws.
– 4.0 mm cancellous bone screws.
– 3.5 mm cortex screws, extra long.
– 3.5 mm reconstruction plate, curved.

7.12.5 Preoperative Planning and Preparation

Timing:
– Surgery is usually delayed until local bleeding has subsided and the patient is fit. Ideally it is performed within 10 days. Vascular or nerve injuries are indications for immediate surgery. Irreducible or unstable posterior dislocation of the femoral head is an indication for urgent surgery.

Positions:
– For the Kocher-Langenbeck approach (fractures type A1, A2, B1): Lateral or prone on a fracture table or a regular table on a vacuum mattress. The leg is draped to be freely mobile. The draping leaves most of the buttock free.
– For the straight lateral and ilio-femoral approach (fracture types A2, A3, B1, B2, C2, C3): Lateral on a fracture table or on regular table on a vacuum mattress The leg is draped freely mobile. The area is draped free to the symphysis pubis, to the

Acetabulum

Implants:
– 4.0 mm cancellous bone screws as lag screws (Fig. 5).

Fracture:
– Shear fracture of the head combined with neck fracture (C3.2, C3.3).

Implants:
– Total hip replacement (THR) or arthrodesis with cobra head plate depending on age (Fig. 6).

Fracture:
– Femoral neck fractures (B2, B3).

Implants:
– Three 7.0 mm cannulated screws, or 6.5 mm cancellous bone screws (Fig. 7).
– 130° angled blade plate (Fig. 8).
– DHS, with separate 6.5 mm cancellous bone screws (Fig. 9).

Fracture:
– Trochanteric- or intertrochanteric fractures.

Implants:
– DHS, in old patients with osteoporotic bone for unstable fractures with smaller fragments (Fig. 10).
– 95° condylar plate, especially in younger patients with large fragment fracture-and good quality bone (A1) (Fig. 11).
– DCS in younger patients (A3) (Fig. 12).

Fracture:
– Subtrochanteric fracture with extension into the trochanteric area.

Implants:
– 95° condylar plate (Fig. 13).
– DCS.

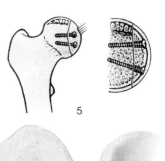

5

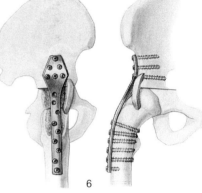

6

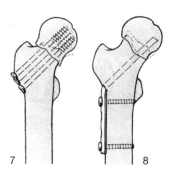

7

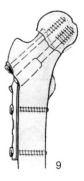

8

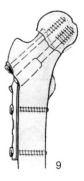

9

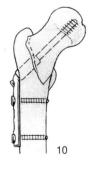

10

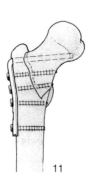

11

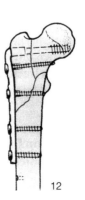

12

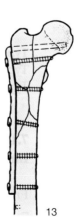

13

7.13.5 Preoperative Planning and Preparation

Timing:
– Open reduction and internal fixation should be performed as an urgent procedure within 6 h because of the risk of damage to the vascular supply of the femoral head.
– Joint replacements are elective procedures, but a displaced femoral head must be repositioned as an emergency manoeuvre prior to any further diagnostic steps.

Positioning:
– Supine with some padding beneath the buttock; the leg is draped so that it can be freely moved. A fracture table is often used to allow easy X-ray control.

Incision:
– A straight incision along a line joining the greater trochanter to a point approximately a handbreadth below the fracture (Fig. 14).

Preparation of instruments:
– Instruments for insertion of 4.0 mm cancellous bone screws (p. 214).
– Instruments for insertion of 7.0 mm cannulated screw (p. 121).
– Instruments of insertion of DHS (p. 150).
– Instruments for insertion of DCS (p. 150).
– Instruments for insertion of 95° condylar plate (p. 172).

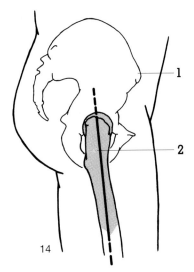

1 Anterior superior iliac spine
2 Greater trochanter

7.13.6 Checklist for Operative Technique

Large shear fractures of the femoral head:
– By drilling 2 mm holes in the main fragment, bleeding will confirm the preservation of the vascular supply.
– Anatomical reduction using for example a small sharp hook.
– Insertion of 4.0 mm cancellous bone screws as lag screws (p. 195).
– Elevation of a depression and bone grafting.

Femoral neck fracture:
– Anterior capsulotomy in line with the neck.
– Removal of the intracapsular haematoma.
– The fracture is exposed with the aid of three retractors; one long-tip 16 mm retractor and two short-tipped retractors. The head can be stabilised with the tip of an 8 mm retractor.
– Fixation with 7.0 mm cannulated screws (p. 117) or 6.5 mm cancellous bone screw (p. 81).
– Fixation with DHS and additional 6.5 mm cancellous bone screws as lag screws to prevent rotation of the head (p. 143).

Proximal Femur

Trochanteric fractures:
– Closed reduction is attempted; light traction, external rotation and abduction, otherwise open reduction and stabilisation with one of the following:
– Fixation with DHS (p. 143).
– Fixation with DCS (p. 150).
– Fixation with 95° condylar plate used with tension device (p. 161).

Subtrochanteric fractures with extension into the trochanteric area:
– Exposure of the fracture.
– Reduction of type A and B fractures before introduction of the condylar plate.
– In multifragmentary fractures (type C): introduction of the condylar blade plate before reduction using indirect reduction technique with the distractor (p. 355).
– Cancellous bone graft may be inserted in multifragmentary fractures.

7.13.7 Special Consideration – Escape Routes

Stable impacted subcapital fractures in older patients do not require internal fixation, unless they disimpact. Evacuation of the haemarthrosis may still be recommended to prevent impairment of the blood supply to the femoral head.

In femoral neck fractures with a vertical fracture plane the shearing force can be transformed into compression force by an intertrochanteric valgus osteotomy of 30° – 40°.

Preoperative drawings and planning of internal fixation for subtrochanteric fractures may help achieve a good result. A reversed X-ray of the normal side is used as a model.

If a 95° condylar blade plate or a DCS is used for the fixation of subtrochanteric fractures, the placement of the window for the seating chisel is of great importance. It is prepared at the junction of the anterior and the middle thirds of the greater trochanter. The seating chisel is inserted into the neck 1 cm below its superior cortex.

The condylar plate is introduced and fixed with a cortex screw in the proximal fragment into the calcar. The plate is then lined up with the shaft and a self-centring bone-holding forceps applied. The distractor is then applied with one bolt through the second plate hole and the other in a predrilled 4.5 mm hole distal to the plate. Slight distraction will enable reduction of the fragments and fixation of the plate first distally, then any lag screws and finally the remaining plate screws. Intraoperative X-ray control is a wise precaution. See also p. 18.

7.13.8 Postoperative Care

- Suction drainage for 24–36 h.
- Postoperative AP and cross-table lateral X-ray views.
- The entire leg is placed in a neutral position in a rubber foam splint.
- Mobilisation in a frame or with crutches on the 1st postoperative day.
- Depending on the stability, partial weight-bearing is allowed. In the elderly this may not be advisable.
- Isometric muscle exercises as soon as possible.
- Proximal femur fractures normally take 3–5 months to heal.

7.13.9 Implant Removal

In young patients implants may be removed after 12–18 months if healing has been uneventful. In the elderly implants are generally left in place if not symptomatic.

7.13.10 Recommended Reading

Mast J, Jakob R, Ganz R (1989) Planning and reduction technique in fracture surgery. Springer, Berlin Heidelberg New York

Müller ME, Allgöwer M, Schneider R, Willenegger H (1991) Manual of internal fixation, 3rd edn. Springer, Berlin Heidelberg New York

Müller ME, Nazarian S, Koch P, Schatzker J (1990) The comprehensive AO classification of fractures of long bones. Springer, Berlin Heidelberg New York

Regazzoni P, Rüedi T, Winquist R, Allgöwer M (1985) The dynamic hip screw implant system. Springer, Berlin Heidelberg New York

Rüedi T, Hochstetter AHC, Schlumpf R (1984) Surgical Approaches for Internal Fixation. Springer, Berlin Heidelberg New York

Schatzker J, Tile M (1987) The rationale of operative fracture care. Springer, Berlin Heidelberg New York

Sequin F, Texhammar R (1981) AO/ASIF instrumentation. Springer, Berlin Heidelberg New York

7.14 Fractures of the Femoral Shaft

Femoral shaft fractures are the result of significant trauma and are often associated with considerable soft tissue damage and with other fractures of the same leg. Urgent stable internal fixation is today the accepted method of treatment. This will reduce the risk of pathophysiological complication, as well as help to prevent permanent impairment of the knee function by early mobilisation. Medullary nailing, with or without locking, is the favoured method. Plating, however, has its place in certain fractures, as has external fixation.

7.14.1 Anatomy

Right femur from the front (Fig. 1a).
Right femur from behind (Fig. 1b).

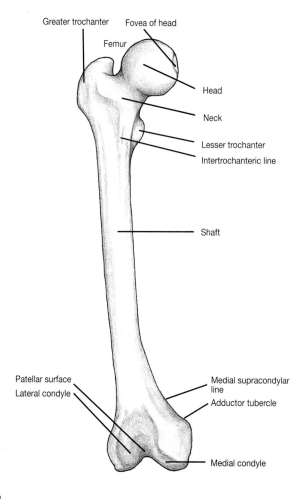

Greater trochanter — Fovea of head
Femur
Head
Neck
Lesser trochanter
Intertrochanteric line
Shaft
Patellar surface
Lateral condyle
Medial supracondylar line
Adductor tubercle
Medial condyle

1a

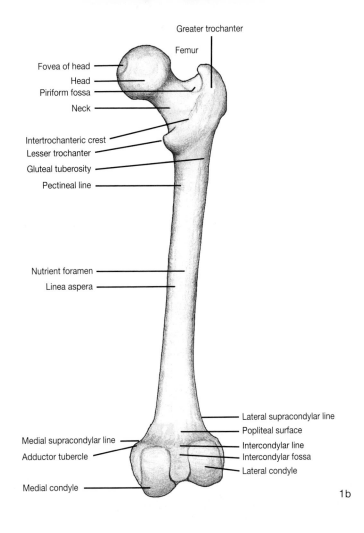

Greater trochanter
Femur
Fovea of head
Head
Piriform fossa
Neck
Intertrochanteric crest
Lesser trochanter
Gluteal tuberosity
Pectineal line

Nutrient foramen
Linea aspera

Lateral supracondylar line
Popliteal surface
Medial supracondylar line
Intercondylar line
Adductor tubercle
Intercondylar fossa
Lateral condyle
Medial condyle

1b

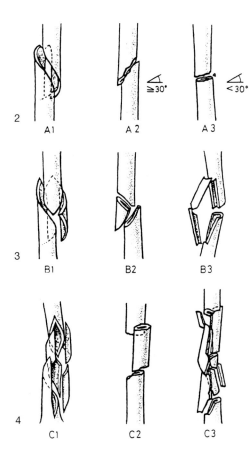

2

A1   A2   A3

3

B1   B2   B3

4

C1   C2   C3

7.14.2 Assessment

Special examination:
– Since these patients are often multiply injured, the general priorities such as respiratory, cardiovascular, cranial, thoracic, and abdominal needs are satisfied.
– The skeletal injuries should be recognised early and treated accordingly.
– Injuries to the knee ligaments may be involved.

Radiography:
– AP view, joints above and below included.

7.14.3 AO Classification

See also Sect. 5.1

Type 32 A: Simple fractures (Fig. 2).
Type 32 B: Wedge fractures (Fig. 3).
Type 32 C: Complex fractures (Fig. 4).

Femoral Shaft

495 ∎

7.14.4 Indications for Osteosynthesis –
Implants of Choice

Fracture:
– High subtrochanteric fracture of the femoral shaft (Types A, B).

Implants:
– 95° condylar plate, 4.5 mm cortex screws as lag screws (Fig. 5).
– DCS, 4.5 mm cortex screws as lag screws.

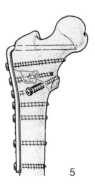

5

Fracture:
– Subtrochanteric fracture of the femoral shaft.

Implants:
– Universal interlocking nail – "closed" method for fractures at least 2 cm distal to the lesser trochanter.
– 95° condylar plate, 4.5 mm cortex screws as lag screws (Fig. 6).

Fracture:
– Transverse or short oblique fracture in the middle third (A2, A3).

Implants:
– Universal interlocking nail, "closed" method.

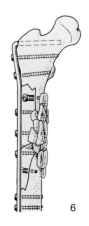

6

Fracture:
– Long spiral or butterfly fracture in the middle of the femur.

Implants:
– Universal interlocking nail, closed method (Fig. 7).
– Broad DCP or LC- DCP, 4.5 mm on the dorsolateral aspect of the bone, with lag screw through the plate if possible, otherwise separate. Bone graft on the medial side.

Fracture:
– Multifragmentary fracture in the middle of the femur (Type C).

Implants:
– Universal interlocking nail.
– Broad DCP or LC-DCP as a bridging plate on the dorsolateral aspect of the bone. The bridging plate is fixed to the intact distal and proximal part of the bone. Only a few 4.5 mm screws are used as lag screws to hold fragments in place.

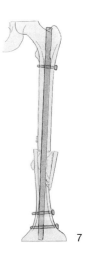

7

Fracture:
– Open fractures grade 2 and 3. (See also p. 43)

Implants:
– External fixator.

Fixation of Various Fractures

7.14.5 Preoperative Planning and Preparation

Timing:
– The associated injuries determine the timing for surgery. Early stabilisation of the fractured femur will, however, enhance the ease and quality of the nursing care, and is an important factor in managing the soft tissue injury.

Positioning:
– Lateral positioning on a vacuum mattress or similar support. The entire leg is disinfected and draped to allow free movement. The ipsilateral iliac crest is included in the preparation as donor site for bone graft.
– Supine position may be necessary for the polytraumatised patient.
– Fracture table, especially for "closed" nailing.

Incision:
– Made on a straight line connecting the greater trochanter with the lateral femoral condyle. The length depends upon the location and extent of the fracture. It also depends on fixation method (nail, plate) (Fig. 8).

Preparation of instruments:
– Instruments for application of 95° condylar plate (p. 172).
– Instruments for insertion of DCS (p. 150).
– Instruments for insertion of universal nail and for interlocking of the nail (pp. 306, 307).
– Instruments for application of DCP, 4.5 mm or LC-DCP, 4.5 mm (p. 112).
– Instruments for application of an external fixator (p. 337).

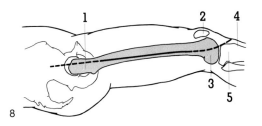

8

1 Greater trochanter
2 Patella
3 Lateral condyle of femur
4 Tuberosity of tibia
5 Tubercle of GERDY

7.14.6 Checklist for Operative Technique

Simple subtrochanteric fractures and fractures with a butterfly fragment:
– After exposure using three Hohmann retractors, the bony landmarks such as the superior of the femoral neck and the rough line of the greater trochanter are identified.
– Atraumatic reduction and fixation of the fracture or the butterfly fragment with 4.5 mm cortex screws as lag screws (p. 77).
– Preparation for and insertion of the 95° condylar plate (p. 161) or the DCS (p. 150) A 4.5 mm cortex screw is inserted through the most proximal plate hole into the calcar to enhance the stability of the fixation.

Complex, multifragmentary high subtrochanteric fractures:
– Exposure and identification of landmarks as above.
– Preparation for and insertion of the condylar plate (p. 161) or the DCS (p. 150) in the proximal fragment. Fixation with a 4.5 mm cortex screw in the calcar.
– Extensive cancellous bone grafting on the medial side. If graft is to be used medially, it should be inserted at this stage through the fracture gaps into the medial soft tissue and before fracture reduction. Inserting the graft after fixation necessitates further soft tissue dissection.
– Application of the distractor with the first bolt through the second proximal plate hole. Distal to the plate the other bolt is inserted through a predrilled 4.5 mm hole (p. 355). Through gentle distraction fragments are reduced indirectly. These should preferably be left undisturbed but may be fixed with lag screws through the plate, provided this does not destroy the soft tissue attachment. Final fixation of the plate. See also p. 18.

Subtrochanteric fractures of the femoral shaft, the fracture line 2 cm below the lesser trochanter and fractures in the middle third:
– For interlocked nailing the patient is positioned either on a regular table or on a fracture table. An image intensifier is necessary and has to be correctly placed and draped.
– Reduction of the fracture may be done with the distractor (p. 355). In "closed" medullary nailing the reduction may be performed with the patient on the fracture table using distal femoral skeletal traction and external manipulation.
– Insertion of the universal interlocking nail (p. 289).
– Application of a broad DCP or LC-DCP as tension band or neutralisation plate with lag screw through the plate (pp. 100, 102).
– Application of a broad DCP or LC-DCP as a bridging plate

Open fractures grade 2 and 3 (see also p. 43).
– Application of an external fixator (p. 331).

7.14.7 Special Consideration – Escape Routes

If open reduction and internal fixation are planned it may be easier to position the patient on a regular table and use the distractor for reduction. With the patient on a fracture table and the extremity in traction, strong tension of the soft tissue makes exposure, visualisation, retraction and manipulation difficult.
If plate fixation is chosen to stabilise a multifragmentary fracture of the shaft, it may be better to delay surgery for 7–10 days. It has been stated that during this interval the blood supply to many of the small fragments will have improved, which may en-

hance the bone healing. If surgery is to be delayed, the fracture is splinted and the extremity placed in skeletal traction. This must be balanced against the disadvantage that 7–10 days of traction can increase the risk of complications such as fat embolism syndrome and adult respiratory distress syndrome (ARDS).

7.14.8 Postoperative Care

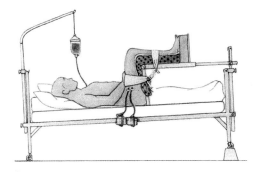

9

– Suction drainage for 24–36 h.
– The patient is positioned for the first 4–5 days with the hip and the knee flexed at 90° in the so-called 90/90/90/position (Fig. 9).
– As for intra-articular fractures, continuous passive motion is beneficial.
– On the 5th postoperative day the patient can sit, and within a day or two can get up using crutches.
– Partial weight-bearing of 10–15 kg may start. Depending on progression of healing further weight-bearing is allowed.

7.14.9 Implant Removal

Implants in weight-bearing bones are in general removed. If fracture healing has taken place without complications nails and plates are removed after 24–36 months.

7.14.10 Recommended Reading

Mast J, Jakob R, Ganz R (1989) Planning and reduction technique in fracture surgery. Springer, Berlin Heidelberg New York
Müller ME, Allgöwer M, Schneider R, Willenegger H (1991) Manual of internal fixation, 3rd edn. Springer, Berlin Heidelberg New York
Müller ME, Nazarian S, Koch P, Schatzker J (1990) The comprehensive AO classification of fractures of long bones. Springer, Berlin Heidelberg New York
Rüedi T, Hochstetter AHC, Schlumpf R (1984) Surgical Approaches for Internal Fixation. Springer, Berlin Heidelberg New York
Schatzker J, Tile M (1987) The rationale of operative fracture care. Springer, Berlin Heidelberg New York

7.15 Fractures of the Distal Femur

Supra- and intercondylar fractures present a challenge in that they are difficult to treat both operatively and conservatively. Younger patients sustain their fractures due to high-energy trauma, with soft tissue injury and other fractures. Older patients often sustain theirs from a simple fall but their osteoporotic bones make stable fixation difficult. Internal fixation may be successful if the fracture can be anatomically reduced and fixed rigidly. This in turn allows early mobilisation which aids articular cartilage healing and helps prevent stiffness of the knee joint.

7.15.1 Anatomy

Distal end of the right femur from the front (Fig. 1 a).
Distal end of the right femur from behind (Fig. 1 b).

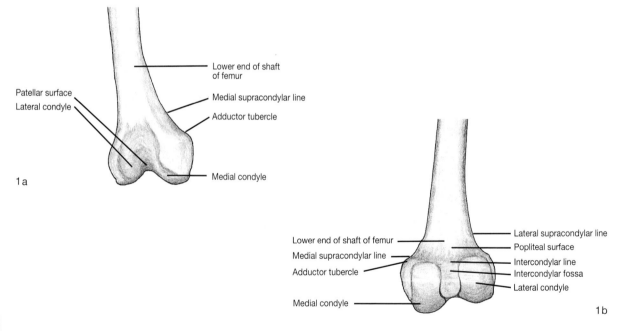

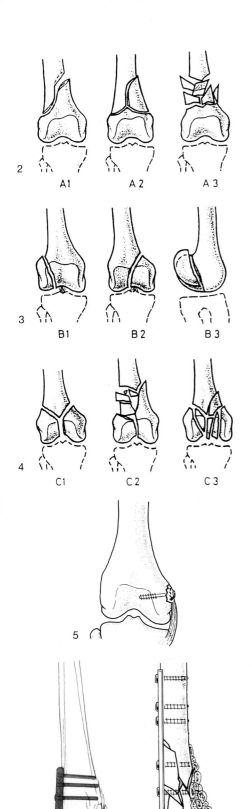

7.15.2 Assessment

Special examination:
– Check for knee ligament injuries. This may have to wait until the femoral fracture has been fixed.

Radiography:
– AP, lateral and oblique views, also of the uninjured side.
– Tomography.
– CT scan in complex injuries.

7.15.3 AO Classification

See also Sect. 5.1

Type 33 A: Extra-articular fracture (Fig. 2).
Type 33 B: Partial articular fracture, lateral or medial condyle, sagittal; partial articular fracture, frontal plane (Fig. 3).
Type 33 C: Complete articular fracture – both condyles separate from shaft (Fig. 4).

7.15.4 Indications for Osteosynthesis – Implants of Choice

Fracture:
– Avulsion of the medial collateral ligament from its proximal insertion together with a piece of bone (A1).

Implant:
– Lag screw fixation with either a small or a large cancellous bone screw combined with the corresponding size spiked washer (Fig. 5).

Fracture:
– Simple supracondylar fracture (A2) or supracondylar fracture combined with complex fracture of the distal shaft (A3).

Implants:
– DCS, bone graft in multifragmentary fractures (Fig. 6).
– 95° condylar plate, bone graft in multifragmentary fractures (Fig. 7).

Fractures:
– Fracture of the lateral condyle (B1).
– Frontal fracture of one or both condyles.
– Tangential posterior fracture (Hoffa fracture) (B3).

Distal Femur

501 ■

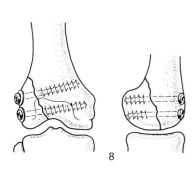
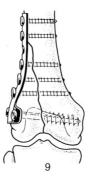

8   9

Implants:
- 6.5 mm cancellous bone screws (Fig. 8).
- 7.0 mm cannulated screws.
- T buttress plate in osteoporotic bone, or with long proximal extension (Fig. 9).

Fracture:
- T or Y fracture (C1).
- Bicondylar fracture with comminution of the distal shaft (C2).

Implants:
- DCS (Fig. 10).
- 95° condylar plate (Fig. 11).

Fracture:
- Bicondylar fracture with complex fracture of the distal femur and additional frontal fracture of one or both condyles.

Implants:
- Condylar buttress plate combined with 7.0 mm cannulated screws, for the frontal fractures (Fig. 12).

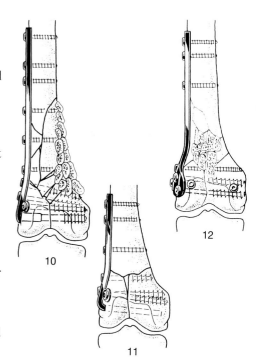

10   11   12

7.15.5 Preoperative Planning and Preparation

Timing:
- The associated injuries determine the timing of surgical intervention, but the sooner the better. If a delay of a few hours is necessary the extremity is placed in a splint in skin traction. Skeletal traction becomes necessary in longer delays.

Positioning:
- Supine with the knee flexed over a roll (60°–90°) to relax the gastrocnemius muscle. Hip and knee are draped free.
- Use of a sterile tourniquet may be indicated.

Incision:
- Incision along a line joining the greater trochanter, the lateral condyle, and the tibial tuberosity (Fig. 13).

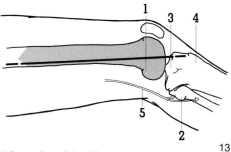

13

1 Lateral condyle of femur
2 Head of fibula
3 Tubercle of GERDY
4 Tuberosity of tibia
5 Common peroneal nerve

Preparation of instruments
- Instruments for insertion of 6.5 mm cancellous bone screws (p. 82).
- Instruments for insertion of 7.0 mm cannulated screws (p. 121).
- Instruments for insertion of 95° condylar plate (p. 172).
- Instruments for insertion of DCS (p. 150).
- Instruments for application of T buttress plate (p. 112).
- Instruments for application of condylar buttress plate (p. 112).

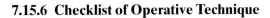

7.15.6 Checklist of Operative Technique

Supracondylar fractures without intra-articular extension (Type A2 and A3):
- Reduction and provisional fixation with Kirschner wires.
- Three further Kirschner wires are inserted. The first is used to determine the axis of the knee joint parallel to the distal articular surface of the femoral condyles (1); the second marks the inclination of the patello-femoral articular surface (2), and the third the direction of DCS or blade insertion (3). This last Kirschner wire should be parallel to the first and to the second Kirschner in the coronal plane[2] (Fig. 14 and 15).
- Preparation and insertion of the 95° condylar plate (p. 164) or DCS (p. 146).
- The fracture is compressed with the aid of the articulated tension device.
- Stability is increased by inserting lag screws across the fracture through the plate.
- In fractures with comminution a cancellous bone graft is applied on the medial side.

Fractures of the lateral condyle, with and without extension into the femoral shaft (B1, B2), tangential fracture of the condyles (B3):
- Anatomical reduction and temporary fixation with Kirschner wires and reduction forceps.
- In young adults fixation with two 6.5 mm cancellous bone screws (p. 81) or two 7.0 mm cannulated screws (p. 117) with 32 mm thread. Washers to prevent the screw head from sinking in.

---

[2] Drawing: Wires 1 and 3 are parallel when viewed from in front of femur, i.e. in the transverse plane. Wires 2 and 3 are parallel when viewed along long axis of femur, i.e. in the coronal plane. In this way wire 3 is parallel both to the plane of the tibio-femoral joint (knee extended) as marked by wire 1, and to the plane of the patellar surface of the femur as marked by wire 2.

Distal Femur

- In tangential fractures the screws are inserted in AP direction at right angles to the femoral shaft axis. They should be as far laterally as possible to avoid the articular cartilage. Counter-sinking for the screw heads may be necessary.
- In osteoporotic bone a T plate is contoured and fixed to the bone (p. 108).

Supracondylar T or Y fracture, bicondylar fracture with comminution of the femoral shaft (C1, C2):
- Careful reduction of the joint fragments and elevation of depressed metaphyseal fragments.
- Temporary fixation with Kirschner wires.
- The entry point of DCS or condylar blade plate is determined.
- Insertion of two 6.5 mm cancellous bone screws with 32 mm thread as lag screws, without obstruction of the site for the DCS or the condylar blade plate. The threads must grip the far condyle only. Washers prevent the screw heads from sinking in.
- Preparation and insertion of the DCS (p. 146) or the 95° condylar plate or (p. 164).
- Extensive cancellous bone graft if there is bone loss medially.

Bicondylar fracture with complex fracture of the distal femoral shaft and frontal fracture of one or both condyles:
- An additional medial parapatellar incision is necessary if the medial condyle is fractured.
- The tangential fracture is reduced and fixed with two 6.5 mm cancellous bone screws (p. 81). The thread length depends on the size of the far fragment.
- Reduction of the condyles and temporary fixation with Kirschner wires or guide wires for 7.0 mm cannulated screws. Insertion of any 6.5 mm cancellous bone screws or 7.0 mm cannulated screws as lag screws (p. 117) that cannot be inserted through the plate.
- Extensive cancellous bone graft is carried out on the medial side.
- The condylar buttress plate is contoured and applied (p. 109). Lag screws through the plate increase the stability.

7.15.7 Special Consideration – Escape Routes

The condylar plate, as well as the DCS, has to be inserted in the anterior part of the femoral condyles. Since this part is of a smaller dimension than the posterior aspect, the length of the condylar plate blade or the DCS screw must be shorter than projected on a radiograph of the distal femur. Too long an implant would penetrate the medial cortex, cause synovitis and damage

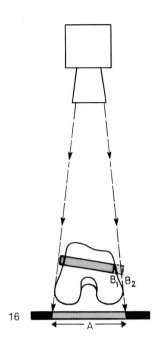

16

the medial capsule, which causes pain and could lead to joint stiffness (Fig. 16).

In young patients with dense, hard cancellous bone it may be very difficult to insert the seating chisel without splitting the supracondylar fragment. Predrilling the slot using a 3.2 mm drill bit would prevent the splitting.

When hammering in the seating chisel in young hard bone one must apply counter pressure on the medial side to avoid driving the previously fixed condyles apart.

To reduce the supracondylar fragments the distractor may be used (p. 355). Place the first bolt distally through a plate hole, the second proximal to the plate. A slight overdistraction facilitates the careful reduction of the fragments. The plate is fixed to the main diaphyseal fragment with 4.5 mm cortex screws.

7.15.8 Postoperative Care

– Suction drainage for 24–36 h.
– Immobilisation of the knee in 90° flexion for 3–4 days. See Fig. 9 in Sect. 7.14). Thereafter active flexion and extension exercises.
– Continuous passive motion for the first 4–7 days is of great advantage. Thereafter active mobilisation in a functional brace.

7.15.9 Implant Removal

In general, implants in weight-bearing bones are removed after an uneventful healing process. For implants in the distal femur the removal may take place after 12–24 months.

7.15.10 Recommended Reading

Mast J, Jakob R, Ganz R (1989) Planning and reduction technique in fracture surgery. Springer, Berlin Heidelberg New York
Müller ME, Allgöwer M, Schneider R, Willenegger H (1991) Manual of internal fixation, 3rd edn. Springer, Berlin Heidelberg New York
Müller ME, Nazarian S, Koch P, Schatzker J (1990) The comprehensive AO classification of fractures of long bones. Springer, Berlin Heidelberg New York
Rüedi T, Hochstetter AHC, Schlumpf R (1984) Surgical Approaches for Internal Fixation. Springer, Berlin Heidelberg New York
Schatzker J, Tile M (1987) The rationale of operative fracture care. Springer, Berlin Heidelberg New York

7.16 Fractures of the Patella

The patella is a sesamoid bone and lies within the tendon of the quadriceps muscle. Any displaced fracture of the patella in the longitudinal axis therefore results in loss of function of the extensor mechanism and should be reduced and internally fixed. Sometimes osteochondral fractures need surgery to remove an intra-articular loose body.

7.16.1 Anatomy

Right femur, tibia, fibula and patella, from the front and the side (Fig. 1).

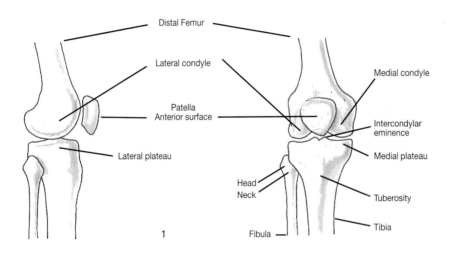

7.16.2 Assessment

Special examination:
– Haemarthrosis with fat globules most likely present in joint aspirate.
– Tenderness when palpating the medial and lateral parapatellar expansions of the quadriceps may indicate that they are torn and might need repair.
– A palpable gap may be present in the patella.

Radiography:
– AP and horizontal beam lateral views. A fluid level between the blood and fat may be seen in the joint on this lateral view indicating an intra-articular fracture.
– Intercondylar notch.
– "Skyline " view.

7.16.3 AO Classification

The patella (together with the mandible, clavicle and scapula) is in region 9. It is classified 9.1.1. Subtypes and subgroups have not yet been defined.

7.16.4 Indication for Osteosynthesis – Implants of Choice

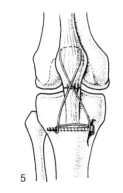

Fracture:
– Avulsion fracture of the distal pole.

Implants:
– 4.0 mm cancellous bone screw as lag screw, or two longitudinal Kirschner wires, in combination with tension band wire (Fig. 2).

Fracture:
– Simple transverse fracture.

Implants:
– Two Kirschner wires and a tension band wire (Fig. 3).

Fracture:
– Complex fractures.

Implants:
– Two or more Kirschner wires and a tension band wire, sometimes in combination with 4.0 mm cancellous bone screws as lag screws. In complex fractures patellectomy is an option (Fig. 4).

Fracture:
– Rupture of the infrapatellar tendon.

Implants:
– Tension band wire and transversely inserted 3.5 mm cortex screw through the tibial tubercle for distal wire anchorage (Fig. 5).

7.16.5 Preoperative Planning and Preparation

Timing:
– As soon as possible, to release haemarthrosis, relieve pain, and to reduce a displaced patella. Internal fixation is performed at the same time.

Positioning:
– Supine with the leg extended.
– Tourniquet.

Patella

Incision:
– Vertical midline or parapatellar lateral incision (Fig. 6).

Preparation of instruments:
– Instruments for insertion of Kirschner wires and
– Instruments for application of tension band wires (p. 369).
– Instruments for insertion of 4.0 mm cancellous bone screws (p. 214).
– Instruments for insertion of 3.5 mm cortex screw (p. 215).

7.16.6 Checklist for Operative Technique

Avulsion fracture of the distal pole:
– Anatomical reduction and temporary fixation with the pointed reduction forceps.
– Insertion of the 4.0 mm cancellous bone screw as a lag screw (p. 195).
– Insertion of Kirschner wires (p. 368).
– Using a curved large-bore needle the tension band wire is first inserted through the quadriceps tendon close to the bone, then through the patellar tendon at the lower pole.
– The wire is tightened while palpating the articular surface and controlling the reduction.
– Flexion of the knee to check compression.

Transverse fractures, simple and complex:
– Elevation of any articular depression and filling of defects with cancellous graft.
– Two parallel longitudinal holes are drilled with the 2.0 mm drill bit in the proximal fragment close to the anterior surface of the patella. A 1.6 mm Kirschner wire inserted in the first drilled hole will ensure that the second is drilled parallel (p. 368).
– Anatomical reduction and temporary fixation with pointed reduction forceps.
– Drilling is continued with the 2.0 mm drill bit through the distal fragment.
– Two 1.6 mm Kirschner wires now bent 180° at the proximal ends are inserted.
– The wire loop is passed around the Kirschner wires and tightened with the wire tightener.
– The bent ends of the Kirschner wires are hammered into the bone and their distal ends cut.
– Fixation of additional fragments with either 4.0 mm cancellous bone screws as lag screws or oblique Kirschner wires.

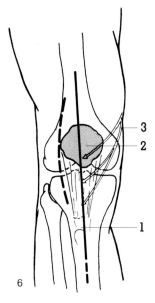

1 Tuberosity of tibia
2 Patellar ligament
3 Infrapatellar branches of saphenous nerve

Rupture of the infrapatellar tendon:
– The tendon is repaired with resorbable sutures.
– Protection of the sutures by adding a figure-of-eight tension band wire: The wire is passed through the quadriceps insertion and the tibial tubercle. In osteoporotic bone, a 3.5 mm cortex screw is inserted transversely through the tibial tubercle and the tension band wire is wound around each end of the screw.

7.16.7 Special Consideration – Escape Routes

A circumferentially placed wire can only hold a fractured patella reduced as long as the knee is not flexed. When flexed, the fracture gap opens and congruency is lost. Only the tension band wire passing over the front of the patella ensures compression across the fracture at all times.

Kirschner wires used to secure fragments must be parallel or impaction or compression will not occur.

Only one end of the Kirschner wire should be bent over or removal will require greater dissection.

When repairing the infrapatellar tendon the correct position of the patella should be checked using preoperative X-ray of the opposite knee. A patella baja (low patella) is otherwise produced.

Before wound closure the range of knee flexion is carefully tested whilst the repair is watched. The safe range is recorded in the operation note.

7.16.8 Postoperative Care

– Suction drainage for 24–36 h.
– If the fixation and the range of motion is satisfactory, active exercises start immediately.
– Continuous passive motion is recommended, with the arc of movement carefully set to the safe range as judged at operation.
– Partial weight-bearing for the first 6 weeks.

7.16.9 Implant Removal

– Usually the implants are removed after consolidation of the fracture at 8–12 months.
– In infrapatellar repair the tension band wire is removed after 6 months.

Heim U, Pfeiffer KM (1988) Internal fixation of small fragments, 3rd edn. Springer, Berlin Heidelberg New York

Müller ME, Allgöwer M, Schneider R, Willenegger H (1991) Manual of internal fixation, 3rd edn. Springer, Berlin Heidelberg New York

Rüedi T, Hochstetter AHC, Schlumpf R (1984) Surgical Approaches for Internal Fixation. Springer, Berlin Heidelberg New York

Schatzker J, Tile M (1987) The rationale of operative fracture care. Springer, Berlin Heidelberg New York

Sequin F, Texhammar R (1981) AO/ASIF instrumentation. Springer, Berlin Heidelberg New York

7.17 Fractures of the Tibial Plateau

Fractures of the tibial plateau are intra-articular fractures of a weight-bearing joint. Any significant disturbance of the joint surface and damage to the articular cartilage can produce post-traumatic osteoarthritis. Reconstruction of the joint surface, axial alignment, internal fixation, and early motion may help prevent this painful complication. The lateral plateau is the one most often involved. Injuries to vessels, nerves, capsule, collateral and cruciate ligaments as well as to the menisci can be associated with these fractures.

7.17.1 Anatomy

Proximal end of the right tibia from the front (Fig. 1).

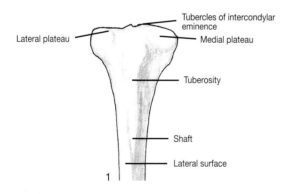

1

Fixation of Various Fractures

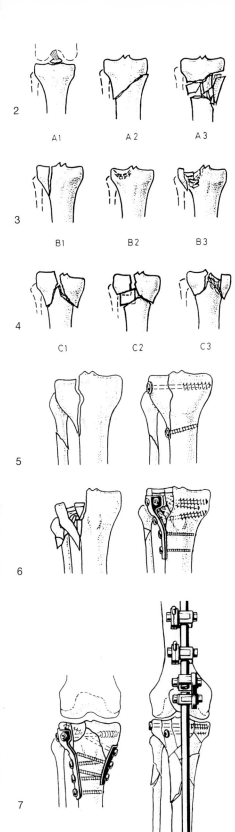

2 A1   A2   A3

3 B1   B2   B3

4 C1   C2   C3

5

6

7

8

7.17.2 Assessment

Special examination:
– Definitive examination is made only after radiography.
– Areas of tenderness.
– The state of the anterior skin (local crushing is common and not always immediately obvious).
– Ligament instability.
– Range of motion, especially abnormal coronal motion.
– Careful neuro-vascular assessment.

Radiography:
– AP, lateral, and internal and external oblique views.
– Tomography, AP and lateral views (degree of depression of the tibial plateau).
– CT scan (comminuted fracture).

7.17.3 AO Classification

See also Sect. 5.1

Type 41 A: Extra-articular fracture, avulsion fractures (Fig. 2).
Type 41 B: Partial articular fracture (Fig. 3).
Type 41 C: Complete articular fracture (Fig. 4).

7.17.4 Indication for Osteosynthesis –
Implants of Choice

Fracture:
– Unicondylar fractures (type B), usually lateral side.

Implants:
– Two 6.5 mm cancellous bone screws or 7.0 mm cannulated screws with washers (in young people) (Fig. 5).
– L or T buttress plate, lateral tibial head buttress plate, DCP, or LC-DCP, 4.5 mm (in older people) (Fig. 6).

Fracture:
– Bicondylar fractures (type C).

Implants:
– L or T buttress plate, DCP, or LC-DCP, 4.5 mm, or lateral tibial head buttress plate sometimes combined with three- or four- hole semi-tubular plate on the medial side as a buttress (Fig. 7).
– 6.5 mm cancellous bone screws or 7.0 mm cannulated screws, combined with external fixator in complex or open fractures (Fig. 8).

Tibial Plateau

7.17.5 Preoperative Planning and Preparation

Timing:
– Immediately, if an open fracture, an acute compartment syndrome, or vascular injury. Simple fractures are also best treated early.
– If a delay of more than 1–2 days is necessary skeletal traction prevents telescoping or further displacement of fragments. Aspiration of haemarthrosis improves comfort.

Positioning:
– Supine with the knee flexed over a roll 50–60°.
– The leg is draped to be freely moved.
– Tourniquet.

Incision:
– Lateral parapatellar approach; with the leg extended the incision starts over the distal head of the vastus lateralis, continues just lateral to the patella and its tendon (Fig. 9).
– For complex fractures a long straight anterior midline incision is used.

Preparation of instruments:
– Instruments for insertion of 6.5 mm cancellous bone screws (p. 82).
– Instruments for insertion of 7.0 mm cannulated screws (p. 121).
– Instruments for application of L or T buttress plates (p. 112).
– Instruments for application of DCP or LC-DCP, 4.5 mm (p. 112).
– Instruments for application of lateral tibial head buttress plates (p. 112).
– Instruments for application of semi-tubular plates (p. 112).
– Instruments for application of external fixator (p. 337).
– Instruments for harvesting and inserting bone graft (p. 369).
– Instruments for application of the femoral distractor (p. 353).

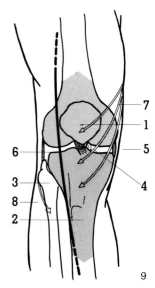

1 Patella
2 Tuberosity of tibia
3 Head of fibula
4 Cruciate ligaments
5 Medial collateral ligament
6 Lateral collateral ligament
7 Infrapatellar branches of saphenous nerve
8 Superficial peroneal nerve

7.17.6 Checklist of Operative Technique

Unicondylar or so-called wedge fracture (type B):
– Anatomical reduction and temporary fixation with Kirschner wires.
– Insertion of two 6.5 mm cancellous bone screws as lag screws with washers (p. 81), or insertion of two 7.0 mm cannulated screws as lag screws with washers (p. 117) in young patients.
– In older patients, application of a L or T buttress plate, (p. 108) DCP, LC-DCP as buttress plate (pp. 101, 106), or lateral tibial head buttress plate with 6.5 mm cancellous bone screws as lag screws through the plate (p. 109).

Unicondylar or wedge fractures with depression (B 2 and 3):
- Reduction of a central depression by fenestrating the anterior cortex just in front of fibula using a bone punch. The defect is packed with cancellous bone.
- In wedge fractures with impaction the large lateral fragment is rotated laterally and the joint reduced.
- Filling of the defect in the metaphysis with cancellous bone graft.
- Temporary fixation of the lateral cortex with Kirschner wires.
- Application of the L or T buttress plate (p. 108) or lateral tibial head buttress plate (p. 109).

Bicondylar fractures (Type C1 and C2):
- Reconstruction of the joint and temporary fixation with pointed reduction forceps or Kirschner wires. Later these are replaced with 7.0 mm cannulated screws (p. 117).
- Filling of the defect with cancellous bone graft.
- The tibial plateau is joined to the shaft using pointed reduction forceps or Kirschner wires.
- Application of a three- or four-hole semi-tubular plate to the medial side (p. 106).
- Application of the L or T buttress plate to the lateral side (p. 108).

Complex bicondylar fractures (C3):
- Reconstruction of the joint with 6.5 mm cancellous bone screws (p. 81), or 7.0 mm cannulated screws (p. 117) as lag screws.
- Bridging of the knee by using an anterior unilateral external fixation frame. Half-pin fixation away from the fracture focus if a later fixation of the fracture is necessary after healing of the soft tissue. Moderate distraction is applied in order to stabilise the soft tissue by ligamentotaxis. The external fixator may be reapplied beneath the knee after 2–3 weeks to allow motion, or internal fixation may be employed as a secondary procedure depending upon the healing of the soft tissues.

7.17.7 Special Consideration – Escape Routes

The distractor is very useful in reduction of most tibial plateau fractures. In lag screw fixation of a lateral wedge fracture, care must be taken not to damage the medial articular surface when inserting the proximal screw. The lateral plateau is higher than the medial.
In bicondylar fractures the reconstruction should begin with the simple fracture, which is usually the medial of the two.

Accurate contouring of the plates is necessary even though some are preshaped. On the medial side the plate is applied to the antero-medial face of the proximal metaphysis deep to the pes anserinus (insertion of the hamstrings into upper tibia) and the anterior fibres of the medial collateral ligament. On the lateral side, the plate is fixed slightly obliquely with its distal end flush to the anterior tibial crest and its proximal end as far postero-lateral as possible.

The menisci must always be tested and repaired if damaged. The collateral and cruciate ligaments are also tested for laxity. Medial collateral repair should be carried out at the same time. Combined cruciate repair is usually not possible.

7.17.8 Postoperative Care

- Suction drainage for 24–36 h.
- Active and passive motion using the continuous passive motion machine starts immediately if the fixation is stable.
- Partial weight-bearing of 10 kg for the first 3–4 months.
- A hinged functional brace is used when the ligaments, and/or menisci have been repaired.

7.17.9 Implant Removal

As a rule implants in weight-bearing bones are removed after complete healing. In tibial plateau fractures implants may be removed after 12–18 months, if causing symptoms.

7.17.10 Recommended Reading

Heim U, Pfeiffer KM (1988) Internal fixation of small fragments, 3rd edn. Springer, Berlin Heidelberg New York

Müller ME, Allgöwer M, Schneider R, Willenegger H (1991) Manual of internal fixation, 3rd edn. Springer, Berlin Heidelberg New York

Müller ME, Nazarian S, Koch P, Schatzker J (1990) The comprehensive AO classification of fractures of long bones. Springer, Berlin Heidelberg New York

Rüedi T, Hochstetter AHC, Schlumpf R (1984) Surgical Approaches for Internal Fixation. Springer, Berlin Heidelberg New York

Schatzker J, Tile M (1987) The rationale of operative fracture care. Springer, Berlin Heidelberg New York

Fixation of Various Fractures

7.18 Fractures of the Tibial Shaft

The treatment of tibial shaft fractures has long been a question of controversy. Experience has shown that nonsurgical management can achieve excellent results especially if the fracture is minimally displaced and reduction can be easily accomplished and maintained. The advent of functional bracing has greatly reduced the cast time in these fractures. In other instances the treatment with plaster cast or brace fixation for some months may result in permanent impairment due to malunion, joint stiffness, and post-thrombotic oedema formation. The AO/ASIF group has shown that, if based on sound biomechanical and biological principles, internal or external fixation has its place in the treatment of tibial shaft fractures.

Fractures with concomitant vessel or nerve injuries, or compartment syndrome, and open fractures are considered absolute indications for surgical stabilisation. Recommended indications for internal or external fixation are e.g.:

- Shaft fractures in polytrauma patients requiring intensive care treatment.
- Unstable fractures with severe displacement of the main fragments.
- Fractures with shortening of more than 1 cm.
- Unstable fractures with interposition of muscle, tendon, or with tilted or rotated bone fragments.
- Segmental fractures.
- Ipsilateral fractures of the femur or severe knee or ankle injuries.
- Short oblique fractures associated with a multifragmentary zone.

Tibial Shaft

7.18.1 Anatomy

Right tibia and fibula from the front (Fig. 1).

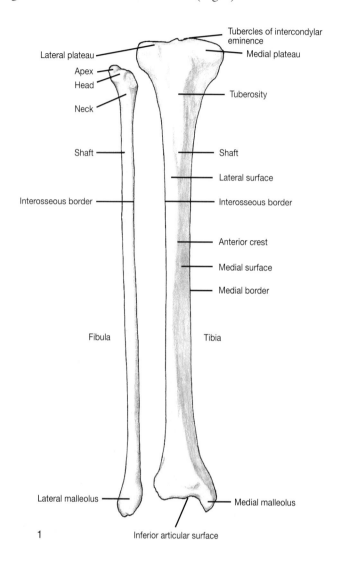

1

Tubercles of intercondylar eminence

Lateral plateau

Medial plateau

Apex

Head

Neck

Tuberosity

Shaft

Shaft

Lateral surface

Interosseous border

Interosseous border

Anterior crest

Medial surface

Medial border

Fibula

Tibia

Lateral malleolus

Medial malleolus

Inferior articular surface

7.18.2 Assessment

Special examination:
- Soft tissue injuries (open fracture?). The state of the skin is crucial to internal fixation. If in doubt, surgery in closed fractures is delayed until signs such as swelling, blisters or contusions are not seen on the skin.
- Neurological and vascular status (repeated examination).
- Anterior or posterior compartment ischaemia.

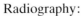

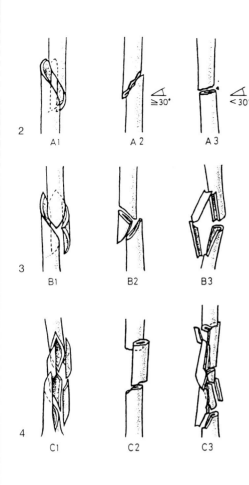

A1   A2   A3

B1   B2   B3

C1   C2   C3

2
3
4

Radiography:
- AP, lateral views, full length.
- Tomography, if joint fracture has been diagnosed.
- Arteriography, if vascular impairment.

7.18.3 AO Classification (Tibia/Fibula Diaphysis)

See also Sect. 5.1

Type 42 A: Simple fracture; spiral, oblique or transverse (Fig. 2).
Type 42 B: Wedge fracture; spiral-, bending-, or fragmented wedge (Fig. 3).
Type 42 C: Complex fracture; spiral, segmented or irregular (Fig. 4).

7.18.4 Indication for Osteosynthesis –
Implants of Choice

Fracture:
- Open fractures of the tibial shaft (see p. 43).

Implants:
- External fixator (Fig. 5).
- Unreamed tibial nail (Fig. 6).

Fracture:
- Transverse or short oblique fractures (A2, A3).

Implants:
- Universal tibial nail, unlocked or locked (Fig. 7).
- Lag screw fixation, 4.5 mm-or 3.5 mm cortex screws, in combination with a 4.5 mm narrow DCP or LC-DCP plate (Fig. 8).

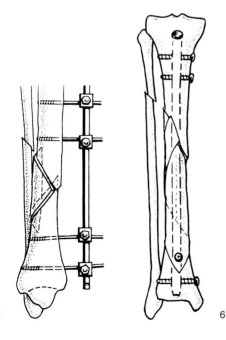

5   6

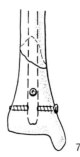
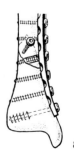

7   8

Tibial Shaft

517

7.18.8 Postoperative Care

- Suction drainage for 24–36 h.
- The leg is elevated on a padded frame with the knee flexed to 45° and the ankle to 90° (Fig. 18).
- If the fracture is stable and no other complication is expected, motion can start early.
- The splint is removed on the second postoperative day and the patient encouraged to move the ankle.

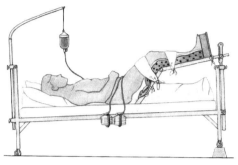

18

7.18.9 Implant Removal

In general, stainless steel implants in weight-bearing bones are removed after an uncomplicated healing process. Separate screws and titanium implants may be left in place if symptomless. The time for removal depends on the fracture type and the course of healing. Medullary nails can be removed after 18–24 months, plates after 12–18 months.

7.18.10 Recommended Reading

Müller ME, Allgöwer M, Schneider R, Willenegger H (1991) Manual of internal fixation, 3rd edn. Springer, Berlin Heidelberg New York

Müller ME, Nazarian S, Koch P, Schatzker J (1990) The comprehensive AO classification of fractures of long bones. Springer, Berlin Heidelberg New York

Rüedi T, Hochstetter AHC, Schlumpf R (1984) Surgical Approaches for Internal Fixation. Springer, Berlin Heidelberg New York

Schatzker J, Tile M (1987) The rationale of operative fracture care. Springer, Berlin Heidelberg New York

Sequin F, Texhammar R (1981) AO/ASIF instrumentation. Springer, Berlin Heidelberg New York

7.19 Fractures of the Distal Tibia "Pilon Fractures"

Both tibia and fibula can be involved in this fracture type. If displaced, these fractures are difficult to treat and present a challenge to the operating team. The fracture is often caused by high energy trauma, for example, a fall from a height, or a motor vehicle accident. It can involve both compressive and shearing forces which can lead to severe impaction of the cancellous bone, disruption of the articular surface, and a fractured fibula. In for example ski injuries the fracture is the result of shearing forces which makes it grossly unstable. The condition of the skin and the soft tissue will also greatly influence the choice of the treatment. Fractures with minimal displacement and an intact joint surface are best treated conservatively in a cast and later a brace, or with an external fixator for a brief initial period before gentle active motion starts at 3–4 weeks.

7.19.1 Anatomy

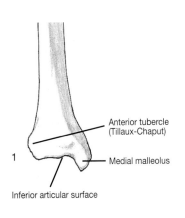

Distal end of the right tibia from the front (Fig. 1).

7.19.2 Assessment

Special examination:
– Neuro-vascular status.
– Skin and soft tissue condition.

Radiography:
– AP, lateral and oblique views.
– AP and lateral tomography.
– CT (articular surface damage).

7.19.3 AO Classification (Tibia/Fibula Distal)

See also Sect. 5.1

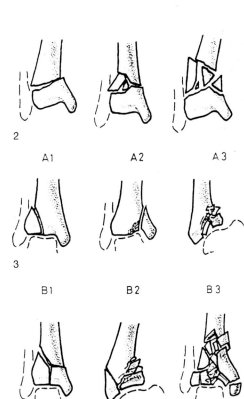

Type 43 A: Extra-articular fracture, metaphyseal simple, wedge, or complex (Fig. 2).
Type 43 B: Partial articular fracture, split and/or depression (Fig. 3).
Type 43 C: Complete articular fracture; simple, multifragmentary (Fig. 4).

7.19.4 Indication for Osteosynthesis – Implants of Choice

Fracture:
– Fibular fracture and explosion fracture of distal tibia (most often young patients) or impaction fracture of distal tibia (mostly elderly).

Implants:
– For the fibular fracture: One-third tubular plate (Fig. 5).
– For the tibial fracture: 4.0 mm cancellous bone screws, or 3.5 mm cannulated screws.
– T plate, cloverleaf plate, DCP or LC-DCP, 4.5 mm
– External fixation, especially if the skin condition is poor (Fig. 6).

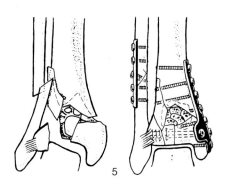

5

7.19.5 Preoperative Planning and Preparation

Timing:
– As soon as possible, before severe soft tissue swelling and fracture blisters occur. If this is the case, the fracture is stabilised with traction or external fixation to maintain length. Surgery is delayed for 7–10 days or until the skin recovers.

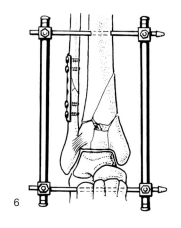

6

Positioning:
– Supine; tourniquet.

Incision:
– Medial side: The incision starts lateral to the anterior crest of the tibia curves around and 1–2 finger widths from the anterior edge of the medial malleolus to a point 1–2 cm distal to the tip of the malleolus (Fig. 7).
– Lateral side: If a second incision is needed there should be a 7 cm skin bridge between the two. The incision is made posteriorly.

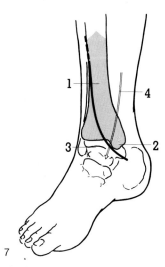

Preparation of instruments:
– Instruments for application of one-third tubular plate (p. 216).
– Instruments for insertion of 4.0 mm cancellous bone screws (p. 214).
– Instruments for insertion of 3.5 mm cannulated screws (p. 134).
– Instruments for application of T plate (p. 112).
– Instruments for application of cloverleaf plate (p. 112 and/or 216).
– Instruments for application of 4.5 mm DCP or LC-DCP (p. 112).
– Instruments for application of external fixator (p. 327).

7

1 Anterior border of tibia
2 Medial malleolus
3 Ankle joint (talocrural joint)
4 Saphenous nerve

7.19.6 Checklist for Operative Technique

With fibula and tibia fractures:
- Anatomical reduction of the fibular fracture. If possible 3.5 mm cortex
screws as lag screws, and then the one-third tubular plate (p. 200).
- Reconstruction and temporary fixation of the joint surface with Kirschner wires.
- Fixation with 4.0 mm cancellous bone screws as lag screws (p. 195), or
- Fixation with 3.5 mm cannulated screws over preplaced guide pins (p. 133).
- Application of cancellous bone graft in bone cavity.
- Application of a medial buttress plate; T plate (p. 108), a cloverleaf plate (p. 212), DCP or LC-DCP (pp. 101, 106). The siting of the plate will depend on the direction in which the joint surface would angulate if deformity occurred. If varus collapse is to be avoided a medial buttress is needed, but if anterior collapse is feared the plate should be on the front of the distal tibia.
- Application of a bilateral external fixator (p. 335).

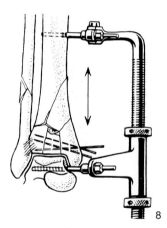

8

7.19.7 Special Consideration – Escape Routes

An X-ray of the intact side for comparison is essential when reconstructing a complex fracture. Restoration of the fibular length is essential. The distractor or the external fixator may facilitate reconstruction of the fracture by ligamentotaxis and indirect reduction. The lower pin is placed in the talar notch (Fig. 8).

When cancellous bone grafting is indicated, harvesting the bone graft is best done before reconstruction of the fracture starts. The operating- and tourniquet time on the pilon fracture can thus be shortened. A cloverleaf plate can be cut to the desired shape for the distal part of the tibia. Newly designed plates are fixed with small fragment screws only. The former design of the cloverleaf plate allowed the use of 4.5 mm cortex screws in the diaphyseal portion of the implant. Many of these older implants are still in use.

The wounds should be closed without tension, or else skin necrosis can cause major surgical disaster. If this is impossible, part of, or the entire, lateral incision is left open for 5–10 days. In old patients with osteoporotic bone, it may be necessary to use bone cement to hold screws.

Distal Tibia

7.19.8 Postoperative Care

- Suction drainage for 24–36 h.
- The leg is placed in a double U-splint with the ankle in 90° to prevent equinus deformity for the first few days (Fig. 9). The extremity is kept elevated to reduce swelling.
- If the fracture is stable, motion is started immediately with dorsiflexion and delayed weight-bearing. In comminuted intra-articular fractures weight-bearing can only start after firm union; that is after 8–12 weeks.
- A walking calliper, which takes the weight off the pilon, is recommended for the long period of reduced or partial weight-bearing. See SYNTHES cataloque

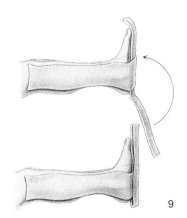

9

7.19.9 Implant Removal

Single screws and titanium implants may be left in place. Other implants can be removed after 12–18 months if the healing process has been uncomplicated.

7.19.10 Recommended Reading

Heim U (1991) Die Pilon-tibial-Fraktur. Springer, Berlin Heidelberg New York

Heim U, Pfeiffer KM (1988) Internal fixation of small fragments, 3rd edn. Springer, Berlin Heidelberg New York

Müller ME, Allgöwer M, Schneider R, Willenegger H (1991) Manual of internal fixation, 3rd edn. Springer, Berlin Heidelberg New York

Müller ME, Nazarian S, Koch P, Schatzker J (1990) The comprehensive AO classification of fractures of long bones. Springer, Berlin Heidelberg New York

Rüedi T, Hochstetter AHC, Schlumpf R (1984) Surgical Approaches for Internal Fixation. Springer, Berlin Heidelberg New York

Schatzker J, Tile M (1987) The rationale of operative fracture care. Springer, Berlin Heidelberg New York

Fixation of Various Fractures

7.20 Malleolar Fractures

Malleolar fractures are among the most common skeletal injuries. They may be caused by direct force but most often they occur with minimal violence resulting from a subluxation or dislocation of the talus out of the ankle mortise. These fractures are often a combination of injuries to the fibula and/or tibia, the joint cartilage, the ligaments, and the capsule.

The operative treatment of malleolar fractures has long been disputed. It is, however, felt that anatomical reduction and exact reconstruction of the ankle mortise is a necessity to avoid a later post-traumatic osteoarthritis in unstable malleolar injuries.

7.20.1 Anatomy

Lower end of the right tibia from the front (Fig. 1).

Two groups of ligaments are involved:
– The inferior tibio-fibular ligamentous complex, consists of three elements:
  The anterior syndesmotic ligament, (anterior tibio-fibular ligament).
  The posterior syndesmotic ligament (posterior tibio-fibular ligament).
  The interosseous membrane (Fig. 2).

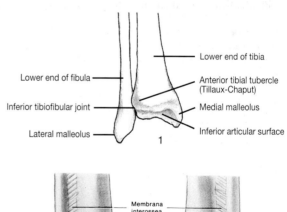

Lower end of fibula — Lower end of tibia
Anterior tibial tubercle (Tillaux-Chaput)
Inferior tibiofibular joint — Medial malleolus
Lateral malleolus — Inferior articular surface

1

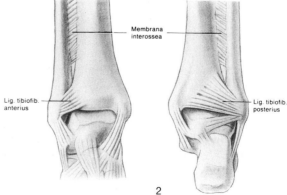

Membrana interossea

Lig. tibiofib. anterius

Lig. tibiofib. posterius

2

The collateral ligaments:
   The lateral collateral ligament, with three divisions (Fig. 3.).
   The medial collateral, or deltoid, ligament, with two divisions.

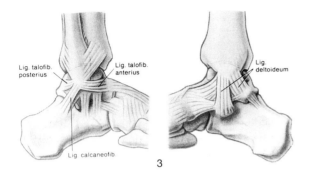

Lig. talofib. posterius   Lig. talofib. anterius   Lig. deltoideum   Lig. calcaneofib.

3

7.20.2 Assessment

Special examination:
– Condition of the skin.
– Points of tenderness. If over a ligament or capsule, injury is
  likely to be present.
– The whole fibular shaft must be palpated for tenderness as in
  some type C injuries the fibular fracture may be in the upper
  third.
– Abnormal motion of the talus in the ankle mortise.

Radiography:
– AP, and lateral views.
– Mortise view, taken at 15° internal rotation for proper view of
  the inferior tibio-fibular syndesmosis, and the talo-fibular articulation.
– Tomograms, to assess the degree of comminution and a possible talar dome fracture.

7.20.3 AO Classification

See also Sect. 5.1

Type 44 A: Infrasyndesmotic fibular lesion with or without
           fracture of the medial malleolus (Fig. 4).
Type 44 B: Transsyndesmotic isolated fibular fracture, with
           medial lesion, and/or with postero-lateral tibia
           (Volkmann's) fracture (Fig. 5).
Type 44 C: Suprasyndesmotic lesion with simple or multifrag-
           mentary diaphyseal fibular fracture, or proximal
           fibular fracture, and with medial disruption (Fig. 6).

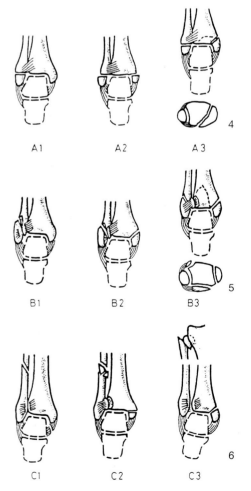

A1   A2   A3   4

B1   B2   B3   5

C1   C2   C3   6

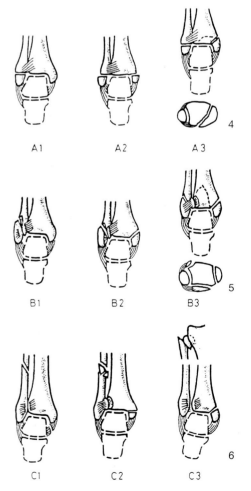

Fixation of Various Fractures

7.20.4 Indication for Osteosynthesis – Implants of Choice

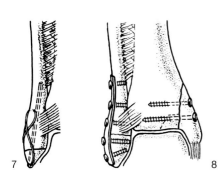

7 8

Fracture:
– Infrasyndesmotic fibular fracture, short oblique or transverse, and vertical fracture of the medial malleolus (type A).

Implants:
– Kirschner wires, 1.6 mm diameter, and figure-of-eight tension band wires, 1.2 mm diameter for fibula (Fig. 7). For a larger fragment a one-third tubular plate.
– 4.0 mm cancellous bone screws, or 4.5 mm cannulated screws as lag screws for medial malleolus (Fig. 8).

Fracture:
– Transsyndesmotic fibular fracture, medial malleolar fracture, postero-lateral tibia fragment (type B).

Implants:
– 3.5 mm cortex screws as lag screws in oblique fractures of the fibula.
– Contoured one-third tubular plate in multifragmentary fibular fracture and to neutralise lag screw fixation
– Kirschner wires, 1.6 mm diameter, and 1.2 mm cerclage wire for tension band wiring of the medial malleolus.
– 4.0 mm cancellous bone screws, or 4.5 mm cannulated screws for lag screw fixation of the medial malleolus and postero-lateral tibia fragment
– 6.5 mm cancellous bone screw for the postero-lateral tibia fragment (Fig. 9).

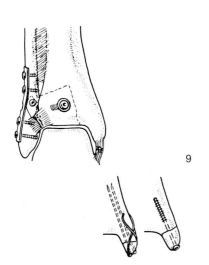

9

Fracture:
– Suprasyndesmotic comminuted fibular fracture, and medial malleolar fracture, postero-lateral tibia fragment.

Implants:
– One-third tubular plate, 8–12 holes, for the fibular fracture.
– 4.0 mm cancellous bone screws, or 4.5 mm cannulated screws for the medial malleolar fracture.
– Kirschner wires, 1.6 mm diameter, and figure of eight wire, 1.2 mm diameter for medial malleolar fracture.
– 6.5 mm cancellous bone screw for the postero-lateral tibia fragment.
– 3.5 mm cortex screw as transfixation screw (Fig. 10).

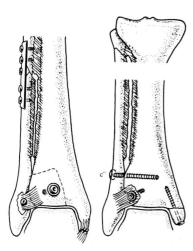

10

7.20.5 Preoperative Planning and Preparation

Timing:
– If possible within 6–8 h following injury. If the skin shows oedema and/or blisters surgery is postponed until skin condition has improved. The fracture is reduced and immobilised in a well-padded plaster cast. The leg is kept elevated. Open reduction is undertaken when the swelling has subsided after 4–6 days.

Positioning:
– Supine, with the leg in slight internal rotation.
– Tourniquet.

Incision:
– Lateral malleolus: A straight or hockey stick incision about 10 cm long is made anteriorly (be careful of the superficial peroneal nerve!) or posterior (be careful of the sural nerve and the small saphenous vein!) to the palpable lateral malleolus (Fig. 11).
– Medial malleolus: The incision curves behind and 1 finger breadths from the posterior edge of the medial malleolus to a point 1–2 cm distal to its tip (Fig. 12).
– For fixation of the Volkmann's fracture: The lateral incision is extended proximally curving it back to the Achilles tendon. Wedge cushion underneath the buttock.

Preparation of instruments:
– Instruments for tension band wiring (p. 369).
– Instruments for application of a one-third tubular plate (p. 216).
– Instruments for insertion of 3.5 mm cortex screws as lag screws (p. 215).
– Instruments for insertion of 4.0 mm cancellous bone screws as lag screws (p. 214).
– Instruments for insertion of 4.5 mm cannulated screws (p. 128).
– Instruments for insertion of 6.5 mm cancellous bone screws as lag screws (p. 82).
– Instruments for insertion of 3.5 mm cortex screws as transfixation screws (p. 215).

7.20.6 Checklist for Operative Technique

Type A and B fractures:
– Anatomical reduction of the fibula and temporary fixation with a pointed reduction forceps.
– Fixation of the fibular fracture by tension band wiring (p. 366), or one-third tubular plate (p. 200).

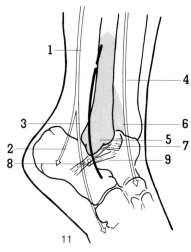

1 Peroneal nerve
2 Lateral calcaneal branches of peroneal nerve
3 Lateral dorsal cutaneous nerve
4 Intermediate dorsal cutaneous nerve
5 Lateral malleolus
6 "Tubercle of Chaput"
7 Anterior talo-fibular ligament
8 Calcaneo-fibular ligament
9 Lateral talo-calcaneal ligament

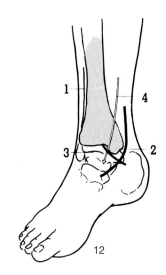

1 Anterior border of tibia
2 Medial malleolus
3 Ankle joint (talocrural joint)
4 Saphenous nerve

- Exposure of the medial malleolus and careful reflexion of any trapped periosteum.
- Reduction of any impaction fracture of the articular surface of the tibia and bone grafting of a resulting cancellous bone defect.
- Fixation of the medial malleolus by tension band wiring (small transverse avulsion fragment), or by 4.0 mm cancellous bone screws as lag screws (large shear fragment) (p. 195), or 4.5 mm cannulated screws (p. 126).
- Reduction and provisional fixation of posterior fragment by Kirschner wire.
- Final fixation by 4.0 mm cancellous bone screws as lag screws in antero-posterior direction.
- Suturing of torn ligaments, usually only the lateral ligament in type A injuries.

Type C fractures:
- Anatomical reduction and fixation of the fibular shaft fracture with 3.5 mm cortex screws as lag screws (p. 196), in combination with a one-third tubular plate (p. 201).
- Exposure of the anterior syndesmosis. Lag screw fixation if avulsed from the bone (tubercle of Tillaux-Chaput), otherwise possible suture of ligament.
- If instability persists, a 3.5 mm cortex screw is inserted as a fibulo-tibial transfixation (positioning)screw about 2–3 cm above the ankle. The screw is inserted obliquely at an angle of $25° – 30°$ starting postero-laterally and aiming antero-medially. Such a screw is threaded in the fibular and tibial cortices. It is not a lag screw (p. 197).
- Fixation of the medial malleolus and any postero-lateral fragment as described for type B fractures.

7.20.7 Special Consideration – Escape Routes

In type C fractures with a very high fibular fracture, exposure may not be necessary. Using a hook or a pointed reduction forceps the fibula is reduced down into its normal position and stabilised here with a Kirschner wire. A transfixation screw is inserted as described above, after checking fibular length and rotation by X-ray and exposure of the anterior syndesmosis.

- A small notch is cut into the dorsum of the metatarsal 1–1.5 cm distal to the joint.
- Insertion of 3.5 mm cortex or cannulated screws as lag screws perpendicularly across the joint (p. 133, 196). The drill hole is placed at the upper end of the notch to prevent splitting the base of the metatarsal. Screws are used for fixation of the first, the second, and possibly of the fifth metatarsals.
- Insertion of Kirschner wires in the third and fourth metatarsals.

Metatarsal fractures:
- Open anatomical reduction of the first and fifth metatarsal.
- Application of a one-third tubular plate straight dorsally or medially on the first metatarsal (p. 200).
- Application of a quarter-tubular plate laterally 2.7 mm DCP on the fifth metatarsal.
- Insertion of Kirschner wires in the third and fourth metatarsals in correct direction to prevent extension deformity: The fracture is opened and the wire run distally just under the dorsal cortex parallel to the axis of the bone (see Fig. 8). The fracture is reduced and the wire driven retrograde beneath the dorsal cortex.

7.21.7 Special Consideration – Escape Routes

In talus fractures it is extremely important that the blood supply be preserved. Any stripping of soft tissue across the dorsum of the neck and head region or in the sinus tarsi must be avoided.

7.21.8 Postoperative Care

- Suction drainage for 24–36 h.
- Talus fractures: A 90° splint is applied if there is doubt about the stability of the fixation and the quality of the bone stock. On the second postoperative day gentle, active motion can start after removal of the splint. The splint is kept during the night.
- Calcaneus fractures: The foot is kept elevated 3–4 days with a bivalved cast at 90° during the night to prevent equinus. Early gentle, active mobilisation with frequent inversion/eversion exercises. Touch weight-bearing is allowed.
- Tarsometatarsal fracture dislocations and metatarsal fractures: Elevation of the foot in a bivalved cast, which allows active motion during the day. This is kept during the night for some weeks. Partial weight-bearing of about 10 kg. After 6–8 weeks full weight bearing can start.

7.21.9 Implant Removal

In talus and calcaneus fractures, screws and plates are removed after 8–12 months if symptomatic. In tarsometatarsal fracture/dislocation the screws are removed after 12–14 weeks, since the joint is not fused and motion will eventually cause the screws to fatigue. In metatarsal fractures the Kirschner wires are removed after 4 weeks. Other implants may be left in if there is no discomfort to the patient.

7.21.10 Recommended Reading

Heim U, Pfeiffer KM (1988) Internal fixation of small fragments, 3rd edn. Springer, Berlin Heidelberg New York

Müller ME, Allgöwer M, Schneider R, Willenegger H (1991) Manual of internal fixation, 3rd edn. Springer, Berlin Heidelberg New York

Schatzker J, Tile M (1987) The rationale of operative fracture care. Springer, Berlin Heidelberg New York

Foot

7.22 References

Colton CL, Hall AJ (1991) Atlas of orthopedic surgical approaches. But-
   terworth – Heinemann, Oxford
Fernandez Dell'Oca (1989) Modular external fixation in emergency with
   the AO tubular system. Intergraf, Montevideo
Heim U (1991) Die Pilon-tibial-Fraktur. Springer, Berlin Heidelberg New
   York
Heim U, Pfeiffer KM (1988) Internal fixation of small fragments, 3rd edn.
   Springer, Berlin Heidelberg New York
Hierholzer G, Rüedi T, Allgöwer M, Schatzker J (1985) Manual on the
   AO/ASIF tubular external fixator. Springer, Berlin Heidelberg New
   York
Mast J, Jakob R, Ganz R (1989) Planning and reduction technique in frac-
   ture surgery. Springer, Berlin Heidelberg New York
Müller ME, Allgöwer M, Schneider R, Willenegger H (1991) Manual of in-
   ternal fixation, 3rd edn. Springer, Berlin Heidelberg New York
Müller ME, Nazarian S, Koch P, Schatzker J (1990) The comprehensive
   AO classification of fractures of long bones. Springer, Berlin Heidelberg
   New York
Regazzoni P, Rüedi T, Winquist R, Allgöwer M (1985) The dynamic hip
   screw implant system. Springer, Berlin Heidelberg New York
Rüedi T, Hochstetter AHC, Schlumpf R (1984) Surgical Approaches for
   Internal Fixation. Springer, Berlin Heidelberg New York
Schatzker J, Tile M (1987) The rationale of operative fracture care.
   Springer, Berlin Heidelberg New York
Sequin F, Texhammar R (1981) AO/ASIF instrumentation. Springer,
   Berlin Heidelberg New York

8 AO/ASIF Technique
in Late Reconstructive Surgery

By R. Hertel

8.1 Post-traumatic Deformities

8.1.1 Malunion

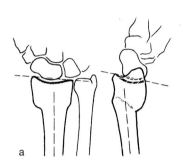

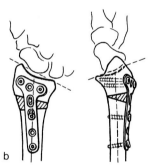

Malunion of the distal radius. **a** Typical deformity after untreated Colles' fracture. There is a dorsal and radial tilt of the articular surface. **b** Osteotomy is performed at the site of deformity. A biplanar corticocancellous wedge is interposed and a 3.5 mm T plate is used to stabilise the reconstructed bone.

A malunited fracture is defined as a fracture which has healed with an abnormal position of the fragments. Depending on its location a malunion may impair function and appearance. The most serious problems are intra-articular malunions with steps in the subchondral bone plate. Untreated, these may lead to joint degeneration. Metaphyseal and diaphyseal malunions may result in shortening, angular or rotational deformities. The deformity itself is often painless, although neighbouring, or even distant, joints may be affected by the resulting unphysiological load distribution, leading to chronic pain and to progressive osteoarthritis.

Malunions are caused by inadequate primary reduction or by unrecognised secondary displacement due to ineffective immobilisation during healing.

In children, post-traumatic deformities may occur despite perfect reduction and healing in an anatomical position. This is especially true when the growth plate is injured, which may lead to a variable degree of growth disturbance.

Treatment is indicated when function is jeopardised and when serious complications can be anticipated. Whenever possible, correction should be done at the site of the deformity. In special cases the correction can best be achieved by creating a second deformity which will counterbalance the first. Fixation is achieved by plate, intramedullary (i. m.) nail or with an external fixator.

Prevention is best achieved by careful primary treatment and close follow-up in cases of relative instability.

541 ■

8.1.2 Delayed Union, Nonunion

The time it takes for a fracture to heal depends on several factors. The most important are the site (metaphyseal or diaphyseal), the type of fracture including the mechanism of injury, the soft tissue injury, the amount of tissue devascularisation, associated trauma, the general condition of the patient, medication such as steroids and anticoagulants and the type of treatment.

Union is considered delayed when healing has not progressed in the average time for a given fracture situation. As a general rule, if a fracture has not healed by 4–6 months there is delayed union. Nonunion is present when consolidation has ceased to progress. This is generally the case after 6–8 months. The final stage may be the development of a frank pseudarthrosis. This false joint may be lined by fibrocartilage and have a joint capsule.

Reasons for nonunion can be summarised as biological and mechanical. Biological factors are an insufficient tissue response, usually due to excessive devascularisation of the bone and soft tissues, the presence of interposed tissue or an infection. Mechanical factors include too much relative motion at the fracture site. It is important to realise that the amount of motion tolerated depends on the type of fixation that has been chosen.

Two types of nonunions can be differentiated: the hypertrophic and the atrophic types. In the first type, the ends of the bone are hypervascular and capable of biological reaction. Radiologically, this type can be recognised by its typical "elephant foot" appearance. In the second type, the bone ends are avascular and characterised by the lack of callus and by a varying degree of resorbtion. Either type of nonunion can be infected or noninfected. Treatment is directed towards improvement of the biological and mechanical environment.

In hypertrophic nonunion, improvement of the biological potential is superfluous. Improving the degree of stability is all that is needed. This can be achieved by compression plating or intramedullary nailing taking care to avoid additional devascularisation due to surgery. In the atrophic type, improvement of the biological potential is necessary. This can usually be achieved by decortication and cancellous bone grafting. Decortication includes resection of dead bone in the proximity of the nonunion. In the case of major defects, reconstruction can be achieved either by segmental bone transport or, for more substantial defects, by microvascular free bone transplantation.

The infected nonunion is a major challenge. As a general rule infection has to be treated first by adequate debridement. Resection of all necrotic tissue is mandatory. Resection of all infected tissue including the bone is desirable but sometimes not feasible. This is especially true for chronic infection where the entire bone may be involved. Debridement and reconstruction

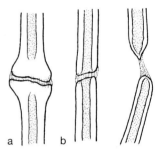

Two types of nonunion. **a** The hypertrophic nonunion has an elephant's foot appearance and is well-vascularised. **b** The atrophic nonunion shows no reaction, eventually resorbtion of the bone ends leads to true defects.

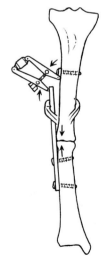

Compression plating of hypertrophic nonunion. Position of the plate is chosen according to the requirements for axial correction. The plate is first fixed to one fragment, then the articulating tension device is mounted. Compression is applied while reduction is forced with a Verbrügge clamp.

are carried out in either one or several stages, depending on the activity and extent of the infection. Reconstruction is performed according to the same principles as above.

Prophylaxis should focus on active prevention of infection by early debridement and soft tissue reconstruction in open fractures and by choosing an adequate, nondevascularising fixation for each given fracture situation

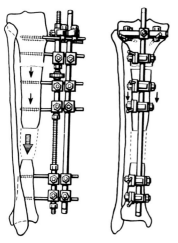

Segment transport for diaphyseal defects. The unilateral tube fixator is provided with a threaded bar on which a short tube slides, driven by a transport nut. After the osteotomy and a lag period of a few days, the transport is started. Transport is carried out at a rate of 1 mm per day.

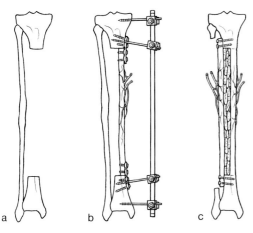

a   b   c

Vascularised bone transplantation. **a** Large segmental defect, where segmental transport is not possible. **b** First step: the contralateral vascularised fibula is transplanted. Excentrical stable fixation is essential for early union of the osteotomies. **c** Second step: 2 months later the vascularised ipsilateral fibula is shifted medially, thus reconstructing the lateral cortex. The gap between the two fibulae is filled with autologous bone graft.

8.1.3 Segmental Bone Defect

Segmental bone defects are true cylindrical gaps in meta- or diaphyseal bone. They can vary in length from 1 cm to more than 30 cm. Generally, they result from fractures or tumours. It is extremely rare to "lose" a segment of bone as a direct consequence of the accident; more often a defect occurs later in the treatment of high energy open or closed trauma. Debridement of necrotic and/or infected bone may lead to the segmental defect.

At present there are available 4 techniques for segmental bone reconstruction:
1. Cancellous bone graft (autologous)
2. Segmental bone transport
3. Vascularised bone transplantation (autologous)
4. Nonvascularised allograft.

Experimental work indicates that cancellous bone graft wrapped with vascularised periosteum is rapidly remodelled to cortical bone and could therefore be an interesting option in the future.

Cancellous bone graft alone is indicated for smaller defects. Probably 5–6 cm is a reasonable limit for this method although clear scientific data are missing.

Segmental bone transport is a fascinating concept which was popularised by Ilizarov. The principle consists in creating an additional osteotomy proximal or distal to the gap. With an external fixation device the intermediate segment is slowly transported, with steps of 1 mm per day. One problem is poor circulation of the transported segment which impairs bone regeneration and healing at the "docking" site.

Vascularised bone transplantation is a very efficient method of reconstruction. The fibula, where a segment of up to 30 cm can be harvested, is the main donor site. For femur and tibia reconstruction two parallel fibulae and additional cancellous bone graft are used. With this method full weight-bearing is generally possible at 6 months, independent of the length of the defect. Problems are related to the feasibility and patency of the microvascular anastomoses.

Allograft is contraindicated in the post-traumatic situation due to its high infection rate. After tumour resection it is a valuable

Post-traumatic Deformities

giography help in further evaluation of anatomical and biological features of the tumour. Finally, biopsy is essential for definitive diagnosis.

The next step is the judgement of the degree of aggressiveness of the tumour followed by multidisciplinary planning of treatment. For malignant tumours, generally a resection in sound tissue several centimetres away from the tumour gives a sufficient margin. A variety of reconstruction techniques are possible, taking advantage of all types of fixation methods. The fine tuning between biology and mechanics remains the key factor for successful reconstruction.

8.3.2 Metastatic Disease

Skeletal metastases are a frequent problem. Often they first present with a spontaneous (pathological) fracture. These fractures occur in the diseased bone without adequate trauma. Metastases can be osteolytic or osteoblastic. Osteolytic metastases are most often due to breast carcinoma, bronchus carcinoma, thyroid carcinoma or hypernephroma. Osteoblastic metastases are mainly due to carcinoma of the prostate.

Treatment is mostly palliative. When pain is the presenting symptom and skeletal weakening is not relevant, radiotherapy is useful. If skeletal weakening is advanced so that an impending fracture can be anticipated, prophylactic stabilisation with composite fixation systems is indicated. When the bone has fractured, intralesional tumour resection and stable composite fixation is aimed at. Composite fixation follows the known principles of open reduction and internal fixation either with plates or i.m. nails. Methylmethacrylate is used to fill the defects, giving primary, medium or long term stability to the composite assembly. Adjunctive radiotherapy and/or chemotherapy is used.

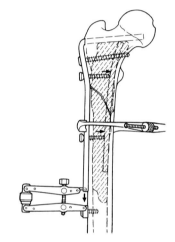

Composite fixation for pathologic fractures in metastatic disease. After intralesional resection of the tumor, the fracture is stabilized with an inner and an outer plate. Push screws help maintaining the correct position of the intramedullary plate while the cavity is filled with pressurized bone cement. The compound is immediatly stable for full weight bearing.

8.4 Congenital Deformities

Congenital deformities are by definition already present at the time of birth. Some are visible, other become apparent within the first years of life. The aetiology is either genetic or due to damage of the fetus during pregnancy, especially in the first 3 months when the fetus is particularly vulnerable to toxic agents. This is the period when organogenesis takes place.

The most frequent localisations are the foot and the hip: about 2% of newborns have a clubfoot, while 1.5% show congenital hip dislocation or dysplasia, although regional differences are

Late Reconstructive Surgery

important. Treatment is primarily conservative. Corrective splints, plasters or orthoses are often sufficient. In the advanced stage surgical correction is necessary.

8.5 Glossary

Allograft: Tissue transplant (i.e. bone) from a donor of the same species but genetically different. Bone is generally transplanted without revascularisation. Histocompatibility studies, as in organ transplantation, are not necessary.

Anastomosis: The anastomosis is the junction between two vessels or tubular structures.

Arthrodesis: Fusion of a joint that was obtained with a surgical procedure.

Ankylosis: Fusion of a joint that occurred spontaneously in the course of a disease.

Biopsy: Excision of tissue, and histological examination to clarify the diagnosis.

Bone Graft: Cortical or cancellous volume of tissue used to reconstruct areas of missing bone.

Buttress. A buttress plate supports the overlying bone.

Callus: During usual fracture healing callus is formed to bridge the defect. It is a calcifying tissue that arises from fracture haematoma and periosteal tissue.

Chemotherapy: Treatment of malignant tumours with intravenous drugs to impair or stop their growth.

Corticotomy: Special osteotomy where the medullary content and the periosteum is not injured while the cortical bone is cut with a chisel.

Debridement: Resection of all avascular tissue.

Deformity: Any anomaly in shape of the locomotor system.

Delayed union: Fracture that does not consolidate after 6 months.

Fibrocartilage: Repair tissue after lesion of the articular cartilage.

Malunion: Consolidation of a fracture in a bad position.

Methylmethacrylate: Polymer generally named bone cement.

Microvascular: Microvascular anastomoses or microvascular tissue transfer is related to the need for an operating microscope to technically do the anastomosis.

Nonunion: Lack of consolidation 9 months after the injury.

Osteoblastic: Producing bone.

Osteolytic: Resorbing bone.

Osteotomy: Controlled fracture of a bone.

Radiotherapy: Treatment of malignant tumours with X-rays.

Reduction: Achieve realignment of a displaced fracture.

Spontaneous Fracture: Fracture that occurs without an adequate trauma.

Synovectomy: Excision of the synovial membrane.

8.6 Recommended Reading

Brunner CF, Weber BG (1981) Besondere Osteosynthesetechniken. Springer, Berlin Heidelberg New York

Mast J, Jakob R, Ganz (1989) Planning and reduction techniques in fracture surgery. Springer, Berlin Heidelberg New York

Müller ME, Allgöwer M, Schneider M, Willenegger H (1990) Manual of internal fixation, Springer, Berlin Heidelberg New York

Weber BG, Cech O (1973) Pseudarthrosen. Pathophysiologie-Biomechanik-Therapie-Ergebnisse. Huber, Bern

9 Surgical Fixation
of the Immature Skeleton

By C. Colton

9.1 Anatomy of Growth

Long bones grow at the cartilaginous growth plates (or physes). These are discs of highly specialised cartilage tissue interposed between the bone ends, or epiphyses, and the shaft of the bone. The portion of the shaft near the physis is called the metaphysis, the main shaft being the diaphysis. The layer of cartilage nearest the epiphysis is nourished by blood vessels which loop down into it from the epiphyseal circulation, and consists of small chondrocytes which gradually increase in number by cell division.

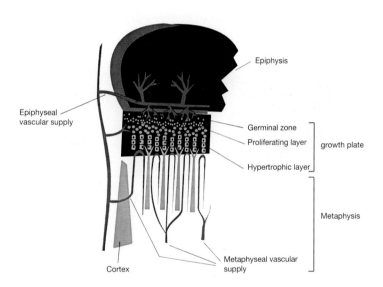

These "parent" chondrocytes form the germinal layer of the physis, and the layer produced by their progeny is the layer or zone of proliferation. After the new cells are produced they start to swell, or hypertrophy, and at the same time line themselves up in columns parallel to the long axis of the bone; it is the increase in diameter of these cells which thickens the growth plate and causes the increase in length. As newer cells continue to be formed by the germinal layer, the older cells in the metaphyseal region of the growth plate, arranged in axial columns, are separated by cylinders of cartilaginous matrix and each cell lies in its own "pocket", or lacuna.

It is in the walls of these cylinders that calcification occurs. In the more mature layers of the growth plate the old hypertrophied cells die (as fine capillary loops from the metaphyseal circulation enter there lacunae) and the cylindrical walls of calcified matrix become covered with new bone, forming primary trabeculae; this is the zone of provisional ossification. These primary trabeculae are then remodelled in the metaphyseal zone to form the normal trabeculae of cancellous bone. Cortical bone is laid down by the periosteum.

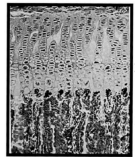

Germinal zone
Proliferation

Hypertrophy

Provisional ossification

Remodelling

9.2 Growth Plate Injuries

The intact growth plate resists axial loads well, provided the membrane bounding the circumference of the cartilaginous disc is intact. The growth plate is, however, less resistant to shearing forces generated either by lateral shift or rotational displacements. The zone of hypertrophy with its bulk of cytoplasm and minimal matrix is the plane along which shearing forces disrupt the physis. There are various patterns of growth plate injury, according to the combinations of epiphyseal and/or metaphyseal fracture that may accompany the growth plate disruption.

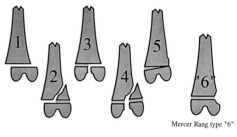

Mercer Rang type "6"

Salter Harris 5 types

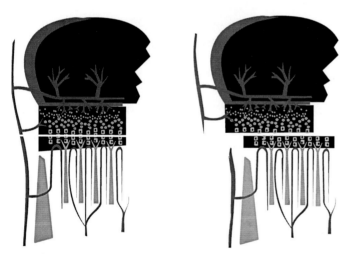

Showing zone of shear and how this leaves the germinal and proliferating layers with intact blood supply.

9.3 Indications for Surgical Fixation

Most children's fractures require only conservative treatment. Fracture disease in the form of joint stiffness, marked muscle wasting, circulatory changes and lymphoedema are not prominent features. Union of fractures is rapid and almost certainly as-

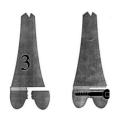

sured. The speed with which union occurs is, however, a limiting factor on the time available to make management decisions – if union is rapid, then malunion will be rapid! Although malunion of a growing bone will remodel in many instances, if the deformity is not in the plane of motion of the nearest joint and/or the child is near to skeletal maturity, remodelling is less likely.

Noncorrectable displacement may require surgical intervention, but no precise indications can be given; it is a matter for experienced clinical judgement. Some growth plate injuries, especially those involving the joint surface (Salter Harris types 3 and 4), will need to be surgically fixed if they are displaced. Any such fixation should avoid further violation of the growth cartilage – implants are usually placed either totally intra-epiphyseally and/or totally within the metaphysis The use of small cannulated screws for this purpose is most helpful. Very occasionally, the bony fragments are too small for screws and Kirschner wires have to be used, although much less secure fixation is afforded and supplementary external splintage will be needed.

If plates are used on growing bones, it has to be remembered that plastic deformation of the bone of a child is possible and less compression can be applied than in adult bone. Also, because the growing bone is highly vascular, and therefore more porous than adult bone, less screw torque can be applied. Considerable surgical experience is required to avoid damaging the bone. Intramedullary nailing is of limited application in the child as it is virtually impossible to insert the nail without risking significant damage to the growth plates. In general terms, the sort of situations where surgical fixation is indicated are as follows:

– Uncontrollable displacement of the fracture fragments due to the nature of the fracture or the nature of the patient (head injury, cerebral palsy, noncompliance for other reasons)
– Displaced physeal injuries, especially involving the joint surface
– Fractures with major vascular compromise
– Multiple fractures in the polytraumatised child
– Severe open fractures, or fractures with adjacent severe soft tissue injury
– Precision osteotomy in reconstructive and orthopaedic surgery
– Certain specific injuries, including:
  Unstable Monteggia injuries
  Unstable pelvic injuries
  Fractures of the femoral neck
  Traumatic separation of the upper femoral epiphysis
  Displaced tibial spine avulsions

9.4 External Fixation

External fixation is useful in children in certain situations. It is rapid and reliable in the polytraumatised child. The "floating knee" can be managed with minimal internal fixation, protected for a short period by a femoro-tibial external fixator. Severe open injuries are a strong indication for external fixation The techniques of external fixation in the child do not differ from those used in the adult, other than the need to respect the growth plate. Union, as stated above, is usually rapid and rarely delayed in children and the fixator can, in most cases, be removed fairly early.

9.5 Glossary

Avulsion: Pulling off

Chondrocytes: These are the active cells of all cartilage, whether articular cartilage, growth cartilage, fibrocartilage, etc. They produce the cartilage matrix, both its collagen and the mucopolysaccharides of the ground substance.

Cytoplasm: The substance of a cell that surrounds its nucleus.

Floating Knee: Fractures of the femur and the tibia in the same limb, resulting in the isolation of the knee joint from the rest of the skeleton.

Lymphoedema: Accumulation of watery fluid in the tissues as a result of poor outflow of the lymph, usually due to the incompetence or obstruction of the lymphatic vessels.

Matrix: The relatively amorphous substance between the cartilage cells. It consists of a network of collagen fibres interspersed with a "jelly" of waterlogged mucopolysaccharide molecules (complex organic chemicals in large molecular chains).

Monteggia Injury: A displaced ulnar fracture associated with a dislocation of the radial head from its articulation with the capitellum. First described in the nineteenth century by Giovanni Battista Monteggia, an Italian physician.

Periosteum: The periosteum is the membrane covering the exterior surface of a bone. The periosteum plays an active part in the blood supply to bone, and bone remodelling:

Plastic Deformation: Change in the shape of a growing bone following the application of a deforming force. The alteration in shape does not "rebound" to the original as the bone has been stressed beyond its elastic limit, but not to the point of breaking. This usually only occurs in young bones.

Polytrauma: Multiple injury. An injury severity score (ISS) of more than 16 is usually taken to indicate polytrauma.

Shear: Shearing forces are those which tend to cause one segment of a body to slide upon another, as opposed to tensile forces which tend to elongate or shorten a body.

Tibial Spine: The area of the proximal tibia lying between the medial and lateral tibial plateaux, which is non-articular and bears the attachments of the horns of the two menisci as well as the tibial ends of the two cruciate ligaments.

Trabecula: The solid bony struts of cancellous bone.

9.6 Recommended Reading

Rang M (ed) (1983) Children's fractures, 2nd edn. Lippincott, Philadelphia

Weber BG, Brunner C, Freuler F (1980) Treatment of fractures in children and adolescents. Springer, Berlin Heidelberg New York

10 Infections After Surgical Fixation

By C. Colton

Infection of bone is a serious complication. It may occur by blood-borne inoculation of hitherto healthy bone as haematogenous osteomyelitis, which is usually a disease of children and not within the scope of this discussion. In the adult, bone infection usually follows either open fracture or occurs as a complication of osteosynthesis. With good surgical care, the infection rates in each of these situations are low. In osteosynthesis of closed fractures, the avoidance of infection relies upon many factors, including:

– Immaculate aseptic procedures by the operating room (OR) staff and surgical team
– Atraumatic soft tissue handling
– Good OR discipline
– The preservation of the blood supply to the bone and the soft tissues
– The achievement of fracture stability
– The timing of surgery

In osteosynthesis of open fractures, there is the added need for careful surgical excision of any nonviable tissue from the injury site and copious lavage. Infection of a fracture site results in the death of tissue locally, including bone. Bone with marginal vascularity is especially susceptible. High-energy injuries, where the tissues are already severely compromised, suffer most if infection supervenes.

Infection is to be suspected if the postoperative pain is more than expected or increases, if the wound area is swollen and unexpectedly tender, or if there is reddening of the skin and/or a rising temperature. Once infection is seriously suspected, the treatment is surgical. "Wait and see" results in progressive tissue death and a worsening of the complication. Early infection demands re-exploration of the fracture site. If there is any dead and infected tissue, it must be removed, even bone. There is a surgical maxim that all dead and infected bone end up in a bucket, one way or another! This may occur by deliberate debridement, dismemberment or death. The former is desirable, the others disastrous.

The surgically debrided site is then washed thoroughly with copious volumes of fluid, preferably Hartmann's solution or Ringer-lactate – dilution is the solution to pollution. A local an-

Infections

tibacterial agent must be delivered to the site of the infection, either by irrigation-suction or by the implantation of a bactericidal preparation, such as antibiotic impregnated polymethyl methacrylate (PMMA) beads. Appropriate systemic antibiotic therapy should be instituted, on the basis of the results from microbiological studies. Early exploration of the infection site yields fluid and tissue for rapid identification of the organism.

The fracture should be stable. If the current implant continues to control the fracture then it should not be removed. If on the other hand, the implant is loose, then the fracture must be restabilised by substitute internal fixation, or an alternative such as external fixation. Once the infection is under control, any soft tissue reconstruction procedures must be undertaken and various techniques, including split skin grafting, local fascio-cutaneous or muscle flaps, or free microvascular tissue transfer, are used in different situations.

The final stage of combating the effects of the infected osteosynthesis, when the infection is controlled and the soft tissue envelope restored, is to proceed to bony union either by closed cancellous bone grafting, open cancellous bone grafting (Papineau technique) or by bone transport techniques.

10.1 Glossary

Antibiotic: Any of various substances, such as penicillin, produced by certain fungi, bacteria, and other organisms, that are effective in inhibiting the growth of, or destroying, microorganisms. They are widely used in the prevention and treatment of infections.
Bactericidal: Capable of killing bacteria.
Haematogenous: Blood-borne.
Inoculation: The instillation, either by accident, or design, of micro-organisms into the tissues or a culture medium.
Osteomyelitis: An acute or chronic inflammatory condition affecting bone and its medullary cavity, usually in relation to bone infection.

Subject Index

M. E. Müller, M. Allgöwer, R. Schneider, H. Willenegger

Manual of Internal Fixation

Techniques Recommended by the AO–ASIF Group

Contribution on Biomechanics by S. M. Perren

Coordinating Editor: M. Allgöwer

3rd, exp. and completely rev. ed. 1991.
XXVIII, 750 pp. 500 figs. mostly in color.
ISBN 3-540-52523-8

The **Manual of Internal Fixation** is well known internationally as a standard work for every specialist dealing with osteosynthesis. Every year hundreds of courses are held for orthopedic surgeons all over the world, so that they may learn the operating techniques according to the AO principles.

Due to the many changes that have taken place in recent years, the authors have completely revised and expanded the manual. This new, third edition reflects today's knowledge and is *the* necessary reference for every AO specialist.

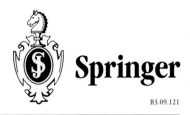

Springer

Preisänderungen vorbehalten.   B3.09.121

M. E. Müller, S. Nazarian, P. Koch, J. Schatzker

The Comprehensive Classification of Fractures of Long Bones

With the collaboration of U. Heim

1990. XIII, 201 pp. 93 figs., mostly in colour. ISBN 3-540-18165-2

This book presents a comprehensive classification of fractures of all long bones. The fundamental principle of this classification is the division of all fractures of a bone segment into three types and the further subdivision into three groups and their subgroups. The groups are arranged in an ascending order of severity according to the morphologic complexities of the fractures, the difficulties inherent in their treatment, and the prognosis. Thus once a surgeon classifies a fracture, he will have determined its severity and will have a guide to its best possible treatment.

U. Heim, K. M. Pfeiffer

Internal Fixation of Small Fractures

Technique Recommended by the ASIF-Group

3rd Edition of Small Fragment Set Manual

In Collaboration with J. Brennwald, C. Geel, R. P. Jakob, T. Rüedi, B. Simmen, H. U. Stäubli

Translated from the German by T. C. Telger

Drawings by K. Oberli

1988. 258 figs. in more than 700 sep. ills. XI, 393 pp. ISBN 3-540-17728-0

Contents: History and Goals. – Implants and Instruments. – General Techniques for the Internal Fixation of Small Fractures. – Preoperative, Operative, and Postoperative Guidelines. – Removal of Implants. – Autogenous Bone Grafts. – Reconstructive Surgery. – Introduction and Overview. – The Shoulder Girdle. – The Elbow. – The Shafts of the Radius and Ulna. – The Wrist and Carpus. – The Hand. – The Knee. – The Tibial Shaft. – The Ankle Joint. – The Foot. – Special Indications. – References. – Subject Index.

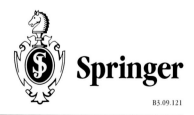

Springer

Preisänderungen vorbehalten.

B3.09.121